Positive Schooling and Child Development

Sibnath Deb
Editor

Positive Schooling and Child Development

International Perspectives

Springer

Editor
Sibnath Deb
Department of Applied Psychology
Pondicherry University
Puducherry
India

ISBN 978-981-13-0076-9 ISBN 978-981-13-0077-6 (eBook)
https://doi.org/10.1007/978-981-13-0077-6

Library of Congress Control Number: 2018941232

Printed on acid-free paper

This Springer imprint is published by the registered company Springer Nature Singapore Pte Ltd.
The registered company address is: 152 Beach Road, #21-01/04 Gateway East, Singapore 189721, Singapore

The book is dedicated to my parents

Sushil Chandra Deb
Sandhya Deb

Foreword

The poet T. S. Eliot asked fundamental questions for his time and our time. In 1934, the information age had barely begun when Eliot published *Choruses from 'The Rock'*. The technological transformation across eight decades since was barely imaginable, but like many great poets, Eliot could see the essence of our evolving human struggle:

> Where is the wisdom we have lost in knowledge?
>
> Where is the knowledge we have lost in information?

The clear truth that *information* $\neq$ *knowledge* $\neq$ *wisdom* should be placed atop boards in our classrooms, in footnotes on our PowerPoint slides, and in banners on our websites. Its meaning should be ingrained into the minds of our teachers and our children. As a form of positive discipline, it should be etched above computer screens and on to the smartphones of the growing numbers of misguided Google scholars who loosely connect factoids rather than understand facts, who eschew deep inquiry for filtered fake news, and whose actions are based on feelings rather than evidence.

Two decades into the twenty-first century, the field of child development is awash with information and opinion. Parents, principals, teachers, children, researchers, psychologists, the media, politicians, administrators; we all have ideas about what makes children healthy, resilient, flexible, and ready for their future. There are many divergent and contested beliefs, but we all have common questions: How are children shaped by their schooling? Why have some been harmed or robbed of their potential? How can schools be made more positive?

We have, in this book, a serious attempt to learn from the deep experience of a broad range of experts on positive schooling and child development in India and globally.

Sibnath Deb guided this work and has done a valuable service for our field. This book captures and interprets important research into children's development, including the adverse effects of heavy academic pressure and bullying, through to the positive outcomes when child protection and safety concepts and extracurricular fun are integrated into teacher training and school resources. The positive impacts that principals, teachers and those who train teachers can have is supported by convincing evidence. When children's resilience, mental health, and well-being are seen as core educational outcomes, we can realize the benefits of multi-tiered strategies to promote psychosocial competence, reduce stigma and social exclusion, and provide psychological support or specialist referral for troubled children. When healthy child development is seen as a fundamental human right, and when the evidence shows that this right has been transgressed by some forms of traditional schooling, we are forced to act to create environments and programmes that are more positive.

Throughout this book, there is a strong focus on action rather than dispassionate analysis. These authors share an ethos of fairness for children, and they envision a better future for our schools. Most of all, they share their wisdom, which is precisely what we need at this time.

Brisbane, Australia/Hue City, Vietnam

Professor Michael Dunne
Queensland University of Technology
The Institute for Community Health Research

Preface

Teaching is a noble and satisfying profession for an individual who possesses a real passion for enlightening minds, as one can see the changes in knowledge and performance of children. There are teachers who are committed to teaching the subject with full interest and making the class more interesting to the students. They also ensure that students participate in the discussion. Any student with average intelligence levels can understand any subject if the subject is presented and taught in an interesting manner. They also become admirers of the teacher in the process. As a result, parents feel more comfortable about the quality of education and safety of their wards. Although a majority of school teachers are responsible, knowledgeable, and committed to teaching, the irresponsible and insensitive behaviour of some teachers and non-teaching staff, especially caretakers, security personnel, school bus drivers and helpers, has become a serious concern for parents and school administrators across the society. The 2017 incident of Ryan International School in Gurugram, India, where a 7-year-old boy was murdered in the washroom in the early hours of school, and other incidents in different schools across the country, raised serious questions about the safety and security of children in the schools. In another incident, a female school teacher slapped a young boy 40 times in two minutes in the classroom in front of all other students for not responding to the attendance roll-call. The CCTV camera had recorded the incident. In another incident, a girl child of Grade V was forced to stand in front of the boys' toilet in a school for not coming to school in proper school uniform. In both the latter cases, it was female teachers who had punished the students. There are many such examples of violence against children in schools across the world, which requires the immediate attention of school authorities and policy makers for corrective measures.

Other major challenges for students in schools include non-availability of teachers, ineffective teaching by some teachers, not addressing the queries of the students, too much home work just before the inspection of the school, not taking classes regularly, improper evaluation, discrimination, differential treatment, and harmful disciplinary measures. The challenges vary from country to country. However, these challenges are part and parcel of school life, given the cultural diversity, lack of commitment and accountability of people in responsible positions, and the magnitude of the population of different countries. Countries with more population experience more challenges. Challenges require joint efforts and cooperation from concerned individuals. Nevertheless, these challenges could be minimized if leaders of educational institutions are sensitive, dynamic, and prone to taking proactive measures involving the teachers. There are some examples of good leadership in some schools where the challenges are reduced. However, for selection of the Principal of a school, seniority should not be the only criteria; it could be just one of the selection criteria. Broad parameters for selecting a Principal of a school could be good academic background, teaching and administrative experience. Most importantly, leadership qualities and passion for administration must be the very essential qualities. In most cases, age becomes an important criteria; that is, a senior teacher who is on the verge of retirement is considered for the post. Generally, a teacher on the verge of retirement becomes more lethargic, psychologically and physically, and thinks twice before introducing a new system. Rather, they worry about a smooth transition to their retirement so that they can leave the school with all the benefits of retirement.

Although the schooling systems in developed countries are much better in terms of teacher–student ratio, salary package of the teachers, student protection policy, flexible curricula, and so on, the present schooling system in developing countries like India requires drastic reforms in all aspects, for creating a better academic environment and producing responsible and skilled manpower. All the stakeholders, right from the Central Government to the local administration, should discharge their responsibilities effectively. When we talk about reforms, it should start with prioritizing education as one of the most important parts of the social and economic development of any country, and allocating more funds to education. Apart from this, the reform requires enforcement of better salary packages for attracting the best candidates for school teaching jobs and making them more accountable. Apart from this, there is an urgent need to revise the curricula periodically, reducing the load of the curricula, and bringing forth uniform curricula with some regional variations, standardization of evaluation process in terms of framing of same question papers for competitive examinations.

Given the above scenario, there is a need to think about positive schooling concepts from the right perspective and evolve student-friendly policies for ensuring healthy and safe academic environment in the school education system.

The broad objective of this document is to present the schooling scenario across the world and its impact on students and children. It intends to share the issues and concerns related to positive schooling with policy makers, school administrators, teachers, academics, researchers, parents and guardians, and students to sensitize them about the relevant issues for improvement of the situation. Further, this document intends to sensitize school administrators for creating student-friendly school environment so that the students can pursue their studies without fear, and grow with knowledge, skills, and good values and contribute towards social development. Highly experienced academics, researchers and professionals from the developed and developing countries contributed chapters to this volume on a wide range of issues related to positive schooling. This is, perhaps, the first volume of such a kind on this important issue.

There are 22 chapters in this volume, on various dimensions of positive schooling. The dimensions include the concept of positive schooling, challenges in ensuring positive schooling environment, safety in the school, students' academic stress, understanding and supporting students' motivation for learning, role of recreational and extra-curricular activities, childhood disability, mental health intervention programmes in schools, life skill education for students, training and motivation of teachers, teacher-student relationships and characteristics of a good principal as a leader.

In Chap. 1, Sibnath Deb elaborates upon the basic concepts of positive schooling and its characteristics. Further, the chapter focuses on the ground reality concerning the schooling system in terms of types of schools, leadership in schools, role of teachers, school infrastructure, selection of qualified teaching staff, teaching methods, students disciplining methods and its impact, school curricula, students' motivation, students' psychological challenges, mental health support services, life skills education including career guidance, importance of extra-curricular activities, safety in school, methods of evaluation of students' performance, and the need for revision of school curricula from time to time. Finally, the chapter proposes a number of remedial measures for the improvement of the school environment and for better academic ambience, in addition to discussing the implications of positive schooling.

Academic stress is a challenge for the students of both developed and developing countries. Cheryl Maykel, Johanna deLeyer-Tiarks, and Melissa A. Bray discuss this issue in Chap. 2 and highlight the ways in which the teachers and the parents can help the students to overcome academic stress. Further, the authors discuss how school-based interventions, such as standardized muscle relaxation, yoga, gratitude writing, and imagery, can help students to overcome academic stress and recommend delivering these support services to the students in the schools.

In Chap. 3, Victoria G. Lidchi raises a very pertinent question based on first-hand clinical experiences of school education in the UK, that is, whether education has lost sight of children. There are many challenges for children and young people in the modern education system, and for the professionals too, who support them. At the end, Victoria G. Lidchi suggests a number of measures for improving the situation.

Motivating students in their studies is very important for their better performance. In Chap. 4, Linda Gilmore highlights the importance of motivation for children's learning and describes the ways in which motivation may be strengthened. Finally, the chapter focuses on strategies for promoting and sustaining motivation. In particular, the chapter emphasizes the importance of providing optimal challenge, experiences of success, and support for autonomy, as well as the benefits of positive strategies for developing self-regulatory skills.

In Chap. 5, Amity Noltemeyer, Erin A. Harper, and Anthony G. James emphasize the need for adopting culturally Responsive Positive Behavioural Interventions for supporting students. Positive Behavioural Interventions and Supports (PBIS) is the main focus of the chapter which emphasizes on a prevention-oriented, data-driven, multi-tier framework for providing a continuum of behavioural supports to enhance student and school outcomes.

People across society are vulnerable to mental health challenges from various stressful situations. Impulsive, irrational, discriminatory, and judgmental behaviour of some teachers causes tremendous trouble for the students as long as these types of teacher are in service. Mental health practitioners view that the teacher's personality is an important determining factor of children's behaviours. Since there is no system of examination of mental health status of teachers, students become the worst sufferers in terms of gaining knowledge and experience other challenges. Nilanjana Sanyal discusses this issue at length in Chap. 6 based on her long clinical experience as a Psychoanalyst.

Psychology, with its strong theoretical background and empirically verified principles, can play an important role in improving the process of education. In Chap. 7, Anjali Gireesan explores the concepts of psychology in the context of improving educational outcomes for all learners based on the ideology of inclusive education. In addition, this chapter presents various existing philosophies like positive psychology and positive schooling in addition to elaborating the innovative teaching-learning methods that can enhance the learning of the students in the Indian context and the policies that facilitate the implementation of these methods. Chapter 8, jointly written by Shikha Soni and Noufal Hameed, discusses, in detail, the concept of mental health promotion, especially strength-based approaches and how schools can play a role in promoting positive mental health among children. Chetna Duggal and Lamia Bagasrawala, in Chap. 9, highlight the significant mental health concerns experienced by adolescents in light of recent research and discuss the potential of the school as a site for mental health advocacy. The authors argue that, as a microcosm of society, schools can create a mentally healthy climate for students by changing the discourse from an illness-based approach to a well-being model. Further, the authors propose the idea of adopting a multi-level approach and mobilizing resources for mental health promotion, prevention, and intervention within schools. For this, the roles and responsibilities of different stakeholders including parents, teachers, school leaders, peers, and mental health professionals are discussed and the importance of collective efforts is emphasized.

Chapter 10, written by Sibnath Deb, is about the efficacy of reproductive and sexual health education for school-going adolescents. The chapter discusses the knowledge and perception of adolescents about various aspects of reproductive and sexual health, in addition to understanding their behaviour, based on the findings of an intervention programme. Further, the chapter suggests evidence-based measures for disseminating information among adolescents about various reproductive and sexual health-related issues in a culture friendly and sensitive manner so that they become receptive and may benefit from the intervention programmes. Life skills education is one of the most accepted preventive and promotional models for dealing with various challenges and for reinforcing positive behaviour among children and adolescents in a volatile environment. This issue has been discussed in Chap. 11 by Subhasis Bhadra based on his first-hand experiences in Gujarat and he explains the usefulness of this intervention strategy for the promotion of communal harmony among the students in the post-riot context of 2002 in Ahmedabad, Gujarat.

In Chap. 12, Shinto Thomas, K. Alphonsa Jose, and P. Aneesh Kumar critically evaluate the school-based child protection programmes and suggest a model of child protection through positive schooling approach. The need for mental health promotion at schools in order to prevent mental illness and promote mental health has been increasingly endorsed and encouraged in recent times, across the globe. Chapter 13 by M. Manjula discusses the needs for mental health promotion at schools, in addition to discussing challenges in implementing mental health promotion programmes at schools. Further, the chapter emphasizes the importance of the role of teachers and counsellors in successful implementation of school-based programmes for the students.

In Chap. 14, Ana Carina Stelko-Pereira, Jessica Elena Valle, and Lucia C. A. Williams review bullying literature, explore important aspects of its definition, as well as its short- and long term-consequences followed by a careful discussion of the importance of recreational activities, such as face-to-face games and online activities to identify bullying involvement and to intervene in the problem. Evidence clearly demonstrates that extra-curricular activities have several indirect and direct benefits in academics as well as in non-academic activities. However, it has not received much attention from the school authorities. Bangalore N. Roopesh, in Chap. 15, highlights the benefits of extra-curricular activities on students' mental and physical health in addition to positive academic outcome based on evidence. In Chap. 16, S. Visaka Devi discusses the major crises on research orientation, to bring about positive amendments in order to keep India secure from the onslaught of social anomalies and offers some suggestions to emerge from the situation.

The role of the Principal in a school is very important in terms of inculcating proper disciplinary methods, creating good academic ambience and motivating the teachers for teaching effectively. Chapter 17, written by Bishakha Majumdar, traces the evolution of research in the field of school leadership to compute the major themes that emerged over the years, along with the important antecedents and outcome variables. Apart from this, the chapter explores the latest developments in the field, with special focus on the Indian educational scenario and identifies future areas for research.

In Chap. 18 Vimala Veeraraghavan focuses on the training of teachers to create the needed positive climate in the school so that there is effective teaching and learning and inculcation of positive values and attitudes in students. The chapter also argues for appropriate selection of students for admission to B.Ed. and M.Ed. programmes through entrance examination and assessments by interview. Further, the chapter states that management and leadership at school have a key role in promoting positive schooling through school climate and recurrent training along the lines mentioned above. Chapter 19, written by Anjali Gireesan, aims to understand the issue of disability in India in the context of various legislations available to different stakeholders and its success in addressing the concerns of the population as well as the management of disability. Also, the chapter aims to understand two types of disabilities, intellectual disability, and learning disability, with respect to their cardinal symptoms, prevalence, assessment, and intervention, to provide a broad understanding of the disabilities, since these are understood to be the most prevalent in classroom settings. Finally, some suggestions are offered that may help in better management of disability across the nation, for children.

In Chap. 20, Ann Farrell examines Australia's national agenda for optimizing children's life chances for health development and learning. Finally, the chapter identifies key enablers and barriers to optimizing children's life chances for their healthy development and learning. Chapter 21, written by Lina Acca Mathew discusses the main highlights of the Right to Education Act, and the relevant literature regarding sexual exploitation of children in schools. The necessity for further measures to ensure positive schooling, free from sexual exploitation of children is highlighted in this chapter. Positive schooling is an approach to education that draws on positive psychology and emphasizes upon individual strengths and personal motivation to promote learning. Chapter 22 by Sridipa Sinha and Sutripta Banerjee seeks to look into the educational features of the schools established by Rabindranath Tagore and Maria Montessori. This chapter also tries to identify the various features of positive schooling as reflected in the institutions. An understanding of the practices of the institutions established by Rabindranath Tagore and Maria Montessori will pave the way for creating a positive climate in schools of the present era.

All the chapters are based on evidence from different countries, and readers will find a lot of information for bringing in positive changes in the school education system for the welfare and well-being of the students. I am thankful to all the contributors for their significant contribution to this volume, despite their busy schedule. I hope that the volume will be beneficial for policy makers, educational administrators, school authorities, teachers, parents, school students, research scholars, and academics.

Puducherry, India Sibnath Deb

Contents

Editor and Contributors

About the Editor

Prof. Sibnath Deb, Ph.D. & D.Sc. is full-time professor of the Department of Applied Psychology, Pondicherry University (A Central University), India. Prof. Deb is also acting as Director (I/C), Directorate of Distance Education and Dean (I/C), School of Law, Pondicherry University. Prior to joining the Pondicherry University, he was teaching in the University of Calcutta. In 1994, Prof. Deb did an intensive course on 'HIV/AIDS and Qualitative Research' from the University of Western Australia. During April 2009 to August 2009, Prof. Deb visited the School of Public Health, Queensland University of Technology (QUT), Brisbane, Australia as Visiting Faculty. Currently he is also Adjunct Professor of the School of Public Health and Social Work, QUT, Australia. During 2004–'08, he served the International Society for Prevention of Child Abuse and Neglect (ISPCAN) as Councillor Member. In brief, he has got 28 years of teaching, research, and administrative experience and has produced 19 Ph.D.'s in addition to publishing more than 100 research articles/book chapters in the leading national and international journals. Prof. Deb has written seven books and edited six books. His latest books titled '*Child Safety, Welfare, and Well-being*' (2016) and '*An Empirical Investigation into Child Abuse and Neglect in India: Burden, Impact and Protective Measures*' (2018) have been published by Springer. His two more books titled '*Social Psychology in Everyday Life*' (Sage) and '*Distance Education: Prospects, Challenges and Way Forward*' (Pearson) are in press. Current areas of research interest of Prof. Deb include child safety, students' mental health, adolescent reproductive health, and applied social psychology.

Contributors

K. Alphonsa Jose is a Maulana Azad National Junior Research Fellow in the Department of Applied Psychology, Pondicherry University, Puducherry, India. She completed her Master's Degree from the Department of Applied Psychology, Pondicherry University in 2015. She has cleared UGC NET, and holds a PG Diploma in Industrial Psychology. Her research in the area of Environmental Psychology attempts to identify the influencing factors behind choosing eco-friendly houses. She has authored six research articles in various peer-reviewed national and international journals, as well as in edited books. She has presented many scientific research papers in international and national conferences, and received the best paper award for "A Study on Incidents of Child Abuse and Neglect" in Puducherry. Funded by Indian Council of Social Science Research (ICSSR), Government of India.

P. Aneesh Kumar is an Assistant Professor at the Department of Psychology, Christ University, Bengaluru. He has worked as project officer for Indian Council for Social Sciences Research (ICSSR) in Pondicherry University and as Head, Department of Psychology, Wadi Huda Institute of Research and Advanced Studies affiliated to Kannur University, Kerala. He did his doctoral research on the topic "burden of child abuse and neglect in Kerala: risk factors and impact". He has published and presented papers in various national and international forums in the area of public health, child and adolescent psychology. Currently he is also involved in various research project including developing a training model for culturally competent and evidence-based mental health care for diverse societies (United States–India Education Foundation), developing character strength among primary school students through classroom teaching, and socialization of emotion and construal of anxiety and depression among mothers (a multi country project). His research interest includes child mental health, public health and school counselling programmes. He teaches papers in child and adolescent counselling, counselling interventions for special population, development psychology, and qualitative research methods.

Lamia Bagasrawala is a clinical psychologist with a keen interest in child and adolescent well-being. Having completed her Masters from TISS, Mumbai, she has been working as a school counsellor in Mumbai for the last two years. As a school counsellor, she has engaged in individual therapy work, small group activities and classroom based interventions for adolescents as well as worked in collaboration with teachers, parents, school leaders, and support staff to promote student well-being.

Sutripta Banerjee is an Assistant Professor in the Department of Education of Saheed Nurul Islam Mahavidyalaya. Sutripta Banerjee has a teaching experience of 7 years. She also served as an Assistant Teacher in Government Aided School for 3 years. She completed her Masters, B.Ed. and M.Phil. programme in Education from the University of Calcutta with specialization in Special education and Mental

Hygiene. Her research areas are Educational Philosophy and Educational Psychology. This year she submitted her thesis from the University of Calcutta. She has also presented papers in various National and International Seminars.

Subhasis Bhadra, MSW, Ph.D. in Psychiatric Social Work, has been working as Associate Professor and Head in the Department of Social Work, School of Social Science, Central University of Rajasthan, Ajmer, Rajasthan, India. Dr. Bhadra started his career from intervention in Gujarat earthquake (2001) and subsequently worked in riots (Gujarat, 2002), Tsunami (2004), Kashmir earthquake and unrest (2005), terrorist attack (Mumbai serial Train Blast, 2006), cyclone Nargis (Myanmar, 2008), Tsunami in Japan (2011), Himalayan Tsunami (Uttarakhand Disaster, 2013) through different organizations, like Care India, American Red Cross, International Federation of Red Cross, Oxfam India, Action Aid, International Medical Corps. He supported psychosocial work in few Asian countries, through training and material development. His research interest includes peace building, life skills education, social work interventions in community, disaster mental health, community & school mental health and psychosocial support. He has delivered lectures in different institutes/universities on invitation; some of them are School of Social Work, University of Denver (Skype Lecture); Department of Psychology, University of Indonesia; Department of Education, Tohoku University. Dr. Bhadra is actively engaged in various disaster response programme and lectures on disaster management issues in NIDM (National Institute of Disaster Management), New Delhi. In his credit there are number of academic articles and book chapters published at national and international levels. E-mail: bhadrasubhasis@gmail.com.

Melissa A. Bray is a Professor and the Director of the School Psychology program within the Neag School of Education at the University of Connecticut, USA. She is a Fellow of both the American Psychological Association and the American Psychological Society. Dr. Bray is an elected member of the Society for the Study of School Psychology. She is licensed as a psychologist in the State of Connecticut, holds national certification in school psychology, state certification in school psychology, and licensure in speech language pathology. Since receiving her doctorate in 1997, she has published or has in press over 175 articles, chapters, and reviews in the professional literature, and has presented over 100 scholarly papers at national and international conferences. Her research interests are in the areas of interventions for communication disorders (mainly stuttering), classroom disruptive behaviour, and physical health and wellness, especially in relation to asthma and cancer.

Johanna deLeyer-Tiarks is a doctoral student at the University of Connecticut in the School Psychology program within the Neag School of Education, USA. Her research interests include minority stress, mind-body health, and culturally responsive school-based practices. Her background is in childhood social development and the study of socio-psychological processes underlying community systems.

S. Visaka Devi is currently employed as Assistant Professor, Department of English, Pondicherry University. She joined the University in 2010 and has served the University since then. Her area of specialization is Comparative Literature and area of interests is Poetry, Translation, and Culture Studies. She has attended several National and International conferences and presented papers related to Translation, Feminist views, Concept of Self, Autobiographies, Memoirs, Culture, and Religion for social change. She has delivered talks on topics of literary interest and social values. Her talks focus on Literature and Life, Children and Children's Literature navigating into Literature in particular as a tool to bring about a positive social change. She has published several research articles to her credit and has contributed articles in edited books focusing in majority on Translation, Feminism, and Socio-Cultural aspects. The subject of both her research articles and creative writing delve into human psyche and holds Literature as the finest therapy that would serve as a social panacea. A published creative writer, she publishes all her creative works under the pen name Vishaka Sajan. She has published a collection of poems titled Twilight Lamps (2012). She has also published a couple of shorts stories and a couple of translations of short stories from Malayalam to English that have been well received by readers. She is basically interested in understanding human nature which forms the basis of her creative writing. Besides this, she was a featured e-card writer for a Hawaii-based website www.passionup.com (2009) and her cards are still afloat the website.

Chetna Duggal is an Assistant Professor in the School of Human Ecology, Tata Institute of Social Sciences (TISS), Mumbai. She has completed her Ph.D. from TISS, Mumbai, and her M.Phil. in Clinical Psychology from NIMHANS, Bangalore. She is a practicing psychotherapist and works with children, adolescents, couples, and families. She is the trustee of Apnishala, an organization working towards making life skills education accessible to children from underprivileged contexts. She has a keen interest in psychological well-being, promotion, and intervention for children and adolescents.

Ann Farrell is Head of the School of Early Childhood and Inclusive education, Faculty of Education, Queensland University of Technology, Brisbane, Australia. Her work in policy research, ethnography, and mixed method evaluation has a focus on the rights of children and young people to provision, protection, and participation in local and global contexts. Authoring more than 100 scholarly works, she publishes in the areas of early childhood education and care; transdisciplinary research in education, health and the law; research ethics; and globalization. She is the Minister's nominee to the Board of the Australian Children's Education and Care Quality Authority, the national body supporting the National Quality Framework for Early Childhood Education and Care. She serves as an expert assessor with the Australian Research Council, Australia's National Health and Medical Research Council, the Social Sciences and Humanities Research Council of Canada and the National Research Foundation, Reviews and Evaluation Directorate of South Africa.

Linda Gilmore is a Professor of Educational and Developmental Psychology at Queensland University of Technology in Brisbane, Australia where she teaches students in psychology and pre-service education programmes. Linda has researched mastery motivation in children, adolescents, and adults for more than 25 years. Much of her research has focused on children with Down syndrome. She has also investigated the motivational profiles of children whose teachers presume they are just "lazy", demonstrating powerfully that unrecognized learning and attention difficulties may underlie students' apparent lack of interest at school. As a psychologist, Linda has worked with many children, families, and schools with the goal of better understanding and supporting their engagement with learning in positive ways. In particular, her research and practice focus on children with developmental disabilities, such as rare chromosome disorders, and community attitudes towards disability.

Anjali Gireesan has been working as Scientist 'B' in the Defence Research and Development Organization (DRDO), Ministry of Home Affairs, Government of India. Prior to that, she was working as Assistant Professor in the Department of Psychology, Amity University, Noida, India. She has six years of full time teaching and research experience. She has published six research papers and written a book chapter titled 'Contexts of Risks and Exploitation' with Prof. Sibnath Deb for an edited book titled '*The SAGE Handbook of Early Childhood Research (2015)', SAGE Publication, Australia.* Her two more chapters, viz., (i) Enhancing Education: Improving Learner Outcomes with Principles of Psychology, and (ii) Children with Disability in India: Policies, Assessment and Management have been accepted for an edited book titled 'Positive Schooling and Child Development: International Perspectives' to be published by Springer in 2018. Her areas of research interest include child development, childhood disability, child abuse and neglect, and student's mental health.

Noufal Hameed is a Rehabilitation Council of India (RCI) registered, licensed Clinical Psychologist. At present, he is pursuing Ph.D. in Clinical Psychology from the Department of Clinical Psychology, National Institute of Mental Health and Neuro Sciences, Bangalore. He holds his Master's degree in Applied Psychology where he specialized in Clinical Psychology. He also has an M.Phil. in Clinical Psychology from Central Institute of Psychiatry, Ranchi. His areas of research interest include positive mental health, mental health promotion, and stigma reduction. As a member of the Positive Psychology Unit, a part of Department of Clinical Psychology, he regularly conducts workshops on topics related to mental illness and health awareness, stigma reduction, inclusion of persons with disabilities, and promotion of safe riding, among many other related topics. His work focuses on people adolescents and young adults. His doctoral thesis involves development of a positive youth development programme for promotion of mental health among college youth.

Erin A. Harper is an Assistant Professor in the School Psychology programme at Miami University. She was a school psychologist in urban public schools for eight years prior to joining the faculty at Miami. Her research focuses on the development, implementation, and evaluation of culturally responsive school mental health supports for underserved youth in the United States and abroad. As a graduate student, Dr. Harper collaborated with faculty and students at the Georgia State University Center for Research on School Safety, School Climate, and Classroom Management to develop Project P.R.E.V.E.N.T (Promoting Respect, Enhancing Value, Establishing New Trust), a research-based, interactive curriculum to promote the healthy development of adolescent girls. Dr. Harper has published research in numerous peer-reviewed journals and has presented her work at numerous professional conferences. She earned a B.A. in Psychology from Spelman College and graduate degrees (M.Ed. and Ed.S.) in School Psychology from Georgia State University.

Anthony G. James is an Assistant Professor in the Department of Family Science and Social Work at Miami University (OH). His scholarly work uses an interdisciplinary approach to understanding social interactions and human development, with an expertise in positive youth development, religion and spirituality, diverse family systems, and family processes. Currently, he is using national data (continental United States) to investigate the role of youths' spirituality in their positive development, focusing specifically on youth conceptions and self-ratings of spirituality. His has been published in referred journals and book chapters, on topics in the areas of youth development and family relations. Dr. James is a certified relationship assessment facilitator through the PREPARE/ENRICH programme and a certified family life educator through the National Council on Family Relations. He earned B.S. sociology (military science minor) from Lincoln University (MO), with graduate degrees (M.S. & Ph.D.) in Human Development and Family Studies (religious studies minor) from the University of Missouri.

Victoria G. Lidchi is a consultant clinical psychologist and systemic psychotherapist, trained in mediation, public health, and social development. She worked at Great Ormond Street Hospital before spending 8 years in South America as a consultant, trainer, and supervisor of mental health professionals working with children, adults, and families in the field of trauma and abuse in Colombia, Argentina, Bolivia, and Brazil. She is an experienced trainer and supervisor. In the UK, she has worked in the Tavistock court service and now manages a local authority service for vulnerable children, young people, and families with complex with mental health, social care, and educational needs. She is also involved in developing an innovative community mental health project commissioned to deal with the aftermath of the Tottenham Riots—"Thinking Space"—bringing together ideas developed at the Tavistock and those underlying community therapy initiatives in Brazil. She has published in four languages in books and journals.

Bishakha Majumdar a Fellow of the Indian Institute of Management Indore, is involved in teaching and research in the areas of Organizational Behaviour, Psychology, and Human Resource Management. She has also conducted several management development programmes with organizations such as Coal India and Oriental Insurance, in the areas of communication, leadership, and employee motivation. She has 12 national and international publications and her works have been recognized with, among others, an Honourable Mention (ISB-Ivey Global Case Competition 2015), the Best Management Research Award 2013 (National Academy of Psychology), Best Publication Award 2012 (Journal of Indian Academy of Applied Psychology), and the Young Scientist Award, 2011 (Indian Academy of Applied Psychology). Bishakha has also taught Psychology at the undergraduate and post-graduate levels in the University of Calcutta, has also been a Master Trainer for HIV/AIDS counsellors under the World Bank GFATM Programme. She is presently an Assistant Professor in OB & HR at FORE School of Management, New Delhi.

M. Manjula, Additional Professor, Department of Clinical Psychology, NIMHANS, has been working as a faculty at Behavioural Medicine Unit of the Department for over 10 years. She completed her M.Phil. and Ph.D. in Clinical Psychology from NIMHANS. Her specialization is in the area of Cognitive behaviour therapies in various psychiatric disorders and health conditions. She has carried out research in the following areas: psychopathology of anxiety, and mood disorders; cognitive behavioural interventions for emotional disorders, personality disorders and sexual dysfunctions and community based interventions in youth for mood disorders, anxiety, suicidality, academic stress, relationship difficulties and emotion regulation. She has guided about eight Ph.D. theses and about 15 M.Phil. Dissertations in the above said topics. She has published about 35 papers in national and international journals, has written book chapters and edited psychology books for Nursing and Bachelor of Education courses. She is a reviewer for national and international journals of psychiatry and psychology. She has completed funded projects on stress management, self-harm behaviours, suicide prevention, and achieving excellence in sports for youth.

Lina Acca Mathew is Assistant Professor at Government Law College, Kozhikode, Kerala, India. She did her Ph.D. from Queensland University of Technology, Brisbane, Australia, in 2017. Her thesis is titled 'Legislative Models of Prosecuting Child Sexual Abuse in India: A Review and Critical Analysis.' She did her LL.M. from the National Law School of India University, Bengaluru, India (2002) and her LL.B. from Government Law College, Thiruvananthapuram (2000), India. She is interested in the areas of information technology laws and child laws, and has published various papers and made presentations on the same.

Cheryl Maykel is an Assistant Professor in the counselling and school psychology programs in the Division of Education at Rivier University in Nashua, New Hampshire, USA. She has authored numerous publications and has presented her work at local, national, and international conferences. Dr. Maykel's research interests are mainly in the areas of mind-body health, including the cognitive and behavioural benefits of physical activity in the classroom.

Amity Noltemeyer is an Associate Professor and coordinator of the School Psychology programme at Miami University in Oxford, Ohio, USA. Her research interests include Positive Behavioural Interventions & Supports (PBIS), child/adolescent resilience, disproportionality in school discipline, bias in school decision-making, and school climate. Noltemeyer has authored many journal articles and book chapters, and has also co-edited a book and guest-edited a journal special issue. She also manages externally funded grants, including her role as co-director of Ohio's School Climate Transformation Grant. Noltemeyer is a Past President of the Ohio School Psychologists Association, and currently serves as Editor of *School Psychology International* journal. She was awarded the Robert H. and Nancy J. Blayney Professorship from the Miami University Office of the Provost in 2013. She earned an M.S. and Ed.S. from Miami University in School Psychology and a Ph.D. from Kent State University in School Psychology. She is a Nationally Certified School Psychologist.

Bangalore N. Roopesh is Assistant Professor in Clinical Psychology, National Institute of Mental Health and Neurosciences (NIMHANS), Bangalore, India. After obtaining Ph.D. from the NIMHANS, he did Post-Doctoral Research in the Downstate Medical Centre, New York, USA. He has published 14 research papers and presented papers in 16 conferences. Till date, he has completed six research projects successfully.

Nilanjana Sanyal is a Professor in the Department of Psychology, University of Calcutta. She has been teaching at the University and has been practicing psychoanalysis and psychodynamic psychotherapy for the last 33 years. Professor Sanyal has imparted training in counselling in various governmental institutions and N.G.O.s., both nationally and internationally, and is consistently involved in mass media programmes for awareness-generation regarding mental health issues. She has to her credit a number of national and international publications and is also a columnist in different national dailies and magazines. She has edited a book and is a co-author of a Test Manual. She has 27 book chapters to her credit till date. Her research interests include personality and clinical psychology, interpersonal relationships, psychoanalysis and psychodynamic psychotherapy. She is a Co-Researcher for the creation of registered assessment methodologies, namely, the Fairy Tale Test (FTT) with Dr. Carina Coulacouglou, University of Athens, Greece, and State Trait Anxiety Inventory—two Children and Adolescents (STAXI—2 C/A) with Dr. Thomas Bruner and Dr. Charles D. Spielberger, University of South Florida, Tampa, USA. She is an Honorary Member of the Fairy Tale Test Society, Greece, apart from her membership in other national and international professional bodies. She is a Gold Medallist of Calcutta University, both at the under-graduate and post-graduate level. She received Jubilee Merit Prize and Jawaharlal Nehru Award from Government of India along with the Suhashini Basu Memorial Prize from Indian Psychoanalytic Society for excellence of a research paper. She is the recipient of Bharat Jyoti Award, 2012 for meritorious achievement and life time contribution to social works, and Prof. Maya Deb Memorial Award from Asiatic Society, Kolkata, 2012 apart from other awards.

Sridipa Sinha is an Associate Professor, in the Department of Education, University of Calcutta, India. Dr. Sridipa Sinha has a teaching experience of 15 years. She has completed some research projects and has about more than 30 publications in reputed journals. Research based paper prepared by her has been presented in many Conferences both at National and International levels. Her research areas include ICT, Mental Health and Guidance, Teacher Education. Her successful guidance has led to the award of M.Phil. and Ph.D. degrees to various candidates. She has also good organization capabilities and has organized various Refresher Course, and National and International Conferences.

Shikha Soni is an RCI licensed Clinical Psychologist, currently a Doctoral Research Scholar in Psychology in Department of Liberal Arts at Indian Institute of Technology, Hyderabad. She has completed her M.Phil. in Clinical Psychology from Central Institute of Psychiatry, Ranchi, Graduation, and Post-graduation in Psychology from Delhi University. She has dealt with various disorders and their treatment. She has been trained in various psychological testing like psycho diagnostics, intelligence tests, neuropsychology, and other tests (disability/psychopathology) and therapies like cognitive behaviour therapy, behaviour therapy, supportive therapy, marital/family therapy, and various other therapies. She has worked as Senior Research Fellow in Department of Clinical psychology in NIMHANS hospital, Bangalore in a project studying Cognitive behaviour therapy in partial responders with OCD: a randomized controlled trail. Her research interests bridge the areas of positive, social, personality, and clinical psychology. Her research focuses on positive psychology, cognitive behaviour therapy in anxiety disorder, mental health, psychotherapy processes, and outcome.

Ana Carina Stelko-Pereira holds a Ph.D. in Psychology from the Federal University of São Carlos (UFSCar) and is Associate Professor of Psychology and Public Health at Ceará State University (*UniversidadeEstadual do Ceará*, UECE), a Member of the Laboratory of Analysis and Prevention of Violence (Laprev/UFSCar). Her main areas of investigation are: school violence, bullying, teacher-student relationship, and games development.

Shinto Thomas has completed his Master's Degree from the Department of Applied Psychology, Pondicherry University (A Central University) in 2013. He also holds a PG Diploma in Industrial Psychology. Currently he is pursuing his doctoral research in the Pondicherry University, India, on risk behaviour of emerging adults. He has published six research papers. His research area includes mental health, risk behaviour, development, characteristics, and issues faced by emerging adults.

Jessica Elena Valle is a Psychologist and a Ph.D. Candidate at the Psychology Graduate Programme at the Federal University of São Carlos (*Universidade Federal de São Carlos,* UFSCar), and an M.A. in Psychology also from the same University. She is has a fellowship from CAPES (Brazil's Ministry of Education Higher Education Department) and is a member of the Laboratory of Analysis and Prevention of Violence (Laprev/UFSCar) where she investigates: bullying, teacher-student relationship and school engagement.

Vimala Veeraraghavan Former Professor of psychology, Delhi University and Emeritus Professor, Indira Gandhi National Open University, has 35 years of teaching and research experience. She has published more than 50 research papers and written a number of books. Few of them have been published by Sage Publication, India.

Lucia C. A. Williams is a Full Professor of Psychology at the Psychology Graduate Programme from the Federal University of São Carlos, Brazil where she founded the award-winning research laboratory Laprev (The Laboratory for Violence Analysis & Prevention) doing research, consultation and community outreach in the areas of family and school violence. She is a research fellow from CNPq (Brazilian National Council for Scientific and Technological Development) and from Sidney Sussex College, University of Cambridge, and a Council Member of ISPCAN (The International Society for the Prevention of Child Abuse & Neglect).

Chapter 1
Positive Schooling: Concept, Characteristics, Situation Analysis and Implications

Sibnath Deb

Abstract The ultimate objective of education is imparting knowledge to students, enhancing their coping skills, helping them in building their character, and, finally, producing skilled and responsible citizens for nation building. Therefore, schools play an important role in achieving the objective of education and in shaping the career of a child. This chapter outlines the basic concepts of positive schooling and its characteristics. Further, the chapter focuses on the ground reality concerning the schooling systems in India in terms of types of schools, leadership in schools, role of teachers, infrastructure of schools, teaching methods, periodic training for teachers, disciplining methods, corporal punishment and its impact, student motivation, students' enrolment and attendance, examination and methods of evaluation of student performance, revision of school curricula from time to time, effective parents-teachers meeting and feedback mechanism, involving larger community in the school management committee and taking their suggestions for better functioning. The chapter also discusses students' safety, their psychological challenges, mental health support services, life skills or adolescent reproductive health education for school students, assessment of students' aptitude and interests for career guidance, importance of extra-curricular activities, students' protection policy in school, and student feedback mechanism. Finally, the chapter focuses on revisiting the selection procedure of the teachers and making school teaching more attractive by providing better salary and other facilities in addition to describing the implication of positive schooling for overall welfare and well-being of students and prescribing some steps based on evidence.

Keywords Positive schooling · Concepts · Students · Teachers · India

S. Deb (✉)
Department of Applied Psychology, Pondicherry University (A Central University), Puducherry, India
e-mail: sibnath23@gmail.com

S. Deb (ed.), *Positive Schooling and Child Development*,
https://doi.org/10.1007/978-981-13-0077-6_1

Introduction

A school is a place for imparting knowledge, developing skills, and imbibing disciplined behaviour and, in turn, producing responsible, potentially productive citizens for building a healthy society. Along with the moral developments, the success of the student depends upon a positive, supportive, congenial, and friendly schooling environment. Evidence suggests that there is a positive association between the success of students and a positive schooling environment. Students are generally more motivated to do well, and to realize their full potential, in schools that have a positive academic climate, where they feel safe, included, and supported. A safe and fear-free environment in the school and in the classroom are two essential prerequisites of positive schooling. A positive schooling climate exists when all members of the school feel safe, included, and accepted, and actively promote positive behaviours and interactions. Principles of equity and inclusive education must be embedded in the learning environment to support a positive schooling climate and a culture of mutual respect. A positive schooling climate is a crucial component for the prevention of inappropriate behaviour and for inculcating responsible behaviour.

The broad objective of this chapter is to discuss about Indian school education system, characteristics of positive schooling and the role of Principal and teachers in creating effective academic ambiance in addition to discussing about other issues and concerns for revamp of the school education system in India.

Types of Schools in India

Indian schools can be broadly categorized on the basis of administering bodies: Government (State and Central), Quasi-government (Army Schools), Model Schools (Jawahar Navodaya Vidayalas [JNVs]), Public, and Private Schools. These schools develop their curriculum and conduct examinations at the state and central levels under different institutional affiliations: Central Board of Secondary Education (CBSE), Council for the Indian School Certificate Examinations (CISCE) and state education boards. Curricula, and methods of teaching and evaluation of students performance, in the different categories of schools vary, which is in violation of the fundamental idea of the Indian Constitution, of equity and equality. In other words, it might be stated that the present schooling system in India does not give equal inputs to all children, which can be done by following broad and uniform curricula and measuring performance using uniform evaluation methods.

The number of private schools is increasing across the world and in India. But still, it is inadequate as compared to the need. Privatization of education—a drive initiated by the Government of India—is a welcome initiative since the government alone cannot cater to the needs of education. However, the government should also ensure that private schools do not exploit people by collecting high tuition fees in the name of school development. At the same time, in accordance with The Rights of Children to Free and Compulsory Education Act, 2009, each school must offer 25% seats to socially backward children.

Characteristics of a Positive School Climate

Some of the essential characteristics of a positive schooling climate for students include safety, acceptance, respectful relationships, trust, and fairness and kindness in the interactions between teachers and students. For teachers, this means a more supportive environment, location of school, availability of adequate facilities of infrastructure, open exchange of ideas and views, inclusive education, punctuality, sincerity and motivation among teachers, updated knowledge in the subject, effective teaching methods, positive disciplining, thus building a positive school climate, and embedding the principles of equity and inclusive education in all aspects of the learning environment. Above all, the school must support the well-being and achievement of all students. These factors are most important to building a positive schooling environment.

Leadership

Effective leadership makes a difference in any institution. In educational institutions like schools, professionally trained teachers should be appointed for careful planning and management of the system. A person with a good educational pedigree might be suitable for effective teaching, but they may not have the required administrative skills for running school administration efficiently. Therefore, an individual with administrative skills and pedigree in management, along with a passion for school administration, should be appointed for leading an academic institution. Not much research is carried out on leadership styles of school principals. However, available findings are quite interesting and they give an idea as to how a school principal should function. For example, according to Hess and Kelly (2007), school leadership is the key to school improvement. In a new era of accountability, where school leaders are expected to demonstrate bottom-line results and use data to drive decisions, the skill and knowledge of principals matter more than ever.

Based on a primary research using an unstructured interview, Blumberg and Greenfield (1986) identified eight types of principals, in terms of their outstanding characteristics, as revealed through analysis of their comments: the Organizer, the Value-Based Juggler, the Authentic Helper, the Broker, the Humanist, the Catalyst, the Rationalist, and the Politician.

Another study pointed out that the heads should have mastery over time and stress management, exercise and practice of cooperation, learning habits should be such that whatever is learned may be translated into aspired for and desired skills. In the light of the analysis of the data and findings of the study, it has been suggested that the selection of potential leaders should not solely be based on academic qualification; selection criteria should also take into account leadership styles, traits, and competencies. Besides modern knowledge, perspectives of leadership should be included in the curriculum of teacher education (Malik et al. 2016). Further, the authors emphasized that leadership in education must be committed to the vision of excellence, with an equal emphasis on knowledge.

Proper understanding and coordination between the principals and teachers are essential for effective functioning of a school. In this regard, Marks and Printy (2003) focused on school leadership relations between principals and teachers, and examined the potential of their active collaboration around instructional matters to enhance the quality of teaching and student performance. The analysis was grounded in two conceptions of leadership: transformational and instructional. The study disclosed that transformational leadership is a necessary but insufficient condition for instructional leadership. When transformational and shared instructional leadership coexisted in an integrated form of leadership, the influence on school performance, measured by the quality of its pedagogy and the achievement of its students, was found to be substantial. In a review-based article, another author highlights the importance of leaders being learners, its implications for leadership development, and the importance of creating and sustaining certain organizational conditions which facilitate instructional leadership (Southworth 2002).

Finally, a school principal should be committed and hardworking with a pleasing personality and management skills in dealing with challenging situations. He must also be knowledgeable, sensitive to teachers and students' issues, open to criticism and any new ideas for bringing a change in the systems within the purview of the rules and regulations of the school, in the best interest of the students.

School Infrastructure

Infrastructure varies from school to school. However, there are visible differences between private and public schools in terms of infrastructure, although some private schools also do not have adequate facilities. Some of the shortcomings of public schools in India include small classrooms, poor seating arrangements, lack of basic facilities like a blackboard, study materials, poor lighting, lack of sanitary facilities, lack of safe drinking water (Devanathan 2014), the lack of a hygienic environment for consumption of food during recess, distance of the school, poor transportation, and so on. However, the infrastructure of public schools located in urban areas is reasonably better compared to public schools located in semi-urban and rural areas. In semi-urban and rural areas, most public schools do not even have safe drinking water and restrooms. Students mostly depend on tube wells for drinking water facilities and the open fields for excretion and urination. For girls, it is extremely embarrassing to go to the open fields to attend to their metabolic needs and, as a result, a large number of girl students suppress nature's call which sometimes results in other physical health problems. This issue drew the attention of the prime minister of India, Narendra Modi, who took a special interest in making arrangements for restrooms in semi-urban and rural schools (Majra and Gur 2010; Meller and Litschig 2016; Muralidharan and Kremer 2006).

There is an urgent need to allocate more budget for creating basic infrastructure facilities for schools: the classroom, ergonomic seating arrangements, sanitation facilities, safe playground and drinking water, especially in the rural and semi-urban areas. If the classrooms are not well-equipped, a teacher will not feel motivated to teach effectively. Without blackboard, chalk, and duster a teacher cannot teach effectively. Seating arrangements in most public schools are not ergonomically suitable which cause back pain for a large number of students. The lack of restroom and safe drinking water are some of the causes for high school dropouts in rural schools in India (Muralidharan and Kremer 2006).

The Role of Teachers

Teachers are role models for their students. A sincere teacher with adequate knowledge in his/her subject, good communication skills and effective teaching methods can develop interest among students about the subject. At the same time, teachers play an important role in modelling positive, inclusive, and respectful language and behaviour, inside and outside classrooms. To help develop and sustain a positive school climate, boards of study and schools should actively promote and support behaviours that reflect their board's code of conduct, equity, and inclusive education policy and character development initiatives. The school authority should also invite members of the broader community to become involved in this effort as a part of the school community.

Teaching Staff

For quality teaching, qualified and experienced teachers are required for every school. There cannot be any compromise in this regard. Only an erudite teacher with good communication skills can impart knowledge among students effectively (Allen et al. 2011; Shulman 1987). However, this is a big challenge for most schools in India, irrespective of the category of schools. There are good teachers in every school who are committed to teaching; teaching is their passion. Students who come in contact with these teachers really enjoy the subject and also develop a special interest in the same subject. If a teacher comes to class with proper preparation and teaches the subject citing simple examples, any student with average intelligence will understand the subject even if it is a difficult subject. So teachers' skills are very important for quality teaching and generating interest among the students on the subject (Darling-Hammond 2000). It makes a big difference, and more importantly, most of the students perform better in the examination. In turn, it makes the school also well known (Kunter et al. 2013; Mainhard 2015; Sharma 2016). However, the reality is different. A large number of teachers nowadays are not interested in teaching. They have neither knowledge nor do they take any initiative to improve their knowledge and skills in the subject. As a result, this category of teachers fails to satisfy the needs of the students and to overcome their own limitations. On the contrary, they create a fearful environment in the classroom and resort to vindictive attitude if any student asks any question in the classroom for clarification. Unfortunately, most Indian Schools do not have any student feedback mechanism about teachers' performance. Therefore, batch after batch, students suffer and gradually develop disinterest towards the subject (de Souza Barros and Elia 1997). It is an irreparable damage to the student's potentials. A large number of schools, irrespective of the category, conduct classes by utilizing contractual teaching staff and most of the contractual teaching staff is underqualified and/or inexperienced and they take their work casually which results in poor teaching and disinterest among students. Most of the contractual teaching staff are not motivated and committed to teaching because of a number of reasons like poor salary, the uncertainty of the job, and lack of reward (Pendergast and Kaplan 2015). Therefore, every school should appoint knowledgeable and experienced candidates, with good communication skills, for teaching. In some cases, a fresh candidate may not be experienced, but if they are erudite and possess good communication skills, they can perform effectively.

Teaching Methods

There are always arguments about the various methods of teaching. One school of thought is of the opinion that the traditional method of teaching using the blackboard is effective; another school of thought believes that the participatory method of teaching and/or practical hands-on training method are very good (Kyriacou 1997). However, all types of teaching methods have their own strengths and limitations. Finally, it depends on the personal skills and personality of a particular teacher (Araujo et al. 2016; Korthagen and Evelein 2016; Rushton et al. 2007). Teachers who are erudite and sensitive to students can present the subject in a simple manner keeping in mind the diverse background of the students in a classroom. Therefore, there is a need to organize periodic training and workshops for the teachers to enhance their teaching skills and update them about the latest advancements in the concerned subject, in addition to sensitizing them about the psychology of students (Mohanna et al. 2016; Sharma 2016). A teacher should match his/her intellectual level with the level of students while teaching, which will be beneficial for the students. Apart from this, a teacher should be amicable and should enter the classroom with a smile. The smiling face of a teacher will create a healthy psychological ambience for teaching, and students can attend classes without fear or anxiety. In this situation, transmission of knowledge will be more effective (Bove et al. 2016). Although evidence is lacking, from personal experience it has been observed that a good number of teachers lack the latest knowledge in the subject, do not reach the class on time, remain inactive in the classroom, discuss irrelevant topics in the classroom without focusing on the assigned subject, ask students to study the subject at home, do not specify the syllabus at the beginning of the session, do not complete the syllabus, and so on. Interestingly, at the time of examination, teachers who are incapable of teaching the subject effectively, and/or those who do not teach at all, are very particular to frame a very difficult question purposefully to create fear in the mind of the students for their own defence.

Evidence indicates that the effect of the teacher's use of cognitive activation strategies has the strongest positive effect on students' mathematical achievement score, followed by the school and classroom climate indicators. Thus, more cognitively activating instruction, and an orderly and peaceful atmosphere in schools and classrooms, encourage students and help to transform existing interests into mathematical achievements (Bove et al. 2016). The findings of another study by Darling-Hammond (2000) suggest that policy investments in the quality of teachers are related to improvements in student performance. Quantitative analyses further indicate that measures of teacher preparation and certification are the strongest correlates of student achievement in reading and mathematics.

In a study, researchers investigated teachers' pedagogical content knowledge, professional beliefs, work-related motivation, and self-regulation as aspects of their professional competence. Specifically, it examined how these aspects impact instruction and, in turn, student outcomes. Two-level structural equation models revealed positive effects of teachers' pedagogical content knowledge, enthusiasm for teaching, and self-regulatory skills, on instructional quality, which in turn affected student outcomes. In contrast, teachers' general academic ability did not affect their instruction (Kunter et al. 2013). Korthagen and Evelein (2016) examined the relation between the fulfilment of the three basic psychological needs of 36 student teachers and their teaching behaviour, based on Self-Determination Theory and the Model for Interpersonal Teacher Behaviour. The findings of the study revealed strong correlations between the fulfillment of the basic psychological needs and teaching behaviour. The significance of the findings is that quantitative relations were established between the 'inner' side of teaching (student teachers' personal experiences) and the 'outer' side of observable teaching behaviour.

If teaching is effective in the school, no students will go for private coaching or appoint private tutors for studying the same subjects. Because of ineffective teaching in the schools in some subjects, every parent appoints private tutors or sends his child for attending extra coaching classes at centres which cost extra money as well as deprive children of recreation after school hours. In other words, school children are deprived of games and sports. One Kolkata-based study disclosed that more than half of the secondary and higher students had 3–4 private tutors (Deb et al. 2015). Therefore, it is very important to ensure effective teaching in the schools by appointing skilled teachers with good communications skills, which will allow children to enjoy their free time after school hours.

Need for Period Training for the Teachers

Orientation Programmes and Refresher Training are required for school teachers for updating and refreshing their knowledge, and enhancement of teaching skills (Lieberman and Pointer Mace 2008) as the programmes of Academic Staff College of a university where every faculty has to undergo at least two orientation programmes and one refresher course. In the case of school teachers, the introduction of this approach will immensely benefit the teachers to have updated knowledge and in turn, transmit the knowledge to students. In this regard, McCutchen and Berninger (1999) undertook a study to understand the efficacy of a model in the case of service training for regular and special education teachers at the kindergarten through the fourth-grade level, with a focus on updating teachers on recent research developments in preventing and treating reading and writing disabilities and on utilizing this knowledge in classroom practice. The model includes a summer teacher training institute, three follow-up sessions during the academic year, and ongoing observation and consultation in teachers' classrooms. The effectiveness of the model has been demonstrated in measures of teacher knowledge, classroom practice, and student learning outcome in comparison to control teachers who have not received training. In particular, McCutchen and Berninger (1999) focused on: (a) the domain of knowledge teachers are taught that relates to understanding the processes of reading and writing acquisition and instructional approaches for reading and writing; (b) the importance of forming researcher–teacher partnerships in which teachers become the experts in translating research knowledge into classroom practice; and (c) the transformations. Researchers observed the enhancement of teachers' knowledge and in turn, how it was reflected in their effective teaching in classrooms. The findings of this study justify the need for intensive teachers' orientation programme for improvement of their teaching skills. The concerned bodies of different boards of school education should take note of the same issue: arranging periodic training programmes for school teachers and taking appropriate measures for the interest of school students since school is the foundation for every child.

School Curricula

School curricula vary across India. The curricula of Central Board of Secondary Education (CBSE), Council for the Indian School Certificate Examinations (CISCE) and state boards across different states in India, are totally different in terms of content, method of implementation of courses, difficulty in the levels of content, styles of setting question papers, and methods of evaluating student performance (Singh 2009). Therefore, the upbringing of students intellectually, morally, and socially, as well as in terms of personality development, knowledge dissemination, and preparation for the future is totally different (Pandey 2014;

Rana et al. 2016), which affects the performance of the students because of differential treatment and inputs. Each and every child has potential; it is the system which grooms them differently (Verma et al. 2014). There is a need to look at the above issues from newer perspectives and bring uniformity in curricula across the country, reducing the load to a great extent. In addition, it is important to pay attention to better methods of teaching and evaluation of students' performance to the greatest possible extent, taking regional characteristics into account (Banks 1994).

The positive schooling concept requires the special attention of the Ministry of Human Resource Development, Government of India, for debates and discussions on the development of a comprehensive National Education Policy, in which emphasis should be given on uniformity of curricula, load of curricula, the periodic review and revision of curricula, students' performance across the country, study materials—prescribed books—and quality of education. A discussion is also required about challenges and advantages of privatization of education.

Motivating Students

The motivation of students towards studies depends upon a number of factors: fear-free environment created in the classroom by the respective subject teacher, teaching styles, presentation of the subject with simple examples, teachers' personality, teachers' updated knowledge about the subject, positive and encouraging school environment, supervision of the ward's education at home by the parents, parents' encouragement, school support to students in solving any difficulties faced by the students in understanding the subject, if any, availability of study materials, and so on. In this regard, Pendergast and Kaplan (2015) stressed three important themes related to teacher-student interactions within instructional contexts: relationships, competence, and agency. Through consultation and systems-level advocacy, school psychologists can use these themes as starting points for improving the instructional context for both students and teachers. In another study, Wentzel (1997) examined the perceptions of adolescents of pedagogical caring, in relation to their motivation, to achieve positive social and academic outcomes in middle school. Findings revealed that the teachers who care were described as demonstrating democratic interaction styles, developing expectations for student behaviour in the light of individual differences, modelling a 'caring' attitude toward their own work, and providing constructive feedback. In other words, it might be stated that a caring attitude of the teacher becomes motivating for students, and promotes better academic outcome.

An early morning school assembly is a very good practice in every school when it does not take a long time; not more than 15–20 min. It should be well planned and it encourages students to read the daily day news or any important information on a rotation basis. In some schools, it takes more than half an hour, and sometimes more; it becomes difficult for students to remain standing in the open ground in the heat. On a number of occasions, some students become unconscious and sometimes half of the time of the first period gets wasted. This issue needs to be taken care of by the school principal. Some school principal or teachers become carried away and deliver long lectures during morning school assembly. It is important to remember that brief advice has a better impact than long and elaborate lectures.

Disciplining Method

It is important to take multiple measures to discipline students in the school in terms of coming to school wearing prescribed uniforms and shoes, getting there on time, attending assembly every day, attending classes attentively, carrying out tasks in the classroom given by the teachers and completing homework, informing school authority if absent for some reason, behaving properly with fellow classmates, sharing information with classmates, participating in group activities and sharing views and opinion with an open mind, and so on (Bear 2015; Jain 2017). In this regard, the role of the class teacher is very important in inculcating the same good habits among students in a positive manner and, if necessary, reinforcement of the same message for the formation of good habits is required, instead of administering corporal punishment and/or humiliating a student by making derogatory comments in front of other students (Elstad and Christophersen 2017; Kennedy et al. 2017). Encouragement by teachers for doing even a minor task well, and/or any other encouragement will have a positive impact in developing good habits among students. Sometimes, especially at an early stage of schooling, students give more value to any advice of teacher than advice given by parents.

Corporal Punishment (CP)

According to the National Commission for Protection of Child Rights (2008), "corporal punishment involves rapping on the knuckles, running on the school ground, kneeling down for hours, standing up for long hours, sitting like a chair, and beating with a scale, pinching and slapping, child sexual abuse, torture, locking up children alone in classrooms, "electric shock" and all other acts leading to insult, humiliation, physical and mental injury, and even death" (NCPCR 2008).

Corporal punishment is a cultural practice in some developing countries like India. The evidence clearly demonstrates that CP and/or psychological abuse of students has an adverse effect on their mental health and personality development (Banzon-Librojo et al. 2017; Gershoff 2017; Ip et al. 2016; Wendland et al. 2017). However, CP has remained a common practice not only in many homes but is also regularly practiced in schools, particularly in low-income countries, as a measure to maintain discipline. In this regard, in a cross-sectional survey targeting preparatory and secondary school students enrolled in mainstream public schools in Alexandria,

Youssef et al. (1998) observed that a substantial proportion of boys (79.96%) and girls (61.53%) incurred physical punishment at the hand of their teachers. Teachers were using their hands, sticks, straps, shoes, and kicks to inflict punishment without sparing any part of their students' body. Physical injuries were reported by a significantly higher percentage of boys; the most common being bumps and contusions, followed by wounds and fractures. Moreover, it was only among boys that serious injuries such as loss of consciousness and concussion were encountered. In yet another study, Hecker et al. (2014) assessed the occurrence of corporal punishment, at home and in school, in Tanzanian primary school students, in addition to examining the association between corporal punishment and externalizing problems. Nearly all children had experienced corporal punishment at some point during their lifetime, both in family and school contexts. Half of the respondents reported having experienced corporal punishment within the last year from a family member. A multiple sequential regression analysis revealed that corporal punishment by parents or by caregivers was positively related to children's externalizing problems. The present study provides evidence that Tanzanian children of primary school were frequently exposed to extreme levels of corporal punishment, with detrimental effects on externalizing behaviour. Another study examined the relationships between race and CP, and gender and CP, and found evidence of race and gender bias, in the administration of CP (Shaw and Braden 1990).

In a recent study in Puducherry India, by Deb and others, the authors found more than half of the students (62%) reported experiencing school CP in the past 12 months, with males, and those attending public schools, being significantly more likely to report school CP than females and those in private schools. Youth who reported school CP reported more anxiety and depression. That relation was more pronounced in youth who reported family tension. Social support and resilience did not moderate the relations. The findings add to the substantial evidence about negative associations regarding the use of CP, but, in a new venue, the school, thus providing some evidence for the need to change how students are disciplined in schools in India and elsewhere (Deb et al. 2016).

The findings of the above studies clearly indicate that CP is a global phenomenon and all the study findings emphasize the need to make parents, teachers, and governmental organizations—especially in low-income countries—aware about the adverse consequences of using corporal punishment, be it at home or at school. The onus of safeguarding children and students from punishment lies with the school teachers, education administration at all levels, as well as all those responsible for management. The National Commission for Protection of Child Rights directs the education departments of all the states in India to ensure the following issues:

1. All children are to be informed through campaigns and publicity drives that they have a right to speak against corporal punishment and bring it to the notice of the authorities. They must be given the confidence to make complaints and not accept punishment as a 'normal' activity of the school.

2. Every school, including hostels, Juvenile Justice Homes, shelter homes, and other public institutions meant for children must have a forum where children can express their views. Such institutions could take the help of an NGO facilitating such an exercise.
3. Further, a box where children can drop their complaints, even if anonymous, has to be provided for in each school.
4. There has to be a monthly meeting of the Parent-Teachers Association (PTAs) or any other body to review the complaints and take action.
5. The PTAs are to be encouraged to act immediately on any complaints made by children without postponement of the issue instead of waiting for a more grave injury to be caused. In other words, the PTAs need not use their discretion to decide on the grievousness of the complaint.
6. Parents, as well as children, are to be empowered to speak out against corporal punishment without any fear that it would have an adverse effect on children's participation in schools.
7. The education departments at all levels—block, district, and State—are to establish procedures for reviewing the responses to the complaints of children and monitoring the action taken on the same suffering from some contagious disease.

Enrolment and Attendance of Students in Schools

Enrolment and attendance of students in rural and urban schools vary. In rural public schools, enrolment and attendance depend upon many factors: the parents' perception of the value of education; economic and social class; school infrastructure; distance of school; and communication facilities.

As per NITI Aayog report (National Institution for Transforming India), Government of India, net school enrolment ratio at the primary level during 2008–09, 2009–10, and 2010–11 were 98.59, 98.28 and 99.89 respectively.

According to the Ministry of Human Resource Development (MHRD) Report, the national dropout rate at the primary level was 4.34% in 2014–15, and it was even higher at the secondary level, at 17.86%. As per the joint report by the Montreal-based UNESCO Institute for Statistics and Global Education Monitoring, India has 47 million youth of secondary and higher secondary school-going age who are dropping out of school, which is highest in the world (Gohain 2016).

There are many reasons for school dropouts in India. They include lack of supervision of children's study at home, the wrong notion about the value of education among parents, poverty, having to care for younger children when parents go for work, non-availability of school in and around the village, migration of families, child marriage, lack of school infrastructure facilities such as drinking water and toilets, poor communication facilities, and lack of accessibility.

Students' school dropout rate at primary and at secondary level varies across the states in India.

Muralidharan and Kremer (2006) present results from a nationally-representative survey of rural private primary schools in India conducted in 2003. The study revealed that about one-fourth (28%) of the population of rural India has access to fee-charging private schools in the same village. Nearly 50% of the rural private schools in the sample category of the study having been established five or fewer years before the time of the survey, suggesting a rapid growth in the number of private schools. Private schools are more common in areas with poor public school performance. Richer states are less likely to have rural private schools. Compared to public schools, private schools pay much lower teacher salaries, have lower pupil-teacher ratios, and less multi-grade teaching. Private school teachers are 2–8% points less likely to be absent than teachers in public schools, and 6–9% points more likely to be engaged in a teaching-related activity at any given point in time. They are more likely to hold a college degree than public-school teachers, but much less likely to have a formal teacher training certificate. Children in private schools have higher attendance rates. They have higher test scores, even after controlling for observable family and school characteristics.

Given the scenario of enrolment and attendance in rural schools in India, local government should take proactive measures sensitizing the parents to admit their ward in school. Thus, a hundred percent enrolment and attendance of children in rural schools can be ensured, justifying the signing the UN Convention on Rights of the Child by the Government of India. The right to education is the fundamental right of a child. The government should establish schools in rural areas where there are no schools, strengthen the school infrastructure where infrastructure is poor, and appoint regular teachers and other staff from nearby places.

Responding quickly to early indicators of a potential dropout—such as absenteeism—by counselling the student and parent, is one strategy for prevention of school drop-out. In this regard, the MHRD has already initiated a new system of tracking drop-out rates by students' Aadhar IDs, so that early intervention can be made to bring the child back to school. The data will be maintained by the National University for Education Planning and Administration (NUEPA).

Addressing Students' Psychological Challenges and Introducing Mental Health Support Services

Like physical health problems, every child is vulnerable to psychological problems during development phase especially common childhood disorder, anxiety, and depression, which require immediate attention. Further, it is relevant to state here that adolescent students' depression not only interferes with emotional, social, and academic functioning but also is a proven risk factor for school absenteeism, educational underachievement, substance abuse, and suicidal behaviour (Verma et al. 2014). Recent evidence indicates that a large number of students experience common childhood disorders, anxiety, and depression (Igbokwe et al. 2016; Preeti et al. 2017; Ranasinghe et al. 2016). For example, one Indian study carried out among Standard 12 students in various Boards of Education in Raipur city, highlights that 40.49% students were mildly depressed while 19% had major depression. Depression was found more in females (59.5%) as compared to males (56.2%). The percentage of depressed students was highest among students of I.C.S.E. board (48.3%). Among the various factors examined for association with depression, statistically significant factors identified were working mothers, students staying away from home, poor relationship with family and self, or parental dissatisfaction with academic achievement. Peer pressure also had a significant association. Having a hobby acted as a protective factor against depression (Verma et al. 2014).

In a multi-national study called the Global School-Based Student Health Survey (GSHS), the analysis of data collected from 7904 middle school students in India, 25.5% reported symptoms of depression, 8.6% reported loneliness, while 7.8% reported anxiety-related insomnia. Both male and female students who reported symptoms of depression had an increased likelihood of poor hand and oral hygiene, including washing their hands rarely or never and brushing their teeth less than daily. In girls, loneliness was also associated with poor hand and oral hygiene. Reduced mental health status in adolescents may lead to worse hygiene behaviours and an increased risk of infections (Ranasinghe et al. 2016).

Mental health support services for school students are essential so that students can pay attention to studies and perform better. Remaining deprived from these facilities when a student requires it might cause depression and anxiety and even suicidal ideation. Eliamani et al. (2014) performed a study to examine the influence of secondary school students' access to guidance and counselling services on school life, attitude towards studies, and career choices. The findings unearthed that "the services offered in the selected schools included: academic, health, moral, and spiritual matters. Although no trained counsellor was found, the services offered proved to be moderately effective in influencing the study life of students; and effective in shaping students' attitude towards studies and career choice. Finally, it was concluded that being able to access guidance and counselling services have an effect in shaping students' attitude towards studies and in career choices."

There is an increasing academic and policy interest in interventions aiming to promote young people's health by ensuring that the school environment supports healthy behaviours. Keeping this background in mind, Morton et al. (2016) did a secondary research with a view to summarizing the current evidence on school-based policy, physical and social-environmental influences on adolescent physical activity and sedentary behaviour. The findings were synthesized using a non-quantitative synthesis and thematic analysis. Ninety-three papers of mixed methodological quality were included. A range of school-based policy (such as recess length), physical (such as facilities) and socio-environmental (such as teacher behaviours) factors were associated with adolescent physical activity, with limited research on sedentary behaviour. The mixed-studies synthesis revealed the importance of specific activity settings (type and location) and intramural sports opportunities for all students. Important physical education-related factors were a mastery-oriented motivational climate and autonomy-supportive teaching behaviours. Qualitative evidence highlighted the influence of the general school climate, while shedding light on the complexities of the associations observed in the quantitative literature.

Unfortunately, in India, this issue has not received much attention from educational administrators and, thereby, hardly any school has appointed a professional or trained psychologist or school counsellor for addressing the mental health challenges of the students. The mental health challenges of students go unnoticed and, afterwards, when it becomes aggravated, parents or teachers look for a psychologist. In most cases, parents first consult a psychiatrist only when they are supposed to visit a psychologist. In India psychiatrists are easily available in the hospitals, while one has to search for a professional psychologist for the same purpose. Non-availability of trained psychologists in developing countries like India is a big challenge. Therefore, there is a need to train students, after completion of their Master's Degree, in psychology or applied psychology for dealing with the mental health of school students professionally. There is also a need to prepare a directory of trained psychologists and make this information available to the general public so that, as and when they require any such help, they can consult a trained and experienced psychologist for professional support.

Life Skills, or Reproductive and Sexual Health, Education for School Students

Life skills, or reproductive and sexual health, education for school students is also necessary to enhance their psychological competence so that they can easily deal with day-to-day challenges on their own. In this regard, the Indian Council of Medical Research (ICMR) did a multi-centric intervention study, developed a need-based curriculum (six modules) for imparting knowledge and skills among adolescent students, and provided inputs to students twice, following classroom lectures by subject-specific experts, through leaflets and question-box approach, and found that the intervention modules were effective in the enhancement of knowledge and skills of adolescent students. The same modules could be replicated in other schools in India (Deb 2006).

Assessing Aptitude and Interest of the Students for Future Career

The natural potential of students varies; some are good in literature, some in social science, and some in mathematics. Differential aptitude and psychological tests help students to identify their aptitude and interest and accordingly, if they are guided, they can perform better. At the initial stage, some students are unable to decide the subject which they would like to pursue for career growth. Therefore, appointing professional psychologists in the educational institutes, the aptitude and interest of the students could be ascertained and they can guided accordingly (de Guzman and Choi 2013; Eliamani et al. 2014; Mehmood et al. 1971).

Encouraging Students for Extra-Curricular Activities

Evidence clearly indicates that extra-curricular activities have a number of benefits for the overall social, psychological, and academic performance of students. For example, in a study, participants in most extra-curricular activities achieved better educational outcomes than non-participants. Participation in social service and religious activities predicted lower rates of alcohol consumption and drug use. Participation in school sports teams predicted both better educational outcomes and higher rates of alcohol consumption (Eccles et al. 2003).

Encouragement using positive words—like 'although you are doing well, you can improve yourself further', 'you can do much better', 'keep up your good performance', and 'you have the potential'—is highly motivating for students. Using encouraging words and creating a supportive environment, teachers can motivate students in studies and ensure their involvement in extra-curricular activities, and in turn, positive words from teachers will improve the overall performance of students (MacMillan et al. 2015; Morton et al. 2016). There is evidence justifying the usefulness of extra-curricular activities for healthy mental and physical development of children. Extra-curricular activities help a student to remain physically fit, active, energetic, and calm, while also enhancing aptitude and concentration in studies; finally, the student feels fresh. In the present CBSE curricula, much emphasis is given to extra-curricular activities and if all the government schools under CBSE follow the same curricula strictly, it would be highly beneficial for the students. The students passing out from these schools are more competent to deal with the challenges of daily life than the students from schools where there are not many extra-curricular activities. Previous findings have confirmed the same notion repeatedly (Eccles et al. 2003; Eccles and Templeton 2002; Larson 1994).

Education related to environment and eco-system is essential for young students so that when they grow they develop a proper understanding of the environment. For saving our ecosystem, environmental values should be inculcated from the beginning of child development; early inspiration influences the attitude of students towards the environment in a positive way as noted by Pandey (2014). In his study, it was found that "boys of science and commerce streams of the Indian Certificate of Secondary Education (ICSE) Board and Central Board of Secondary Education (CBSE) Board have a similar environmental attitude, whereas, in the case of girls, it was seen that girls belonging to the science and commerce streams of CBSE board have a better environmental attitude than those of ICSE board."

As far as students' creativity is concerned, Rana et al. (2016) examined the influence of home and school environment on the creativity of adolescent students of Hisar city in Haryana (India) in which students from five schools from three educational boards—Hisar Board of Secondary Education (HBSE), Central Board of Secondary Education (CBSE) and Indian Certificate of Secondary Education (ICSE)—participated. Adolescents were assessed for their creativity by divergent production abilities scale. The creativity was found to be highest among CBSE and ICSE board students while HBSE students had a high level of originality. The study highlighted that though the home environment of the child partially influences the creativity of adolescents, the school environment was found to be a significant factor in determining the level of creativity among adolescents.

Ensuring Safety in School

Safety in schools is essential for creating a student-friendly environment. If the school environment is a non-threatening, congenial, and student-friendly one, every child would like to attend the school and pursue their studies with satisfaction. Safety, not only from corporal punishment and sexual abuse, but also from psychological discomfort is necessary. Although the majority of the teachers are student-friendly, some teachers create an intimidating environment in the classroom so that students do not present any queries for clarification (Deb et al. 2016; Youssef et al. 1998). Some teachers even feel offended if a student asks a question. Sometimes they stop a student saying 'don't ask silly questions' even a maths teacher of Standard 11. A query about science or maths might be a silly one to a teacher, but for a student, it is necessary to obtain clarity. Otherwise, the student will not understand the next step. Insensitivity on the part of some teachers causes disinterest and de-motivation among some students and for which a particular teacher is responsible (Shaw and Braden 1990). The issue needs to be taken up by the school authority every year (Daral et al. 2016; Hecker et al. 2014; Lang et al. 2013).

In a study, Banzon-Librojo et al. (2017) examined how the experience of harsh discipline from teachers is related to students' experience of bullying victimization in a Philippine high school. The findings suggested that school discipline strategies may have repercussions on students' behaviour and relationships, highlighting the teacher's role in modelling and setting norms for teachers' acceptable behaviour.

Examination and Methods of Evaluation of Student Performance

Examinations, the setting of question papers, and methods of evaluation vary from board to board. In the case of some State Board of Secondary and Higher Secondary Education, there is an instruction from the competent authority that most of the questions should be given from the prescribed questions provided at the end of each chapter of a book of a prescribed syllabus. As a result, a large number of students get a full percentage in almost all the subjects. On the contrary, in the Central Board of Secondary Education, popularly known as CBSE, there is no set boundary for a question paper, as long as it is within the curriculum. As a result, the performance of the students in CBSE is average or below average compared to some State Boards. Therefore, this issue requires the attention of the MHRD for bringing uniformity in terms of curricula, methods of teaching, method of setting question papers and evaluation, for upholding justice to all children. Otherwise, in the present schooling system in India, it is a gross violation of child rights.

Regarding question paper setting of CBSE, it has been observed that three to four sets of question papers are prepared and randomly distributed to students in the same examination centre and the difficulty levels of the question paper vary greatly because each set of question paper is prepared by different examiners. Obviously, one or two sets will be easy while the others might be difficult; accordingly, the performance of students will vary. Is it justifiable to test the merit or performance of the students of same curricula of the same academic session using four different sets of question papers without ensuring parity in difficulty level? Is there any procedure to normalize the scores of four different sets of question papers? If the philosophy and/or rationale behind setting four sets of question papers for each subject, for the same group of students of the same region, are to avoid copying, the questions of one set could be reshuffled and made into two to three sets of question papers in the larger interest of the students, to uphold justice. This apart, proper invigilation will ensure proper conduct of examinations, free from coping. And, if necessary, the examination may be monitored strictly by using CCTV surveillance. However, the present method of evaluation raises a number of questions in the minds of parents and teaching community.

First, is it not unfair for the students, writing an examination for a subject, answering a difficult question paper, which will invariably result in comparatively poor performance, especially when the performance determines the possibility of admission of the students at the next level?

Second, is it not demoralizing for the group of students who are answering a difficult question paper? Who would be responsible if the experience is traumatic?

Third, is there any method to ensure parity of difficulty between different sets of question papers for the same subject? If there is, what happened in the case of one physics question paper in 2017, which was more difficult than the other sets?

Fourth, who sets the question papers? Senior School Teachers or College Professors? While going through the question papers of Standard 12 of CBSE Examination of 2017, it was well clear that the question paper setter tried his/her level best to prove his/her own knowledge, disregarding the students' level of maturity.

Ideally, any examination should be based on one question paper set. Only then the assessment of students' performance will be reasonably uniform. Region-wise question papers might vary, but it does not necessarily mean different sets of question papers need to be used in the same region and even in the same school. This will lead to academic stress, anxiety, and depression among some school students.

This is absolutely the wrong approach. This approach will cause discrimination and demoralization which will adversely affect the motivation and mental health of students and, in turn, the nation will lose a potential human resource.

While preparing the question paper, one needs to set about 50% of the questions keeping average students in mind, the standard of 25% questions can be higher and the remaining 25% may be difficult or very difficult. When examiners set question papers for university examinations and/or national level entrance tests, this is the normal procedure.

Student Protection Committee and Students Feedback Mechanism

Student Protection Committee is a common body in all industrial countries for ensuring student safety, registering students' complaints, and listening to their voices. In India, the approach is missing. Every school should form a Student Protection Committee, comprising of teacher representatives, student representatives, and psychologists, representatives from NGOs and Child Welfare Committees, and one legal professional. This approach will help the school administration to understand the issues and concerns of students from the right perspective, particularly related to students' perception of classroom teaching, any difficulty related to understanding the subject taught by a particular teacher, punctuality of taking classes, completion of syllabus by the respective subject teacher, safety issues—such as corporal punishment, sexual abuse, bullying by senior students—students' preferences for extra-curricular activities, educational tour and any new idea from the students and taking corrective measures for the interest of students.

Effective Parent-Teacher Meeting and Feedback Mechanism

A Parent-Teacher meeting has a special significance in terms of giving feedback about a student to their parents in a sensitive manner so that parents can guide the student in proper manner (Fan 2001; Fehrmann et al. 1987; LaRocque et al. 2011; Zellman and Waterman 1998). This is the platform which can be most effectively utilized by the school authority in the interest of the students, by sensitizing the parents about various issues like academic stress experienced by the students from the parents, by informing them about how to motivate a child in studies at home, listening to children's voices, not applying corporal punishment at home, but making a child understand in an amicable manner, familial violence and its impact on children's mental health, the necessity of supportive environment at home, quality parenting, and so on. Special lectures on the above issues could be arranged in a school, inviting knowledgeable resource persons on the day of the parents-teachers meeting. Normally, in most schools on the day of the parents-teachers meeting, parents come to the school and collect the report card and teachers encourage parents to write a good remark about the teacher in the attendance sheet for the teacher's benefit. Therefore, this sort of parents-teachers meeting is not very beneficial.

Involving Larger Community in the School Management Committee

School Management Committee should be a composition of representatives of school teachers, an educationist from outside or other higher learning institutes, parents' representative, a representative from an NGO and one legal and one medical professional and a students' representative. This should be a platform to discuss various development-related issues of the school with an open mind and all the members of management committee should be encouraged to attend all the meetings and participate actively in the meeting without any prejudice, for the betterment of the school (Epstein 1995; Fullan and Hargreaves 1991). In reality, in most of the cases, this is more of a formality. In other words, members of a management committee are chosen based on an understanding that these members would never bring up any issue for discussion which needs attention and corrective measures. Even if they raise any important issue related to ineffective teaching by a few teachers, students safety issues, non-availability of safe drinking water, poor maintenance of washroom and so on, in a number of cases, it has been observed that the Principal of the School has not paid any attention and has preferred to remain indifferent because of a perceived non-co-operation from the teachers. However, there are schools where the Principal encourages all the members of the management committee to provide their suggestions and take proactive measures instead of defending mistakes and/or lapses on the part of some of the teachers. Accepting mistakes and/or shortcomings, if genuine, and taking corrective measures for improving the situation in school should be the approach in every school and only then would the management committee members be encouraged to participate in the meeting and contribute significantly (Kruse and Louis 1997; Southworth 2002).

Revisiting Teachers Selection Procedure and Making School Teaching Job More Attractive Providing Better Salary and Other Facilities

There is a need to look at the teaching profession at school level from a different perspective. As of today, the school teaching profession in India is not conducive for attracting meritorious candidates with good academic performance because of the low salary, and the poor social status attached to the school teaching profession. A small number of candidates with good academic background come to teaching because of their passion. But, a sizeable number of candidates who land up in school teaching profession, are ones who have failed to get any other job; they are capable of neither teaching effectively, nor do they have any desire to improve themselves. As a result, in most schools, about one-third of the teachers of this category fail to justify their role as a teacher and students suffer. Therefore, it is essential to ensure that qualified and skilled candidates are recruited for the teaching profession and under no circumstances even a single unqualified and unskilled candidate be appointed as teacher in a school. The selection of just one wrong candidate in teaching could have a long-term negative impact on student performance.

The low social perception about school teaching as a profession should be altered for the best interest of the students and of national prosperity. Improving the salary and offering better service benefits will attract the best candidates to the school teaching profession and, in turn, the system and students will be benefited. In fact, teaching at the school level is very difficult because of the diverse nature and background of the students with varying intellectual capacities. Primary, middle school, secondary and higher secondary level education is very important for building a good foundation for each student. Therefore, school education policy-makers should think about how to strengthen the school education system with quality manpower, by offering an attractive salary and other good service benefits, and allocating more budget for education (Lavy 2007). The moment the service benefits for teaching professionals improve, it will attract the best candidates and thereby this profession will have a better social status, as salary and other service benefits are the determinant factors for the social status of a worker. In turn, this positivity about school teaching as a profession will encourage positive schooling and will benefit the students. Thus, the country will get well-nurtured human resources for building the nation's prosperity.

Parental Involvement

Parental involvement in supervision of academic activities of children at home is considered to be an important influence in their academic progress. Positive schooling concept cannot be materialized without parental quality involvement in students' upbringing. Along with school inputs, parents should spend quality time with their children and supervise their studies regularly. Time spent on homework and in leisure has an important effect on academic learning. Keeping this in mind, one study examined the indirect effect of such involvement on grades through analysing TV-viewing time and time spent on homework. Parental involvement was found to be an important direct, positive effect on grades of school students. Additionally, parental involvement also led to increased time spent on homework, which in turn had a positive effect on grades (Fehrmann et al. 1987).

Conclusion and Implications

Multiple measures are to be adopted for creating a positive schooling environment, starting from basic infrastructure facilities including proper classroom seating arrangements, proper lighting with basic educational materials for teaching, hygienic sanitation facilities, and safe drinking water. Most importantly, appointing an effective Principal and qualified teachers, and sensitizing them about the importance of teaching with passion, using innovative methods to make studies enjoyable, are some of the prerequisites. Although the majority of the teachers are good and they teach with interest matching the needs of the students, there are a significant number of teachers who need to improve their knowledge and teaching skills in addition to becoming student friendly. Periodic orientation programmes for school teachers on pedagogy, teaching skills, individual differences, child psychology, common childhood disorders, and child rights, will be beneficial for teachers. The rewarding system in terms of promotion for teachers should be introduced for motivating them in teaching and also as an example for motivating other teachers to teach effectively. Mental health support services should be made available in every school to help students to overcome any challenges. At the same time, there is a need to revisit the school teaching profession as a novel profession with better service benefits for ensuring the appointment of highly qualified candidates who can ensure quality teaching. Care should be taken to ensure that not a single unqualified and unskilled candidate is selected in school for teaching profession. Selection of even one unqualified and unskilled candidate in the teaching profession will have a long-term adverse impact on students. The school is the foundation for every child. If the foundation is strong, the country will get skilled human resource for faster national growth and social prosperity.

Ensuring positive schooling ambience will have multiple implications. A safe environment in the school will allow the student to grow with positive mental health; the student will enjoy the school life, and in turn, they would like to come to school regularly with full preparation. Encouraging words from teachers can have a powerful positive effect on each student in terms of creating a fear-free environment and encouraging students to clarify their queries. A healthy student-friendly school environment will motivate students in studies and will result in good performance. Parents will also remain free from anxiety because of the safety and quality educational standards maintained in the school.

References

Allen, J. P., Pianta, R. C., Gregory, A., Mikami, A. Y., & Lun, J. (2011). An interaction-based approach to enhancing secondary school instruction and student achievement. *Science, 333* (6045), 1034–1037.

Araujo, M. C., Carneiro, P., Cruz-Aguayo, Y., & Schady, N. (2016). Teacher quality and learning outcomes in kindergarten. *The Quarterly Journal of Economics, 131*(3), 1415–1453.

Banks, J. A. (1994). *An introduction to multicultural education*. ERIC.
Banzon-Librojo, L. A., Garabiles, M. R., & Alampay, L. P. (2017). Brief report: Relations between harsh discipline from teachers, perceived teacher support, and bullying victimization among high school students. *Journal of Adolescence, 57,* 18–22. https://doi.org/10.1016/j.adolescence.2017.03.001.
Bear, G. G. (2015). Preventive and classroom-based strategies. In *Handbook of classroom management* (pp. 15–39).
Blumberg, A., & Greenfield, W. (1986). *The effective principal: Perspectives on school leadership*. ERIC.
Bove, G., Marella, D., & Vitale, V. (2016). Influences of school climate and teacher's behavior on student's competencies in mathematics and the territorial gap between Italian macro-areas in PISA 2012. *Journal of Educational, Cultural and Psychological Studies (ECPS Journal), 1*(13), 63–96.
Daral, S., Khokhar, A., & Pradhan, S. K. (2016). Barriers to disclosure of child maltreatment among school-going adolescent girls of a semi-urban area of Delhi, India. *International Journal of Adolescent Medicine and Health.*
Darling-Hammond, L. (2000). Teacher quality and student achievement. *Education Policy Analysis Archives, 8,* 1.
de Guzman, A. B., & Choi, K. O. (2013). The relations of employability skills to career adaptability among technical school students. *Journal of Vocational Behavior, 82*(3), 199–207.
de Souza Barros, S., & Elia, M. F. (1997). Physics teacher's attitudes: How do they affect the reality of the classroom and models for change? *Connecting Research in Physics Education with Teacher Education.*
Deb, S. (2006). *Report of a study on ICMR task force project titled a study on reproductive and sexual health education for adolescents—A multi centric study (2006)*. New Delhi: Funded by the Indian Council of Social Science Research.
Deb, S., Kumar, A., Holden, G. W., & Simpson Rowe, L. (2016). School corporal punishment, family tension, and students' internalizing problems: Evidence from India. *School Psychology International,* 0143034316681378.
Deb, S., Strodl, E., & Sun, J. (2015). Academic stress, parental pressure, anxiety and mental health among Indian high school students. *International Journal of Psychology and Behavioural Sciences, 5*(1), 26–34.
Devanathan, V. (2014). *Safe drinking water in govt schools still a distant dream* |TNN| June 25, 2014, 02.24 AM IST. http://timesofindia.indiatimes.com/city/madurai/Safe-drinking-water-in-govt-schools-still-a-distant-dream/articleshow/37145182.cms.
Eccles, J. S., Barber, B. L., Stone, M., & Hunt, J. (2003). Extracurricular activities and adolescent development. *Journal of Social Issues, 59*(4), 865–889.
Eccles, J. S., & Templeton, J. (2002). Extracurricular and other after-school activities for youth (Chap. 4). *Review of Research in Education, 26*(1), 113–180.
Eliamani, M. P., Richard, M. L., & Peter, B. (2014). Access to guidance and counseling services and its influence on Students' school life and career choice. *African Journal of Guidance and Counselling, 1*(1), 007–015.
Elstad, E., & Christophersen, K.-A. (2017). Teachers' self-efficacy at maintaining order and discipline in technology-rich classrooms with relation to strain factors. *International Journal of Learning, Teaching and Educational Research, 16*(1).
Epstein, J. L. (1995). School/family/community partnerships. *Phi Delta Kappan, 76*(9), 701.
Fan, X. (2001). Parental involvement and students' academic achievement: A growth modeling analysis. *The Journal of Experimental Education, 70*(1), 27–61.
Fehrmann, P. G., Keith, T. Z., & Reimers, T. M. (1987). Home influence on school learning: Direct and indirect effects of parental involvement on high school grades. *The Journal of Educational Research, 80*(6), 330–337.
Fullan, M. G., & Hargreaves, A. (1991). *What's worth fighting for? Working together for your school*. ERIC.

Gershoff, E. T. (2017). School corporal punishment in global perspective: Prevalence, outcomes, and efforts at intervention. *Psychology, Health & Medicine,* (1).

Gohain, M.P. (2016, July 15). At 47 million, India has the most adolescent school dropouts. *The Times of India*, Tamil Nadu Edition.

Hecker, T., Hermenau, K., Isele, D., & Elbert, T. (2014). Corporal punishment and children's externalizing problems: A cross-sectional study of Tanzanian primary school aged children. *Child Abuse and Neglect, 38*(5), 884–892.

Hess, F. M., & Kelly, A. P. (2007). Learning to lead: What gets taught in principal-preparation programs. *Teachers College Record, 109*(1), 244–274.

Igbokwe, D., Ola, B., & Ndom, R. (2016). Gender differences in the manifestation of brain fag, depression and indices of anxiety among secondary school students in Nigeria. *European Psychiatry, 33,* S154.

Ip, P., Wong, R. S., Li, S. L., Chan, K. L., Ho, F. K., & Chow, C.-B. (2016). Mental health consequences of childhood physical abuse in Chinese populations: A meta-analysis. *Trauma, Violence, & Abuse, 17*(5), 571–584.

Jain, P. (2017). A study about student discipline approach of teachers in schools. *Global Journal For Research Analysis, 5*(11).

Kennedy, B. L., Murphy, A. S., & Jordan, A. (2017). Title I middle school administrators' beliefs and choices about using corporal punishment and exclusionary discipline. *American Journal of Education, 123*(2).

Korthagen, F. A. J., & Evelein, F. G. (2016). Relations between student teachers' basic needs fulfillment and their teaching behaviour. *Teaching and Teacher Education, 60,* 234–244. https://doi.org/10.1016/j.tate.2016.08.021.

Kruse, S. D., & Louis, K. S. (1997). Teacher teaming in middle schools: Dilemmas for a schoolwide community. *Educational Administration Quarterly, 33*(3), 261–289.

Kunter, M., Klusmann, U., Baumert, J., Richter, D., Voss, T., & Hachfeld, A. (2013). Professional competence of teachers: Effects on instructional quality and student development. *Journal of Educational Psychology, 105*(3), 805.

Kyriacou, C. (1997). *Effective teaching in schools: Theory and practice*. Nelson Thornes.

Lang, I. A., Marlow, R., Goodman, R., Meltzer, H., & Ford, T. (2013). Influence of problematic child-teacher relationships on future psychiatric disorder: Population survey with 3-year follow-up. *The British Journal of Psychiatry, 202*(5), 336–341.

LaRocque, M., Kleiman, I., & Darling, S. M. (2011). Parental involvement: The missing link in school achievement. *Preventing School Failure, 55*(3), 115–122.

Larson, R. (1994). Youth organizations, hobbies, and sports as developmental contexts. In *Adolescence in context: The interplay of family, school, peers, and work in adjustment* (pp. 46–65).

Lavy, V. (2007). Using performance-based pay to improve the quality of teachers. *The Future of Children,* 87–109.

Lieberman, A., & Pointer Mace, D. H. (2008). Teacher learning: The key to educational reform. *Journal of Teacher Education, 59*(3), 226–234.

MacMillan, F., Kirk, A., Mutrie, N., Moola, F., & Robertson, K. (2015). Supporting participation in physical education at school in youth with type 1 diabetes: Perceptions of teachers, youth with type 1 diabetes, parents and diabetes professionals. *European Physical Education Review, 21*(1), 3–30.

Mainhard, T. (2015). Liking a tough teacher: Interpersonal characteristics of teaching and students' achievement goals. *School Psychology International, 36*(6), 559–574. https://doi.org/10.1177/0143034315608235.

Majra, J., & Gur, A. (2010). School environment and sanitation in rural India. *Journal of Global Infectious Diseases, 2*(2), 109.

Malik, A., Butt, Z. I., Rashid, K., Saeed, N., Adnan, M. A. J., & Butt, R. H. (2016). Identification of leadership styles, traits and competencies of secondary school heads. *Journal of Science International.*

Marks, H. M., & Printy, S. M. (2003). Principal leadership and school performance: An integration of transformational and instructional leadership. *Educational Administration Quarterly, 39*(3), 370–397.

McCutchen, D., & Berninger, V. W. (1999). Those who know, teach well: Helping teachers master literacy-related subject-matter knowledge. *Learning Disabilities Research & Practice, 14*(4), 215–226. https://doi.org/10.1207/sldrp1404_3.

Mehmood, S. I., Kumar, A., Borleffs, J. C., & Tio, R. A. (1971). Predictors of performance in a medical school. *Selection of Medical Students and Their Specialty Choices,* 15.

Meller, M., & Litschig, S. (2016). Adapting the supply of education to the needs of girls: Evidence from a policy experiment in Rural India. *Journal of Human Resources, 51*(3), 760–802.

Mohanna, K., Chambers, R., & Wall, D. (2016). *Your teaching style: A practical guide to understanding, developing and improving*. CRC Press.

Morton, K., Atkin, A., Corder, K., Suhrcke, M., & Sluijs, E. (2016). The school environment and adolescent physical activity and sedentary behaviour: A mixed-studies systematic review. *Obesity Reviews, 17*(2), 142–158.

Muralidharan, K., & Kremer, M. (2006). Public and private schools in rural India. *Harvard University, Department of Economics, Cambridge, MA.*

The National Commission for the Protection of Child Rights (NCPCR), Delhi. (December 2008). Protection of Children against Corporal Punishment in Schools and Institutions, Summary discussions by the Working Group on Corporal Punishment. http://harprathmik.gov.in/pdf/rte/corporal%20punishment%20ncpcr.pdf.

Pandey, C. (2014). Environmental attitude of science and commerce students belonging to ICSE and CBSE Boards. *Shikshan Anveshika, 4*(2), 101–104.

Pendergast, L. L., & Kaplan, A. (2015). Instructional context and student motivation, learning, and development: Commentary and implications for school psychologists. *School Psychology International, 36*(6), 638–647.

Preeti, B., Singh, K., & Kumar, R. (2017). Study of depression, anxiety and stress among school going adolescents. *Indian Journal of Psychiatric Social Work, 8*(1), 6–9.

Rana, S., Singh, C., & Rana, S. (2016). Relationship of creativity with human ecological factors across different educational boards. *Imperial Journal of Interdisciplinary Research, 2*(10).

Ranasinghe, S., Ramesh, S., & Jacobsen, K. H. (2016). Hygiene and mental health among middle school students in India and 11 other countries. *Journal of Infection and Public Health, 9*(4), 429–435. https://doi.org/10.1016/j.jiph.2015.11.007.

Rushton, S., Morgan, J., & Richard, M. (2007). Teacher's Myers-Briggs personality profiles: Identifying effective teacher personality traits. *Teaching and Teacher Education, 23*(4), 432–441.

Sharma, A. (2016). Professional development of teachers and teacher educators. *Indian Journal of Applied Research, 6*(4).

Shaw, S. R., & Braden, J. P. (1990). Race and gender bias in the administration of corporal punishment. *School Psychology Review, 19*(3), 378–383.

Shulman, L. (1987). Knowledge and teaching: Foundations of the new reform. *Harvard Educational Review, 57*(1), 1–23.

Singh, J. (2009). Status of school library development in India. *Sri Lankan Journal of Librarianship and Information Management, 1*(1).

Southworth, G. (2002). Instructional leadership in schools: Reflections and empirical evidence. *School Leadership & Management, 22*(1), 73–91.

Verma, N., Jain, M., & Roy, P. (2014). Assessment of magnitude and grades of depression among adolescents in Raipur City, India. *International Research Journal of Medical Sciences, 2*(5), 10–13.

Wendland, J., Lebert, A., de Oliveira, C., & Boujut, E. (2017). Links between maltreatment during childhood or adolescence and risk-related substance use among young adults. *L'Évolution Psychiatrique*. https://doi.org/10.1016/j.evopsy.2016.12.002.

Wentzel, K. R. (1997). Student motivation in middle school: The role of perceived pedagogical caring. *Journal of Educational Psychology, 89*(3), 411–419. https://doi.org/10.1037/0022-0663.89.3.411.

Youssef, R. M., Attia, M. S.-E.-D., & Kamel, M. I. (1998). Children experiencing violence II: Prevalence and determinants of corporal punishment in schools. *Child Abuse and Neglect, 22* (10), 975–985. https://doi.org/10.1016/S0145-2134(98)00084-2.

Zellman, G. L., & Waterman, J. M. (1998). Understanding the impact of parent school involvement on children's educational outcomes. *The Journal of Educational Research, 91*(6), 370–380. https://doi.org/10.1080/00220679809597566.

Websites

http://www.oecd.org/pisa/pisaproducts/pisainfocus/50328990.pdf. Does performance-based pay improve teaching? OECD, 2012. Teachers' pay should be based on performance, not years worked: report.

CAROLINE ALPHONSO. http://www.theglobeandmail.com/news/national/education/teachers-pay-should-be-based-on-performance-not-years-worked-report/article16471184/.

Chapter 2
Academic Stress: What Is the Problem and What Can Educators and Parents Do to Help?

Cheryl Maykel, Johanna deLeyer-Tiarks and Melissa A. Bray

Abstract In the educational environment, students of all ages across cultures experience various stressors, including those related to academic achievement. Children as young as preschool-age are being identified with various psychopathologies—such as anxiety and depression—that stem from the pressure that they experience to succeed academically. Fortunately, there are empirical approaches to combating stress, and both educators and parents can make a positive difference. School-based interventions such as standardized muscle relaxation, yoga, gratitude writing, and guided imagery have been demonstrated to have positive effect.

Keywords Academic stress · School · Students · Parents · Teachers

Introduction

"The bar is being set higher, and the start line earlier, all the time" (Yang 2015). Students across the globe experience a significant amount of academic stress, and the highest-achieving students have been found to experience the greatest amount of strain (Banks & Smyth 2015). Academic stress has been described as the mental distress that is associated with the anticipated frustration of an academic failure (Lal 2014). The countless sources of stress that students experience include: academic, social, family, and health. This chapter will focus on academic stress, such as that which results from increased homework, test scores, rigorous course schedules, as well as competition amongst students, parental pressure, and other demands. Academic pressure on students to achieve is not a new phenomenon, though it is becoming an increasingly substantial global concern, as are the increases in

C. Maykel (✉)
Rivier University, Nashua, USA
e-mail: cherylmaykel@gmail.com

J. deLeyer-Tiarks · M. A. Bray
University of Connecticut, Storrs, USA

S. Deb (ed.), *Positive Schooling and Child Development*,
https://doi.org/10.1007/978-981-13-0077-6_2

concomitant mental and physical health issues. These negative outcomes can be long-lasting—into adulthood—and have a significant impact on overall wellbeing (Sleek 2017).

Impact of School Environment on Academic Stress

Although the stress that students experience is often internally driven and related to their own aspirations for the future (Banks and Smyth 2015), the school environment can serve to intensify the academic stress that students experience. For instance, students who perceived that academic achievement was greatly emphasized in their classrooms were more likely to experience depression resulting from academic stress (Liu and Lu 2011). It was also found that student–teacher and peer–peer interactions significantly impacted student academic stress (Banks and Smyth 2015). Further, according to students, teachers can serve to intensify the academic stress students already experience by placing additional emphasis on the importance of the college entrance exam, talking about it too far in advance, or by bringing it up too often (Banks and Smyth 2015).

Many different countries around the world require students to complete some form of college entrance exam that plays a large role in determining student futures, and which, therefore, puts a significant amount of stress on students (see Banks and Smyth 2015). While the Chinese educational culture has resulted in top scores on the Programme for International Student Assessment (PISA), which makes it appealing internationally, this high-pressure environment has also resulted in fierce competition at every level, and has placed a significant burden on students to perform (Zhao et al. 2015). Although the Chinese government has taken steps to address this issue, it seems that this culture of competition is resistant to change: schools continue to emphasize test scores and assign copious amounts of homework, and parents continue to send their children to tutors for additional instruction on top of their already rigorous schoolwork (Zhao et al. 2015). The main reason that this competitive educational environment is so resistant to change, despite its negative outcomes, is possibly because the college entrance exam, the *gaokao*, is the only criterion used in determining acceptance to college (Zhao et al. 2015). The scores on this exam are, therefore, emphasized immensely. Similarly, parents are concerned about their children gaining admission to the university, and later being hired, which motivates them to continue to provide their children with additional tutoring (Zhao et al. 2015). Another reason cited is that teachers are resistant to change in curriculum, since many still feel they must prepare students for the *gaokao*, and that they too will be evaluated based on student performance in this exam (Zhao et al. 2015).

Academic stress can impact other areas of the students' life, such as interpersonal relationships. This includes student-to-student (such as bullying) or student-to-teacher (such as teacher expectations and biases) relational issues in the school environment. In other words, as pressure to achieve in school increases, so does the stress that students experience in other areas of their lives. Even students who seem to be successful in the social arena may experience stress related to achieving positive social experiences, in the face of stressors such as competition for favour by the teacher or school administration. Lack of interpersonal support—in aspects such as feeling safe and accepted by peers and school staff—can exacerbate an already stressful experience in the academic environment (Barnes et al. 1983). This is especially so when students feel they are not given the necessary tools to cope (Barnes et al. 1983). These pressures in the academic environment become particularly stressful when contextualized within the broader life-stressors that school-aged children may face.

Other Relevant Sources of Stress

Non-academic stressors can divert a student's attention, making it hard for a student experiencing these stressors to perform on the same level as peers who are not affected (Masten et al. 1988; Pianta et al. 1990). Civil unrest, poor health, and pressure to perform in extra-curricular activities, are all non-academic stressors that can inform the experience of stress within the school, by dividing the attention of students who are likely to also be experiencing academic stress. Children who experience poverty are more likely to experience multiple stressors and it is less likely that they will arrive at school with their basic needs having been met. In addition, these children are less likely to have proper material resources, such as notebooks and pencils. Students who experience childhood poverty are also less likely to be provided with an academically enriching environment in the home. Without the experience of an enriching home environment, students who are facing childhood poverty are less able than their fiscally stable peers to have access to resources to reinforce their classroom learning. These academic stressors related to poverty can intensify feelings of academic stress, placing these students at a disadvantage, as compared to their school peers.

The literature indicates that individuals who identify as a member of a group not considered to be in the representative majority (for example, a group without power in society) are at an increased risk for stress (Meyer 1995). Minority stress theory suggests that those who identify with an oppressed minority status—ethnic, racial, and religious minorities, women, sexual and gender minorities, or those belonging to a less-privileged class or socioeconomic group—can experience more stress than their peers who belong to a privileged group of individuals. Children who identify with one or more minority group are likely to experience even greater stress than their peers. Minority stressors can be seen, in an academic setting, as fear of bullying or harassment in the school, worry surrounding potential discrimination from teachers, administration, or other students, or as exclusion from activities. Minority stress experienced by students can contribute to academic stress by placing students at a social and structural disadvantage within the school system, as a result of bullying and discrimination.

Perfectionism

While perfectionism is not synonymous with academic stress, many people who experience academic stress might be considered perfectionists and many perfectionists likely experience academic stress. Maladaptive perfectionists are those who constantly feel that their substantial efforts fall short of their own extremely high standards (Flett and Hewitt 2014). Maladaptive perfectionism is very common, and is even on the rise, though perfectionist youth are unlikely to seek help as this may be viewed as an admission of failure (Flett and Hewitt 2014). Further, as a result of the immense pressure these youth experience and the lack of help received, perfectionism is associated with an increased risk of suicide among adolescents (Flett and Hewitt 2014).

Academic stress can also lead to academic dishonesty as students struggle to compete. In a study conducted among Hong Kong university students and faculty, it was found that the top two reasons students report engaging in academic dishonesty are that they have too much work and that they feel pressure to achieve high grades (Kwong et al. 2010). Interestingly, the study found that faculty tend to attribute academic dishonesty to student laziness, and that students and faculty had a different understanding of what types of things were, or were not, examples of academic dishonesty, as well as of the seriousness of the infraction (Kwong et al. 2010). This study is interesting in that it demonstrates the lengths that students will go to in order to maintain the facade of success. Also, that students had a different idea about what constitutes cheating or plagiarism than faculty suggests that the moral culture among students may be influenced by academic stress, such that either students feel these behaviours are more acceptable or they are able to justify their dishonesty in light of the pressure they feel to earn high marks.

Stress related to pressure to achieve is not limited to the academic environment. Societies across many cultures place a high value on achievement in areas including career prestige, salary, family, and parenting success, interpersonal relationships, physical presentation, and health (Chen and Uttal 1988; Salili 1994). The pressure to perform well in a myriad of areas can lead to chronic stress across the lifespan. These stressors can be seen across cultures and among adults as well, such as in the experience of wanting to achieve various things: having the nicest house in the neighbourhood; getting a promotion or a pay raise at work; being the most well-liked or influential within an interpersonal circle; or striving to achieve physical standards of beauty. These stressors are not uncommon but stem from a systemic, cross-cultural, desire to achieve.

Parenting

There is a significant amount of research in support of various models that explain perfectionism as largely developing as a result of parenting and parent characteristics (Flett et al. 2002). Several experts have written about parental attempts to provide opportunities for their children, and the resultant increased emphasis on achievement in yet another domain of life (such as, sports, music, language), while also taking additional time away from what might otherwise be family time or downtime (see Luthar 2003). The multiplicative-stress model posits that individuals are more likely to experience negative outcomes according to the quantity of stressors experienced, rather than the size or scope of stressors experienced (Schneiderman et al. 2005; Young 2016; Langner and Michael 1963). Therefore, it seems logical that engagement in too many extracurricular activities can cause students to experience additional stress.

Many older children and adolescents spend a large proportion of their time outside of school unsupervised, or in isolation from parents (Luthar 2003). The isolation many youth experience, coupled with the pressure to achieve in multiple aspects of one's life, can lead to anxiety and depression, as well as substance abuse, even among seemingly low-risk suburban youth from socio-economically comfortable families (Luthar 2003). Among middle-school students from an affluent community, however, males and females who reported being closer to their mothers also reported significantly less distress and substance use (Luthar and Becker 2002).

Parenting style has also been studied in regards to perfectionism. The authoritarian parenting style (first described by Baumrind 1966) is described as being high in demandingness and low in warmth or responsiveness. Among college students reflecting on their upbringing, the authoritarian parenting style was associated with perceptions of higher parental expectations and criticism, and as a result, more doubts about abilities (Hibbard and Walton 2014). Among males in this study, the authoritarian parenting style was also associated with more concerns about making mistakes. The neglectful parenting style, described as being low in demandingness and low in warmth, was also associated with feelings of criticism (Hibbard and Walton 2014). Children of parents who have both high expectations of their children and who show their children much affection, or those who espouse the authoritative parenting style, typically have the most positive outcomes, though there are important cultural differences that need to be taken into consideration when interpreting research on parenting styles.

Negative Impact of Stress on Health

It has been shown that stress exists on a curve where a small amount of stress can be beneficial, in that it is motivating, but too much stress is debilitating (Hebb 1955). For example, if a student did not feel any stress about an upcoming exam, they might feel they do not need to study. In this way, the small amount of stress about doing well is motivating to the student. However, when the amount of stress tips over to the other side of the curve, such as if the student was not able to sleep due to worry about their performance on the exam, it becomes evident that too much stress impedes one's ability to perform at an optimal level. Importantly, over time, living with this increased level of stress can put an individual at risk for various health issues. When these issues begin in young children and adolescents who are still developing, it will likely mean worse long-term health, unless intervention occurs.

Physical Health

Chronic stress has a substantial impact on physical health. Long-standing stress sources such as unemployment, physical abuse, caring for an ill child, and even chronic academic stress are likely to result in telomere erosion, which is essentially premature ageing at the cellular level (Sleek 2017). Stress initiates and exacerbates a myriad of physical health conditions such as diabetes (Menzies et al. 2014), sleep disorders (Perfect et al. 2010), asthma, heart disease, arthritis, cancer, chronic pain, and epilepsy (as discussed in Peck et al. 2003). These health impairments are often due to immune system issues, including stress hormones like norepinephrine and epinephrine, as they are shown to be associated with destruction of the cellular matrices. This is particularly a problem in relation to the metastasis of cancerous ovarian cells (Cole and Sood 2011; Sood et al. 2006). Further, catecholamines and cortisol are linked to the recurrence of cancer (Melhem-Bertrandt et al. 2011). Other health conditions including high blood pressure and obesity have also been linked with chronically high levels of cortisol, the hormone secreted when stress is experienced (Bose et al. 2009).

Stress and anxiety are also related to the lung functioning of asthmatics (Bray et al. 2017). In a group of students with asthma, lung functioning improved, as measured by standardized spirometry, at the same time that anxiety, stress, and depression was reduced (Bray et al. 2017). A similar finding has been noted among diabetics, as sugar levels are associated with stress (Sleek 2017). Likewise, cardiovascular disease is affected by physiological states through changes in blood pressure and heart rate (Esler 2017). Further, sleep and various states of mind affect, and are affected, by one another (Perfect et al. 2010). There is simply a great deal of empirical support for the relationship between various physical conditions and mental states.

Mental Health

Research supports that rates of poor mental health outcomes associated with stress have increased dramatically in recent years. Mental health conditions such as depression, anxiety, suicide and suicidal behaviour, as well as other psychopathologies, have been connected to stress in the literature (Langner and Michael 1963; Portier et al. 2010). Mental and physical health are intertwined, yet there is still a stigma associated mental health issues and with receiving help for mental health concerns.

Academic stress, specifically, has been shown to have a severe negative impact on overall well-being. Students' perceived academic stress resulting from a lack of achievement was a significant predictor of depressive symptoms among 90% of Chinese sophomores (Liu and Lu 2011). Indian and Malaysian adolescents who were from low-income families scored higher on measures of academic stress and suicidal ideation than their peers (Khan et al. 2016). Males in the same study had significantly higher levels of suicidal ideation than females, which the authors attributed to the social pressures on males in these cultures to provide for everyone in the family (Khan et al. 2016). However, others have reported that females tend to report more academic stress—among Irish adolescents (Banks and Smyth 2015)—and to experience more stress-related depression—among Chinese adolescents (Liu and Lu 2011)—than males. In either case, it is clear that both male and female adolescents experience a significant amount of stress related to academic achievement, and that this stress can have a significant, negative, impact on mental health. It is important to consider these issues, as being aware of the negative health effects of stress is likely more of a motivation for change, for both the individual and their parents, than the discomfort of living with stress itself. Further, spreading awareness of the degree to which these issues are affecting youth globally should motivate policy changes to reduce the pressure adolescent's experience.

Negative Impact of Stress on Society

While poor health and the detrimental individual impact are commonly cited in reference to the outcomes associated with stress, the negative effects of chronic stress on the functioning of society have also been documented. Social phenomena such as the increasing rates of divorce and marital dissatisfaction (Randall and Bodenmann 2009), incarceration within specific communities (Aaron and Dallaire 2010), rates of alcohol and drug addiction (Hawkins et al. 1992), rates of xenophobia, racism, sexism, and religious intolerance (Jackson and Inglehart 1995) have all been associated with stress.

The social effects of stress are certainly not limited to the adult population. Among school-aged children, phenomena such as bullying (Konishi and Hymel 2008), decreased satisfaction in school (Karatzias et al. 2010), negative social interactions (Konishi and Hymel 2008), and decreased enthusiasm for school and extracurricular activities (Karatzias et al. 2010) have also been associated with stress.

Recommendations for Educators and Parents

Students who experience academic stress are not without hope. Educators and parents can aid in reducing stress among students in the school setting and at home. Various practices can be implemented and encouraged at the universal level, to benefit all students, including those who experience significant academic stress. Others are best suited for working with small groups or individual students. In addition, parents can change some of their own practices outside of school, and parents can support the interventions going on at school.

Universal School-Based Recommendations to Reduce Stress

It has been recommended that prevention programmes aimed at preventing perfectionism focus on universal efforts to develop students' strengths (Flett and Hewitt 2014). An intervention based on cognitive behavioural principles and implemented grade-wide to target perfectionism resulted in lower self-judgment and negative affect at six months—but not at 12—after intervention, among participating Australian adolescents (Nehmy and Wade 2015). Unhelpful perfectionism, though, remained significantly lower in the intervention group even 12 months later than among controls (Nehmy and Wade 2015). Therefore, while the cognitive behavioural strategies were initially effective at reducing self-judgment and negative affect, additional booster sessions and closer monitoring following the completion of the intervention may be warranted.

Ginsburg et al. (2008) investigated the usefulness of a universally administered CBT programme within inner city schools with students who had anxiety disorders. The modular CBT treatment was successful in students with respect to no longer having a formal diagnosis of anxiety at the follow-ups. Reduced levels of parenting stress were also associated with better outcomes in the child; this finding has been supported by previous literature (Burstein et al. 2010). This is an important finding, as parenting style is affected by various psychopathologies, including personality and mood disorders (Kopala-Sibley 2017) and, as noted above, parents can be very influential in increasing or reducing stress.

Other strategies that show promise for addressing student stress and anxiety, and that could be implemented among several students at a time, include yoga (Bray et al. 2012) and progressive muscle relaxation and guided imagery (Dobson et al. 2005), which involves actively tensing and relaxing muscle groups while imagining calming or positive scenes. Each of these strategies has been implemented successfully in the school setting. Two other simple intervention strategies, with a successful track record against stress and anxiety, that could be easily implemented in schools, include written emotional expression, which can be an outlet for writing about positive or negative events, and gratitude writing, which involves expressing one's gratefulness and focusing on the positives in life through writing (Bray et al. 2003).

Generally, a school climate that is supportive of student growth and development will be most beneficial to all students as a preventative measure against various types of stressors. A school that supports overall health, such as by promoting physical activity can also positively impact students' healthy habits (Donnelly et al. 2009) and encourage the use of a positive outlet for stress reduction. Further, research shows that students having positive relationships with teachers can serve as a protective factor (Longobardi et al. 2016). Schools should also promote a growth mind-set (Flett and Hewitt 2014) that encourages students to challenge themselves and to learn from their mistakes, rather than one that holds the unreasonable expectation that students will avoid making mistakes altogether as they learn.

Recommendations for Addressing Stress with Individual Students or Small Groups

Cognitive behavioural strategies that target student's maladaptive thinking patterns may also be the most effective strategy when working with individuals. In a study among college students, researchers provided feedback and encouraged discussion with those indicated as maladaptive perfectionists. They noted reductions in global symptomatic distress as well as emotional reactivity and further suggest that feedback of this kind might facilitate or encourage more intensive cognitive therapy (Aldea et al. 2010).

The so-called third generation behavioural strategies involve mindfulness, or actively maintaining one's mind in the present moment, and acceptance, which has to do with accepting one's present experience without judgment (as described in Corey 2016). Mindfulness has had some promising effects on addressing student anxiety (Semple et al. 2005) and there is considerable research to support its use among adults with anxiety (Arch et al. 2013).

Mindfulness-based cognitive therapy, a combination of mindfulness training and cognitive restructuring, has also been successfully implemented in a school setting to improve attention problems and to reduce anxiety and behaviour problems among students with the most anxiety pre-intervention (Semple et al. 2005). Loving kindness meditation, which involves developing kindness and compassion for the self and others, also shows promise among students. Seven weeks of this practice resulted in significant reductions in self-criticism and depressive symptoms, as well as significant increases in self-compassion and positive emotions, even at three months post-intervention, among highly self-critical adults (Shahar et al. 2015).

Recommendations for Parents Outside of School

It is well-known that in order to maximize the benefits of school-based interventions home–school collaboration with parents who support and even bring the intervention into the home is very important. In addition to practicing these strategies at home, parents are also encouraged to model a growth mind-set, such as by displaying a calm response and self-compassion after parents themselves make a mistake (Flett and Hewitt 2014). Additionally, and perhaps most importantly, parents are asked to consider which after-school activities are beneficial and which are either not necessary or even harmful to their children. Parents might consider when they might be able to build more family time into their busy schedules and remain accessible, should they be needed. Generally, parents should strive to stay connected with their children, and find the balance between providing opportunities and adding more stress or expectations to their child's life.

Conclusion

As the global job market becomes more competitive, so does the competition to become accepted at universities, which has the effect of increasing the pressure on high school students to perform in higher classes, which also increases the pressure on elementary students to perform so that they are placed in more advanced courses in high school. There are never enough jobs, enough openings at the university, or enough spots in the top-level secondary classes for everyone, or even for everyone who is hardworking and capable. At the same time, it seems that more and more goes into raising a successful member of society each year: even after spending four or more years away from home earning a college degree, young adults are returning home to continue to prepare to become independent contributors to society, or to continue their education even more, and only then to become fully independent. In short, there is no simple answer or easy route to having it all, for most people, and both school and home environments play a big role in the amount of stress young people experience.

Research continues to collect in favour of early childhood enrichment experiences while parents scramble to provide their child with all of the advantages that they can, hoping to give them the very best start in life. Yet, the pressure that parents feel to provide opportunities for their children in order for them to be successful as adults may, unfortunately, be transferred onto the child and result in pressure that the child experiences to succeed, effectively robbing them of their childhood. So-called enrichment activities are heavily marketed to parents who fall victim to the belief that they must provide all of these things to their child in order for them to be successful (Luthar 2003). Further, an overscheduled family and this 'hurried lifestyle' can result in parents spending less time with their children, parents spending much of their already limited time with children bringing them to and from activities, and children spending less time engaged in creative free-play activities (Luthar 2003). Also, this lifestyle has the effect of teaching people from a very young age that they should always be striving for some future gain, as opposed to teaching children to enjoy the activity that they are engaged in at the moment, for what it's worth and the company they are in, and truly benefitting from the experience.

Schools and the larger cultural context, including policies that schools function within, can also affect the amount of stress students experience. Teachers and others in the schools should seek to find the right balance between preparing students for college entrance exams or other aspects of their future, and emphasizing the importance of academic success so much that they help to tip the stress scale to the point that students become overwhelmed. It is also important for educators to recognize that this tipping point is different for all students. Educators, just like parents, should seek to form and maintain strong positive relationships with students so that they feel accepted and empowered, and are able to overcome shortcomings to reach their full potential.

In addition to setting reasonable expectations for our youth and teaching them how to do the same for themselves, with this pervasive emphasis on constant striving, it seems that now, more than ever, we ought to focus our efforts on teaching young people about mindfulness and acceptance, and how to live more in the present moment. The first step may be increasing awareness of the impacts of, and influences on, stress and generating conversation at all age-levels and across all globalized cultures. We can also push for policy changes, such as the inclusion of criteria other than scores in a single test for determining college acceptance. We can work with students who experience academic stress, as well as preventatively with those who are not yet affected by these issues, and teach them ways to manage their response to stressful situations. The issue of academic stress is a pervasive feature of student life in many societies; it did not reach this point overnight, and we cannot expect to be able to adequately address it in as little time. There is much work to be done by all who help to shape the futures of our youth.

References

Aaron, L., & Dallaire, D. H. (2010). Parental incarceration and multiple risk experiences: Effects on family dynamics and children's delinquency. *Journal of Youth and Adolescence, 39*(12), 1471–1484.

Aldea, M. A., Rice, K. G., Gormley, B., & Rojas, A. (2010). Telling perfectionists about their perfectionism: Effects of providing feedback on emotional reactivity and psychological symptoms. *Behavior Research and Therapy, 48,* 1194–1203.

Arch, J., Ayers, C., Baker, A., Almklov, E., Dean, D., & Craske, M. (2013). Randomized clinical trial of adapted mindfulness-based stress reduction versus group cognitive behavioral therapy for heterogeneous anxiety disorders. *Behavior Research and Therapy, 51,* 185–196. https://doi.org/10.1016/j.brat.2013.01.003.

Banks, J., & Smyth, E. (2015). 'Your whole life depends on it': Academic stress and high-stakes testing in Ireland. *Journal of Youth Studies, 18*(5), 598–616.

Barnes, V., Potter, E., Fiedler, F., & Guion, Robert. (1983). Effect of interpersonal stress on the prediction of academic performance. *Journal of Applied Psychology, 68*(4), 686–697.

Baumrind, D. (1966). Effects of authoritative parental control on child behavior. *Child Development,* 887–907.

Bose, M., Oliván, B., & Laferrère, B. (2009). Stress and obesity: The role of the hypothalamic–pituitary–adrenal axis in metabolic disease. *Current opinion in Endocrinology, Diabetes, and Obesity, 16*(5), 340.

Bray, M. A., Kehle, T. J., Theodore, L. A., & Bracken, B. A. (2017). Interventions for children with asthma. In L. A. Theodore (Ed.), *Handbook of evidence-based interventions for children and adolescents* (pp. 447–456). New York: Springer Publishing Company.

Bray, M. A., Sassu, K. A., Kapoor, V., Margiano, S., Peck, H. L., Kehle, T. J., et al. (2012). Yoga as an intervention for asthma. *School Psychology Forum: Research in Practice, 6*(2), 39–49.

Bray, M. A., Theodore, L. A., Patwa, S. S., Margiano, S. E., Alric, J. M., & Peck, H. L. (2003). Written emotional expression as an intervention for asthma. *Psychology in the Schools, 40*(2), 193–207. https://doi.org/10.1002/pits.10078.

Burstein, M., Ginsburg, G., & Tein, S. (2010). Parental anxiety and child symptomatology: An examination of additive and interactive effects of parent psychopathology. *Journal of Abnormal Child Psychology, 38*(7), 897–909.

Chen, C., & Uttal, D. H. (1988). Cultural values, parents' beliefs, and children's achievement in the United States and China. *Human Development, 31,* 351–358.

Cole, S., & Sood, A. K. (2011). Molecular pathways: Beta-adrenergic signaling incancer. *Clinical Cancer Research, 18,* 1202–1206.

Corey, G. (2016). *Theory and practice of counseling and psychotherapy*. Boston, MA: Cengage Learning.

Dobson, R. L., Bray, M. A., Kehle, T. J., Theodore, L. A., & Peck, H. L. (2005). Relaxation and guided imagery as an intervention for children with asthma: A replication. *Psychology in the Schools, 42,* 707–720. https://doi.org/10.1002/pits.20119.

Donnelly, J., Greene, J., Gibson, C., Smith, B., Washburn, R., Sullivan, D., et al. (2009). Physical activity across the curriculum (PAAC): A randomized controlled trial to promote physical activity and diminish overweight and obesity in elementary school children. *Preventive Medicine, 49,* 336–341. https://doi.org/10.1016/j.ypmed.2009.07.022.

Esler, M. (2017). Mental stress and human cardiovascular disease. *Neuroscience and Biobehavioral Reviews, 74,* 269–276.

Flett, G. L., & Hewitt, P. L. (2014). A proposed framework for preventing perfectionism and promoting resilience and mental health among vulnerable children and adolescents. *Psychology in the Schools, 51*(9), 899–912. https://doi.org/10.1002/pits.21792.

Flett, G. L., Hewitt, P. L., Oliver, J. M., & Macdonald, S. (2002). Perfectionism in children and their parents: A developmental analysis. In G. L. Flett & P. L. Hewitt (Eds.), *Perfectionism: Theory, research, and treatment* (pp. 89–132). Washington, DC: American Psychological Association.

Ginsburg, G. S., Becker, K. D., & Nichols, T. (2008). Transporting CBT for childhood anxiety disorders into inner-city school-based mental health clinics. *Cognitive and Behavioral Practice, 15*(2), 148–158.

Hawkins, J. D., Catalano, R. F., & Miller, J. Y. (1992). Risk and protective factors for alcohol and other drug problems in adolescence and early adulthood: Implications for substance abuse and prevention. *Psychological Bulletin, 112*(1), 64–105.

Hebb, D. O. (1955). Drives and the C.N.S. (conceptual nervous system). *Psychological Review, 62* (4), 243–254.

Hibbard, D. R., & Walton, G. E. (2014). Exploring the development of perfectionism: The influence of parenting style and gender. *Social Behavior and Personality, 42*(2), 269–278.

Jackson, J. S., & Inglehart, M. R. (1995). Reverberation theory: Stress and racism in hierarchically structured communities. In S. E. Hobfall & M. W. de Vries (Eds.), *Extreme stress and communities: Impact and intervention* (pp. 353–373). New York, NY: Kluwer Academic/ Plenum Publishers.

Karatzias, A. K., Power, K. G., Flemming, J., Lennan, F., & Swanson, V. (2010). The role of demographics, personality variables and school stress on predicting school satisfaction/ dissatisfaction: Review of the literature research findings. *Educational Psychology, 22*(1), 33–50.

Khan, A., Hamdan, A. R., Ahmad, R., Mustaffa, M. S., & Mahalle, S. (2016). Problem-solving coping and social support as mediators of academic stress and suicidal ideation among Malaysian and Indian adolescents. *Community Mental Health Journal, 52,* 245–250. https:// doi.org/10.1007/s10597-015-9937-6.

Konishi, C., & Hymel, S. (2008). Bullying and stress in early adolescence: The role of coping and social support. *The Journal of Early Adolescence, 29*(3), 333–356.

Kopala-Sibley, D. C. (2017). Parental depressive history, parenting styles, and child psychopathology over 6 years: The contribution of each parent's depressive history to the other's parenting styles. *Development and Psychopathology*, 1–14. https://doi.org/10.1017/s0954579417000396.

Kwong, T., Ng, H. M., Mark, K. P., & Wong, E. (2010). Students' and faculty's perception of academic integrity in Hong Kong. *Campus-Wide Information Systems, 27*(5), 341–355.

Lal, K. (2014). Academic stress among adolescents in relation to intelligence and demographic factors. *American International Journal of Research in Humanities, Arts, and Social Sciences, 5*(1), 123–129.

Langner, T. S., & Michael, S. T. (1963). *Life stress and mental health: II. The midtown Manhattan study*. Oxford: Free Press Glencoe.

Liu, Y., & Lu, Z. (2011). Chinese high school students' academic stress and depressive symptoms: Gender and school climate as moderators. *Stress & Health, 28,* 340–346.

Longobardi, C., Prino, L. E., Marengo, D., & Settani, M. (2016). Student-teacher relationships as a protective factor for school adjustment during the transition from middle to high school. *Frontiers in Psychology, 7.* https://doi.org/10.3389/fpsyg.2016.01988.

Luthar, S. S. (2003). The culture of affluence: Psychological costs of material wealth. *Child Development, 74*(6), 1581–1593.

Luthar, S. S., & Becker, B. E. (2002). Privileged but pressured? A study of affluent youth. *Child Development, 73*(5), 1593–1610.

Masten, A. S., Garmezy, N., Tellegen, A., Pellegrini, D. S., Larkin, K., & Larsen, A. (1988). Competence and stress in school children: The moderating effects of individual and family qualities. *Journal of Child Psychology and Psychiatry, 29*(6), 745–764.

Melhem-Bertrandt, A., Chavez-Macgregor, M., Lei, X., Brown, E., Lee, R., Meric-Berstam, F., et al. (2011). Beta-blocker use is associated with improved relapse-free survival in patients with triple-negative breast cancer. *Journal of Clinical Oncology, 29*(19), 2645–2652.

Menzies, V., Lyon, D. E., Elswick, R. K., McCain, N. L., & Gray, D. P. (2014). Effects of guided imagery on biobehavioral factors in women with fibromyalgia. *Journal of Behavioral Medicine, 37*(1), 70–80.

Meyer, I. H. (1995). Minority stress and mental health in gay men. *Journal of Health and Social Behavior, 36*(1), 38–56.

Nehmy, T. J., & Wade, T. D. (2015). Reducing the onset of negative affect in adolescents: Evaluation of a perfectionism program in a universal prevention setting. *Behaviour Research and Therapy, 67,* 55–63.

Peck, H. L., Bray, M. A., & Kehle, T. J. (2003). Relaxation and guided imagery: A school based intervention for children with asthma. *Psychology in the Schools, 40,* 657–675. https://doi.org/10.1002/pits.10127.

Perfect, M., Elkins, G., Haynes, P. L., & Bootzin, R. R. (2010). Cognitive–behavioral therapy and hypnotic relaxation to treat sleep problems in an adolescent with diabetes. *Journal of Clinical Psychology, 66*(11), 1205–1215.

Pianta, R. C., Egeland, B., & Sroufe, L. A. (1990). Maternal stress and children's development: Prediction of school outcomes and identification of protective factors. In J. Rolf, A. S. Masten, D. Cicchetti, K. H. Nuechterlein, & S. Weintraub (Eds.), *Risk and protective factors in the development of psychopathology* (pp. 215–235). Cambridge: Cambridge University Press.

Portier, C. J., Thigpen, Tart K., Carter, S. R., Dilworth, C. H., Grambsch, A. E., Gohlke, J., et al. (2010). *A human health perspective on climate change: A report outlining the research needs on the human health effects of climate change*. Research Triangle Park, NC: Environmental Health Perspectives/National Institute of Environmental Health Sciences.

Randall, A. K., & Bodenmann, G. (2009). The role of stress on close relationships and marital satisfaction. *Clinical Psychology Review, 29*(2), 105–115.

Salili, F. (1994). Age, sex, and cultural differences in the meaning and dimensions of achievement. *Personality and Social Psychology Bulletin, 20,* 635–648.

Schneiderman, N., Ironson, G., & Siegel, S. D. (2005). Stress and health: Psychological, behavioral, and biological determinants. *Annual Review of Clinical Psychology, 1,* 607–628.

Semple, R. J., Reid, E. F. G., & Miller, L. (2005). Treating anxiety with mindfulness: An open trial of mindfulness training for anxious children. *Journal of Cognitive Psychotherapy, 19*(4), 379–392.

Shahar, B., Szsepsenwol, O., Zilcha-Mano, S., Haim, N., Zamir, O., Levi-Yeshuvi, S., et al. (2015). A wait-list randomized controlled trial of loving-kindness meditation program for Self-criticism. *Clinical Psychology & Psychotherapy, 22,* 346–356. https://doi.org/10.1002/cpp.1893.

Sleek, S. (2017). The long and the short of it: Chronic stress measured at the cellular level. *APA Observer, 27,* 15–19.

Sood, A. K., Bhatty, R., Kamat, A. A., Landen, C. N., Han, L., Tahker, P. H., et al. (2006). Stress hormone mediated invasion of ovarian cancer cells. *Clinical Cancer Research, 12,* 369–375.

Yang, J. (2015, July 2). *Do Asian students face too much academic pressure?* CNN. Retrieved from http://www.cnn.com/2015/07/02/opinions/yang-genius-girl/.

Young, G. (2016). *Unifying causality and psychology: Being, brain, and behavior*. Switzerland: Springer International Publishing.

Zhao, X., Selman, R. L., & Haste, H. (2015). Academic stress in Chinese schools and a proposed preventive intervention program. *Cogent Education, 2,* 1000477.

Chapter 3
Has Education Lost Sight of Children?

Victoria G. Lidchi

Abstract The reflections presented in this chapter are informed by clinical and personal experiences of school education in the UK. There are many challenges for children and young people in the modern education system and for the professionals who support them. In the UK, there are significant gaps between the highly selective education provided to those who pay privately for it and to the majority of those educated in the state-funded system. Though literacy rates have improved around the world, many children, particularly boys, do not finish their education for reasons such as boredom, behavioural difficulties or because education does not 'pay'. Violence, bullying, and sexual harassment are issues faced by many children in schools and there are disturbing trends of excluding children who present with behavioural problems at school whose origins are not explored. Excluded children are then educated with other children who may also have multiple problems which often just make the situation worse. The experience of clinicians suggests that school-related mental health problems are increasing in severity. Are mental health services dealing with the consequences of an education system that is not meeting children's needs? An education system that is testing- and performance-based may not be serving many children well if it is driving important decisions about them at increasingly younger ages. Labelling of children and setting them on educational career paths can occur well before they reach secondary schools, limiting potential very early on in their developmental trajectory. Furthermore, the emphasis at school on testing may come at the expense of creativity and other forms of intelligence, which are also valuable and important. Meanwhile the employment marketplace requires people with widely different skills, with an emphasis on innovation, creativity, and problem solving. Is education losing sight of the children it is educating?

Keywords School · Education · Children · Violence · Bullying
Sexual harassment · United Kingdom

V. G. Lidchi (✉)
The Tavistock and Portman NHS Foundation Trust, London, UK
e-mail: victorialidchi@terra.com.br

S. Deb (ed.), *Positive Schooling and Child Development*,
https://doi.org/10.1007/978-981-13-0077-6_3

Introduction

This chapter has been inspired by my experiences not only as a clinician (clinical child psychologist and family therapist) but also as the parent of a child in the English Education system. It is designed to be critical, but is from the perspective of a mental health practitioner who is troubled by the number of children and young people who are referred to Child and Adolescent Mental Health Services because of problems related to their schooling. The schooling system in UK has an international reputation, mostly founded on highly regarded private schools, some with histories of over 400 years (for example Eton and Winchester), and a tradition of providing education to the elite. This contrasts with figures in the Equity and Quality in Education (OECD) report which placed Britain 25th out of 35 countries in terms of the number of adults who failed to stay in education up to the age of 18.

The education system has its strengths and weaknesses. Although the system reflects the large social divide in the country among children and young people, my experience in mental health suggest that children across both the private and state system are experiencing similar stresses. Education in the UK has become driven by outcomes and focused on assessments. Children are classified and labelled at increasingly younger ages and, in striving for excellence, the education system is less effective for those who have entered at a disadvantage, many of whom drop out and find other ways to operate in society. In this chapter, I argue that a failing of the British education system is that it focuses too much on outcomes and academic ability, making learning irrelevant to some young people and stressful to others. I outline research that an inclusive education requires a holistic developmental and ecological approach that can appreciate diversity of skills, thus maximizing potential and providing the marketplace with people with the different skills it needs.

Education System in Britain

The History of Schooling in the UK

While the chapter will focus on my experience of schooling in England, the systems in the UK, Wales, and Northern Ireland are similar. Scotland has its own system. England is unique in the differences in the quality of education available in the public and private school systems, and its history is tied to social reform, betraying strong philanthropic roots. Governments of different political persuasion modify the education systems in line with the vision of whichever government is in power, although there has been a consistent concern with standards and academic ability, with successive governments pushing to improve access to higher education, which has been achieved (Hansen and Vignoles 2005). Although, for a long time, the UK spending on education was below the OECD average, it is now above average, but still behind many European countries including the other two biggest European economies, France and Germany, with a greater proportion of investment coming from private sources (Breakspear 2012).

In order to improve the skills of the workforce in the post-war period, the 1960s and 1970s saw a change in the education system to widen access to schools. For the first time, students were taught in mixed ability 'comprehensive schools' introduced by the Labour government. Prior to this, children were categorized in terms of their ability, with the more academically able being selected to pass the 11+ exam and access Grammar School, and other children undertaking vocational training. The categorizing of students according to ability remains a feature of the British education system, with children, in comprehensive and private schools alike, being divided into sets or streams (Machin and Vignole 2006).

In the 1980s an important reform occurred, with children of all academic abilities taking the same examinations, GCSEs at 16. The exam assesses children of a broad range of abilities. The prior system of O levels were also graded on a relative basis using a statistical reference with respect to competing candidates, while GCSEs were intended to be graded with greater reference to absolute standards. O levels were thereby replaced by the more accessible GCSEs, introduced to allow all students to leave with some qualification (Hansen and Vignoles 2005)

After education was made more inclusive, in this way, by the Labour Government, there has been an ongoing concern about standards. An increased emphasis on improved quality and academic achievement in the state sector has led to the introduction of market forces in the education arena in the form of: (1) accountability and transparency in results; and, (2) creation of schools that are allowed to control their own budget and administration. These measures have resulted in a demand for transparency, increasing central comparison of schooling through ranking schools and the trend to devolve powers to high performing schools. The 'surveillance' model of state schooling relies on all schools following a national curriculum and schools being rated in 'league tables' according to their student's results on SAT (Standard Aptitude Tests) and other national exams. Schools attaining good or outstanding rating gain the right to more autonomy.

The private and state-funded parts of the system in England differ also in resourcing. The resources and privileges in the private system are generally above those in state schools, with the resources that the private sector is able to collect being in sharp contrast to the financial constraints faced by the state education system. Although the proportion of pupils in private education has remained constant since the 1970s, private expenditure on education has risen due to the increase in fees. Private school can only be afforded by upper middle and upper classes, with fees ranging from 15,000 to 40,000 lb per year for top boarding schools. The pupil-to-teacher is much lower in the private system, standards are higher and results are better; 60% of pupils schooled through the private system in the 1980s and 1990s attained degrees, while only 16% of state school pupils were able to do so. Higher education in the UK is viewed as a success story, based on figures suggesting that participation is rising. However, these figures mask that higher education remains more accessible to the higher social classes and that, in the

1990s, the gap in higher education participation widened (Machin and Vignole 2006). This means that although poorer students are more likely to go on to higher education than they were in the past, the likelihood of them doing so relative to their richer peers is actually lower than was the case in earlier decades.

The Structure of the UK Education System

State schools are obliged to follow the national curriculum, private independent (non-maintained) schools (and academies) are not required to follow the syllabus, but do have to cover the subjects to allow students to pass the nationally set exams. The National Curriculum handbook for primary teachers in England (1999) reflects the influence of Article 29 of the UNCRC (United Nations 1989) that sees a central role for education, at home and at school, as key in children's well-being including physical and mental development. Early education is seen as fundamental to social mobility and the development of the economy. The framework sets out the minimum educational entitlement for all children of compulsory school age and is organized in key stages with the final year of primary school being the final year of key stage 2. At the end of key stage 1, children mandatorily take national assessments in English and mathematics and, at the end of key stage 2, they to sit in English, Mathematics and Science.

At the end of Key Stage 4, pupils sit the GCSE (General Certificate of Secondary Education) examinations in a variety of subjects. At the end of Year 12, the students take AS (Advanced Subsidiary) level examinations followed by A (Advanced) level examinations at the end of Year 13 which are the basis for access to university courses. Some vocational certificates can be gained at the end of Year 11 for those who are not academically inclined.

In the private system, children enter pre-preparatory school at 4/5 years and then preparatory school at 7/8 years where boys can stay until they are 13 and girls until they are 11. Some boys, and all girls, take 11+ exams to gain entry into top independent schools. Other boys gain entry through common entrance exams at 13. For the top schools however, there can be up to two pre-selection stages to earn the right to take the Common Entrance Exam at 13 for entry into the top day or boarding schools. The English language, educational reputation, and amenities in the top private schools in the UK have proven attractive to parents of children from many parts of the world, and competition for places is intense. The assessment before 11 focuses mostly on verbal and non-verbal reasoning abilities, maths, English and science. At 13, the assessments are focused on a range of subjects.

The UK system is academically focused with schools being regularly inspected either by (1) OFSTED (Office for Standards in Education) in the state system, or (2) ISI, the Independent School Inspectorate. In the state system, schools are rated Outstanding, Good, or Inadequate, and an important part of the judgment is made on the basis of students' performance, how this is tracked and maximized. The Independent Schools Inspectorate has a similar focus but private schools enjoy a greater freedom by not having to focus on the National Curriculum. This academic focus however does not best serve everyone, with the UK education system neglecting the under-achievers who leave school at 16 with few or no educational qualifications, due to a lack of good vocational training. Successive reforms have not managed to achieve what Hansen and Vignole (2005) refer to as parity of esteem between vocational and academic education.

In the UK, 48% of young people from professional, managerial, and skilled non-manual backgrounds enter university, whilst only 18% from a skilled manual or unskilled background do so. The gap in participation at University between rich and poor is a consequence of the system's elitism. and poor performance in ensuring social mobility (Goldthorpe 2007). The OECD PISA (Program for International Student Assessment) suggests that the UK performs well in terms of the number of students graduating from higher education, and skills displayed by secondary school students, as reflected in the OECD and PISA data. However, ISCED (International Standard Classification of Education) figures suggest that the UK produces a lot more workers with the lowest levels of education relative to other major economies in Europe. The other data that suggest that the National Curriculum may failing in its objective of promoting social mobility is the link between parental background and educational achievement (Machin and Vingole 2006). With a large proportion of parents who value education sending their children to private schools a consequence is that "vocal and committed parents are out of the state education system, with potential consequences for standards in the state sector" (Hanson and Vingnole 2005, 6).

Schools and Well-Being

Focusing on academic achievement at the expense of other skills has had several consequences. A high drop-out rate and lack of skills in parts of the work force are two consequences, but another serious one, which may also be contributing to or resulting from the above, is the impact of the education system on children and young people's well-being. Some vignettes of the types of cases referred to Child and Adolescent Mental Health (CAMHS) are illustrated below although for confidentiality reasons no real details are cited:

A 16 years old boy is referred by the GP (general practitioner doctor) from a private selective secondary school. The parents and school are worried because he had not performed as well as predicted in his recent exams. Since becoming aware of this under performance, the schools have noticed other aspects of his functioning including that he is very socially isolated and not integrated into his peer group. He has been at the school for 5 years, and the clinician who sees him thinks he may be a high functioning autistic child.

A mother insists on a GP referral to CAMHS for her 9 years old daughter. Her daughter has an intense dislike of school, feel the teachers think she is stupid and the mother is struggling to get her into school every morning. Her daughter is struggling to learn, does have support from a classroom assistant, but her current reading age is at year 1 level (she is currently in year 5) and she struggles to spell word lists given to children in year 2. Her mother fears she has "dyslexia" but has been told by the educational psychologist that the difficulties are emotional. The mother believes that her daughter has low self-esteem because of repeated educational failure and is worried about how her daughter is going to transition into secondary school at the end of year 6.

A 12 years old girl attendance at school is falling. She has become excessively pre-occupied with her homework, and whether she is doing enough. Her anxiety around homework has led her to refuse to go to school in the morning as she fears her performance at school is also dropping. Her parents are very keen that she does well at school, and there is no indication from school that she is not.

A 15 years old boy is currently refusing to go school and stays in bed all day refusing to see anyone. He tells his mother he will not go back to school as he has been bullied and victimized by boys for the past 3 years. The mother contacts child and adolescent mental health services in a state as the educational welfare officer has got in touch and is threatening to take her to court as he son is not attending school. The school were not aware of the problem and do not seem to have the necessary resources to deal with it. They are dealing with changes in the exam system which is taking up their time.

A boy of 13 years old is expelled from school for being in possession of a knife. The reason that boy was carrying the knife was that he was being bullied on a regular basis. He was excluded and now is placed in a pupil referral unit where he is coming into contact with boys with more extreme anti-social behavior. He is being coerced into performing anti-social acts including a boy who has got him into selling drugs in exchange for protection. The other day he was beaten up outside the school for reasons that are unknown.

It is these scenarios and others which have led the UK government to take child and adolescent mental health seriously, and schools are seen as key to building resilience in children and young people. Some boroughs have commissioned mental health professionals specializing in child and adolescent health to work from the school and there are many helpful tools to support schools in their efforts to build support young people (Young Minds 2017). In the borough where I work, a CAMHS in-school program was set up, to improve joint working between school settings and CAMHS teams, so that children, young people, and their parents could access timely and appropriate specialist mental health and well-being support. Additional aims of this program were to ensure that resources are being used in an efficient manner, and to support Camden school staff to become more confident in dealing with mental health and emotional well-being issues amongst young people. The CAMHS provision is delivered by specialist clinicians who are based in the multidisciplinary CAMHS teams and are commissioned jointly by the Clinical Commissioning group and the Council.

Conclusions

The CAMHS resources that are commissioned are limited and, in some cases, are being used to deal with the systemic weaknesses of an education system that is not in a position to build resilience. Both teachers and students are focused on assessments and attainments, which leaves little space to develop other aspects of children and young people's development, including how to use education as a vehicle to equip young people for life outside school and improve their prospects. The Joseph Rowntree foundation has recommended that to reduce inequalities there needs to be: (1) an improvement in the quality of early years childcare; (2) continuing professional development to promote good teaching; and (3) good quality apprenticeships. Good teaching and good teaching methods are essential to this process (Landry et al. 2009; Normak et al. 2012).

Is Performance the Way to Go?

Performance measurement as a way to generate improvement will always be important. However, what constitutes performance for a school and how to measure it is a continuing debate as it partly depends on values. The recommendations of the Joseph Rowntree foundation are only slowly being heeded but only as an addition to the ongoing outcome- and assessment-focused mainstream of education. The efforts to improve standards the UK education system still focus on performance.

The Cognitive Hypothesis

Education in England is an example of a culture system saturated by the "cognitive hypothesis" (Tough 2014). This is the belief that success depends on "cognitive" or intellectual skills (Deary et al. 2007). The cognitive hypothesis in England is supported by research used to inform documents such 'Every Child Matters' and 'No Child Left Behind'. In these, the government proposed that education is key in reducing inequalities and ensuring that all children irrespective of their background or circumstances maximize their potential, enjoy and achieve, and contribute productively to society. The way to do this seems to be to make sure that children are prepared to make full use of the education they are offered and this is by developing cognitive skills.

The focus on intelligence as a predictor of academic success dates back to the beginning of the century and the work of psychologists such as Binet and Simon (1911), (1916) and Spearman (1927). The focus of Binet's original testing work was to identify those children who struggled in school and needed special educational interventions. Most scholastic assessments now assess intellectual ability associated with the concept of "g" as developed by Spearman (1927), a measure of problem solving ability. Remedial testing, if anything, is underutilized in the

English education system, with a result that children with specific learning problems are often only diagnosed after persistent failure. The reluctance to identify relates to the cost of remedial interventions.

In the British cohort study (1970), being in the bottom quartile of cognitive assessments scores at age 5 were related to higher probability of having low qualifications and experiencing unemployment by the age of 30 (Feinstein and Bynner 2004). Reading, Maths, and attention skills predict later school achievement (Duncan et al. 2007). Research suggests that children from privileged environments are more prepared for school. Parents in more privileged settings have the resources to support their children's development by spending more money, but also more time in cognitively enriching activities. Price (2010) finds an additional year of daily mother-child reading increase children's reading test scores in the early school grades by 41%.

Data from the USA, which has a similar system in terms of the difference between state and private education shows how several factors influence academic success not only results on academic tests. The General Educational Development Program (GED) focused on certification of high school children who had dropped out of school, providing they had acquired the knowledge required to access higher education. A study by Heckman (2000) found, however, that only 3% of the GED's students accessed higher education compared to 46% of students who actually finished school. Heckman suggested that psychological traits, such as persistence and delayed gratification with a tendency to follow through on a plan, had helped the high school finishers persist with their education. This suggestion is supported by findings of the Perry Programme, a study that examined the lives of 123 children born in poverty and at high risk of failing in school. From 1962–1967, at ages 3 and 4, the subjects were randomly divided into a programme group that entered a high-quality preschool programme, and compared the outcomes with a comparison group who received no preschool programme. The study found that adults at age 40 who underwent the preschool programme had higher earnings, committed fewer crimes, were more likely to hold a job, and were more likely to have graduated from high school than adults who did not have a preschool education. However, whilst the scores on the cognitive tests were significantly better in the preschool group when at nursery, these were not maintained over time. The positive outcomes were due to other social and emotional factors developed during preschool that helped them succeed.

The Importance of Social and Emotional Development

Interest in the emotional factors that promote readiness for school is running alongside the research on cognitive development. Early care giving and parenting are important to an infant's social and emotional well-being and cognitive development (Belsky 2005; Toth et al. 2006) Parenting is seen as one of the most important drivers of social inequality (Waldfogel and Washbrook 2010), with good parenting conferring resilience on young children (Gutman and Feinstein 2007). Children from disadvantaged or stressed backgrounds often do not enjoy the sensitive care and stimulation which then compromises early social and emotional development and then affects cognitive development and later school attainment (Moulin et al. 2014; Hanson et al. 2013; NICE 2006; Caspi et al. 1998), and is also linked to behaviour problems and delinquency.

There is much research supporting the importance of the early care-giving relationship, and how sensitive, attuned, and warm early relationships not only optimize development but confer resilience against emotional and behavioural problems (Belsky and Fearon 2002; Hoeve et al. 2012; Moulin et al. 2014). Developments in neuroscience have helped to explain the relationship between sensitive care, affect regulation, and later cognitive, social, emotional difficulties. Emotional regulation is a developmental process that unfolds over time. Infants and young children lack the capacity to regulate their own emotions, and thus are initially reliant on sensitive parenting and the attachment relationship to help them to manage stress (Gerhardt 2004; Shonkoff and Garner 2012). Without this, infants are at risk from toxic stress, that is, prolonged or excessive activation of neurobiological stress response.

Typically, developing children develop the capacity to regulate their own emotions around the age of four, by internalizing emotional regulation strategies (Siegel and Hartzell 2003; Barlow and Svanberg 2009). However, exposure to toxic stress during the sensitive period of infancy and early childhood is thought to affect the development of the brain. Neural circuits and hormonal systems that enable the child to cope with novel or potentially threatening situations may develop to be over or under reactive, resulting in lifelong difficulties in managing every day stressors (National Scientific Council on the Developing Child 2005/2014). Toxic stress has also been linked to the under production of neural connections in areas of the brain associated with planning, reasoning, and behavioural control (Perry 1995; Schore 2003), while prolonged exposure to the stress hormone cortisol may result in damage to the hippocampus, which is important for learning and memory (Shonkoff 2012).

Studies show the impact of poor attachment relationship on cognitive as well as emotional development including executive functioning, language development, and working memory (Carlivati 2001; Duchesne et al. 2009; Bradbury et al. 2012). Sensitive early care, manifested in secure early attachments, enables children to manage their negative feelings and behaviour, whilst insecurely attached children whose parents are rejecting of their child's negative emotions, learn to repress/minimize their expression or exaggerate the expression of emotion when their care giver responds unpredictably. The insecure attachments this produces has been linked to: (1) an increase in externalizing behaviour problems; (2) poorer language development and executive functioning; and (3) reduced resilience when faced with adverse circumstances such as poverty and marginalization (Moulin et al. 2014). Egeland et al. (2005) presented evidence that attachment at age 3 predicted whether children graduated from high school. Other research suggests that attachment relationships influence children's relationships with teachers and peers, and that school may best explain teenagers' satisfaction with school and performance in the academic environment (Carlivati 2001).

Early adversity is linked to self-control and negative behaviours which compromise the children's early years at school. A sensitive attuned parent helps a child regulate negative emotions, a capacity which eventually is internalized and allows the child to cope with stress and danger, and learn the positive aspects of relationships. As Gerhardt (2004) says warm pleasurable interactions with care givers get the baby hooked on social interactions itself by making it highly pleasurable, and this pleasure in social interactions will then translate into pleasurable interactions with other adults such as teachers.

Impact of the Cognitive Hypothesis for Teaching Methods

One of the consequences of the cognitive hypothesis is that children in the UK start school earlier than other countries in Europe (4–5 years old), the argument being that young children are capable of learning the more formal skills inherent in the school curriculum at an early age. Starting early is seen as giving children a head start and provides for children from disadvantaged backgrounds to make up for the deficits in their academic skills. Most children in European countries start school at 6 and in Finland, which is seen as having one of the best education systems, children start at 7. In the UK, children of 7 in the state school system, have already sat standard aptitude tests (SATs) in English and Maths and in the private system have sat competitive exams at 7+ to go from pre-preparatory schools to preparatory schools. While there are no randomized control trials to determine whether early or late school entry is better best, there is some evidence to suggest that any initial advantage of early schooling is not maintained (Elley 1992) and that early introduction to formal academic settings may increase anxiety and impact on self- esteem and motivation to learn (Elkind 1996; Elkind and Whithurst 2001; Sharp et al. 2002).

Even if the assumption (based on the cognitive hypothesis) that children are capable of learning formal skills at an early age, was correct, the question remains whether the didactic style of UK teaching helps children learn skills in a developmentally appropriate fashion Elkind's (1996) research would suggest not. Children enter reception in large classes where they are expected to sit and take in information with low adult-to-child ratios. They are not free to engage in activities of their choice, explore or be physically active and develop supportive relationships with teachers, the significant people in structuring their early learning. In inner city schools, a lack of space may further impact the ability of young children to be physically active.

Development psychology does not seem to inform much of the teaching and learning in UK schools, yet Piaget and Vygostky, two important figures in the field, may help understand why English early school does not confer noticeable advantages in comparison to schooling in other European countries despite early initiation into formal education. Children enter school aged 4 which we have seen is the age at which they begin to self-regulate emotionally. Whilst there has been much criticism of Piaget's theory, his concept of developmental stages reminds us that teaching children should take into account that learning depends on stage of development. One of Piaget‘s (1950, 1952) central messages is the importance of a child's interaction with the environment to promote conceptual learning until secondary school. In the UK, children at 4 are being subjected to didactic teaching with curriculum emphasis on the acquisition of abstract and symbolic systems such as number, reading, and writing (as opposed to an emphasis on play and the development of conceptual, memory, oral and social skills).

Vygotsky (1978) did not assume that there were phases of development. He focuses on the social aspect of learning through interaction with adults, specifically how language is internalized and helped the child structure his activities. Private speech or talking to oneself, Vygotsky thought, was essential in helping children problem solve. The second aspect of Vygotsky's cognitive theory was the zone of proximal development, a level of development instantly above the child's present level and this links to the final component in Vygotsky's theory: scaffolding, the process used to explain how to encourage children to learn. Scaffolding involves assisting and encouraging children through giving advice or suggestions that they can use and understand to help the child master a new concept which is in their zone of proximal development. Learning through interaction with adults who are sensitive to zones of proximal development, is very difficult for children who find themselves in a classroom with high child to adult ratios, like 30 peers and one adult.

Piaget and Vygotsky shared the assumption that children learn by interacting with their environment and how children mentally grow plays a vital role in their learning processes. Research suggests that child-initiated activities may be important in contributing to children's greater task-involvement, independence, and persistence. Sharp (2002) cites evidence from a longitudinal study in the UK that progress in the early years was associated with teaching styles such as ‘sustained shared thinking’ between pupils and adults, an equal balance between child- and adult-initiated activities, and staff who encouraged children in activities with high cognitive challenge. The conclusion was that effective settings balance a teacher-directed approach, and an approach with an adult supporting children's learning, where children are allowed to access to a range of learning environments. Successful education settings included differentiation and feedback, adult support for children in talking through conflict situations, and parental partnership centred on developing the educational environment at home. This way of teaching requires time and individual attention which is very difficult in a class of 30 or more youngsters typical of schools in metropolitan areas.

Conclusions

There is a powerful argument for looking beyond cognition at how education promotes the skills and the ‘traits’ that will help children succeed at school and subsequently (Hayes 1989; Hoerr 1992). These include self-esteem, self-efficacy, planning, motivation, and the confidence or character to learn from failures, as opposed to giving up (Tough 2014). Emotional resilience is as important to school performance as cognitive skills, and, while there is a stress on early intervention and school readiness, there are critical stages of development when these skills can be developed, providing the right teaching methods are used. Executive functioning is controlled by the pre-frontal context which remains responsive to interventions at least into adolescence.

Traditionally, UK 'Public Schools' (private schools) have been known for their development of character. Students develop self-confidence and self-efficacy outside the class room which they then can draw on inside it. These include characteristics that students in the GEDS study did not possess and to which were attributed the reasons why they did not persist with their studies despite having the cognitive skills. The attitudes and mind-sets developed by children educated in privileged private school environments may have been part of their success (Heckman 2011). Dweck's (2008) research shows that people who believe that they can improve their intelligence actually do improve their intelligence. To develop a successful attitude to learning, children should not be praised for being intelligent but for trying their best that they can. Children need to be supported to see the long-term picture when they are frustrated and angry but failure also is helpful in developing a 'learning from failure' attitude which leads to persistence and long term success (Tough 2014).

In the UK's private system there is still considerable interest in children's achievements outside the classroom, and in developing areas of sport, musical and artistic interest that foster experiences of mastery, self-control, discipline, and motivation to do well (Tough 2014). However, private schools have also been excessively influenced by the cognitive hypothesis with a preparatory school headmaster recently decrying the lack of educational benefit "in doing what we are doing, focusing on excessive testing, taking children way beyond where they need to go at the expense of all else, with all its commensurate social problems" (Tait June 2015). He adds "at the very least, schools should view their selection process in a more enlightened and socially responsible way by adopting different criteria for entry". Studies by Luthar and Latendress (2005) showed high rates of mental health difficulties (anxiety and depression) amongst wealthy students especially in adolescence, with one of the main causes of these difficulties being the excessive pressure to achieve, and low levels of physical and emotional closeness. Striving to always be successful can sometimes be experienced as a burden that stifles creativity and can lead children and young people to opt out as opposed to the shame of not meeting other's expectations (Tough 2014).

An Ecological Approach to Education

Understanding children's attitudes to learning, and fostering a healthy approach, require time, interest, and involvement of the child as an actor in his own learning pathway. The UK education system's emphasis on assessment and outcomes risks losing sight of the needs of the children and young people that it is educating.

Factors Interact to Determine Educational Success

Success in school is determined by a complex set of factors. These also interact to determine which children and young people grow up to function well in society. There is a need for a model of education informed by child development, and the impact of social, relationship and individual factors on children and young people's functioning, a contextualized understanding of skills development. Cognitive stimulation is important in language development and educational outcomes, but the child's every day experience in perceiving and interacting with the physical world is enough for robust development of visuo-spatial skills making them insensitive to differences to socio-economic status (Sheridan and McLaughlin 2016).

Children and young people accessing private education enjoy a range of privileges at home that generally, correlate with better outcomes later in life (Duncan et al. 2005; Machin and Vignole 2006; Duncan and Murnance 2011; Tough 2014). This is not only because of the school they access but because of the homes they come from. Language development is one of the skills related to educational outcomes; it is influenced by a number of social, contextual and relationship factors. Children from homes where they are exposed to books, and to adults who enjoy reading, tend to read earlier. This may also be because children who are exposed to books come from different social environments, with parents who have greater social and cultural capital, understand the aims and objectives of the school system, and know what to do to prepare children for school (Bourdieu 1973).

The Ecological Model

The ecological model allows for a holistic developmental approach to education and learning, promoting an understanding of factors impacting on a child's educational journey. Bronfenbrenner's (1979) ecological model (Fig. 3.1) considers the multifaceted and multi-layered nature of influences on development over the life course, a child's temperament, school preparedness, and peer relationships academic performance. The ecological model explores the influences on human behaviour as a system of nested contexts: (1) individual (biological, genetic, personality); (2) interpersonal (family, friends, peers, and partners); and (3) Community (the social context of relationships) (Sameroff et al. 1993; Owens and Shaw 2003).

Bronfenbrenner's' model described in detail the different types of systems, institutions and groups that most immediately and directly impact the child's development. The school and the family are examples of 'micro-systems' that have significant impact on development. Others include religious institutions, neighbourhood. The interconnection between these micro-systems is termed 'meso-system', which refers to the interconnections between the family and teachers, family and the peers. These in turn are impacted by 'ecosystems', social

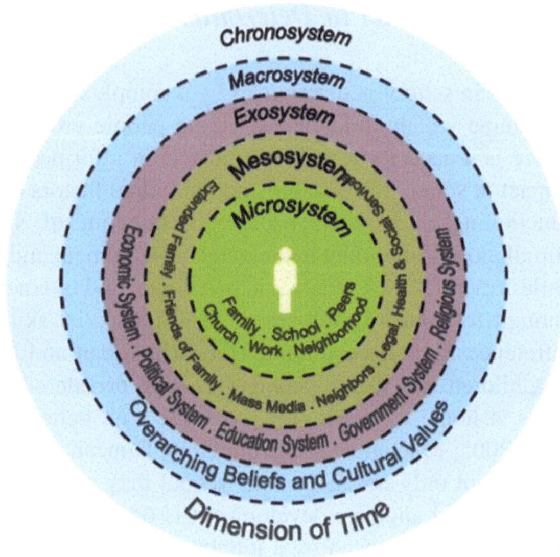

Fig. 3.1 Bronfenbrenner's ecological model

settings in which the individual does not have an active role, such as the impact of a parent's work place on family dynamics, due to changes in working hours, promotion, or redundancies. All these systems are influenced by the 'macro-system' which is the socio-cultural context in which individuals live. Children, their parents, their school, and the workplace are part of a cultural context with an identity, heritage, and values which do change over time but remain shared by specific groups of people. Indeed, education is one of the main mechanisms through which these values are transmitted which is why it is such an important of the systemic context of child development. The ecological model helps unpick all the factors that need to be addressed to help move forward to a more positive form of schooling (Stivaros 2007).

An Ecological Understanding of Education in the UK: Macro-, Exo- and Meso- Systemic Factors

Educational systems reflect the values of the societies (macro-systems) of which they are part, with education being one of the ways the dominant cultural values are communicated. As outlined, the system in the UK is focused on outcomes and reflects a class division, limiting social mobility, with rich and middle class parents accessing expensive private schools, and other parents relying on places in state-maintained schools and competing to attend the best of these. A system focused on results and ratings, discourages children who are failing academically to continue with their education instead of offering and valuing alternative vocational routes to be explored.

With state education operating in an ever-changing context, teachers are under pressure to keep 'standards high', by focusing on what they need to teach to achieve the outcome measurements on which performance is ranked. With a more diverse population of children in many city areas, with differing levels of English, stretched teachers have little time to think of the holistic needs of their charges. Children often come from homes with financial and emotional problems, where the stress on performance is irrelevant for their life experiences. Often ill-prepared and unable to cope with the demands of the classroom, this is yet another pressure on teachers whose options are to fight for support for the child or ignore the needs until they become problematic and the child is excluded.

Children and young people on the other hand are faced with greater pressures to succeed. Bullying in all its forms (direct and more recently cyber bullying) is a pressure, as is peer pressure to consume drugs and alcohol. Young people, who struggle with the system, often have not had a good start, and go on to see school as irrelevant to life plans. Such children lose sight of why they are at school and leave, disillusioned and angry, taking refuge in activities that are considered anti-social (gangs) or are signs of maladjustment (refuge in the virtual world of gaming). Schools also have an incentive to be risk-averse, by excluding children who behave and perform badly because they affect outcome measures.

Children's performance at school is affected by their home and community life and the relationship between family and school (exo- and meso-systems), with good communication between families and school is essential to supporting young people. There are other influences on home life that contribute to children and young people doing well at school (Brooks-Gunn et al. 2000; Smyth et al. 2010). Poverty and scarcity have negative effects on the development of children, and the mechanisms that contribute to such disadvantage are increasingly being understood (Bernier et al. 2012). Executive functioning skills, more specifically working memory, is affected by how much time children had spent in poverty, and correlates with the amount of cortisol in children's blood stream, with the conclusion being that the impact of poverty was mediated by the stress associated with living in poverty (Evans and Schamberg 2009).

Parents, like teachers, are often dealing with busy and complex lives, and parents need to be supporting in parenting children in order that they benefit from education (Brooks-Gunn 2011). At times of economic austerity, impacts on parenting affect children's well-being, which in turn impacts children's ability to function at school. Parents work longer hours, come home tired and stressed, with increased tension in family relationships, relationships break up and there is less time to devote to assisting children. Robson's (2010) youth panel data in Britain over 15 years suggest that there is a decrease in self-esteem, happiness, and income when transitioning out of a two-parent household to a one-parent household. Movement into step-families also decreased happiness, although household income usually increases. Amato (2000) found that divorce was associated with worse academic achievements, conduct, well-being, and social relations. Scott (2004) used 6 years of BHPS panel, and found that educational attainment among young people from intact families was better than in step-families.

Changing gender roles have led to women experiencing conflict and feeling judged regarding about how much time they spend on working outside the home and their parental role, which, in turn, impacts on their experience of motherhood, leading to problems in early relationships with their children, linked to anxiety and depression. There are very few good quality supports to parents that are cost-neutral, yet supporting parents in their home and work environment, to bring up children in a sensitive and caring manner, is likely to provide children with the skills they need to manage learning once they enter the formal school setting.

Micro Systemic Factors

Good (enough) parenting can foster resilience in young children (Gutman and Feinstein 2007), while an absence of sensitive care giving may interfere with a young child's capacity to learn from others through the erosion of "epistemic trust" (Fonagy et al. 2004) Consistent emotional responses of a sensitive caregiver trigger a special mode of learning in the infant, enabling him or her to absorb and assimilate knowledge from this trusted source. If this epistemic trust breaks down—for example, through attachment trauma—the individual's capacity to internalize available knowledge is greatly reduced.

Parents in more privileged settings have the resources to support their children's development by spending more money, but also more time in cognitively enriching activities. The living environments parents provide is also different, more ordered, with higher levels of emotional support and consistent discipline (Kalil 2012). Disparities in parental time are important, as this is shown to have a direct and causal effect on children's cognitive test scores (Villena-Rodan and Rios-Aguilar 2011; Hanson et al. 2013). Educated middle class parents adapt their parenting to the child's developmental stages, and when children are in pre-school, college educated mothers focus on reading and problem solving, moving to managing their children's lives outside school when they are in the middle-school years. Kalil (2012) maintains that those gaps in children's skills could be narrowed if less-advantaged parents could adopt the parenting practice of their more advantaged peers.

Rather than blaming the parents themselves, Kalil (2012) identifies factors that need to be addressed in parenting programmes to help disadvantaged parents improve their parenting skills, and points to the lack of programme effectiveness in doing this to date. He points to research that shows that, as the economic disparity between the most advantaged and disadvantaged families has increased, so has the gap in educational performance (Reardon 2011). Socio-economic gaps in children's cognition and behaviour open early in life and remain constant through the school years (Duncan and Murnance 2011). Parenting programmes need to help parents unlearn and then learn new skills (Duncan et al. 2005). They need to consider incentives and address the impact of cognitive scarcity among low-income parents, stemming from past exposure to toxic stress (Shonkoff and Garner 2012; Shonkoff 2012). Programmes need to understand the impact of daily stressors that place demands on low-income families and the impact on cognitive and emotional functioning that results from this, limiting their capacity for goal-directed and purposeful activity. More focus needs to be given within parenting programmes to addressing parents' own difficulties in executive functioning, including working memory, decision-making, and mindful attention, in order that they can help their children. Promising programmes include coaching multi-media, multi-tasking skills, impulse control, organization, problem solving (Babcock 2014), and mindfulness, meditation, mind–body exercises, and brain games, to increase mental health and parenting (Davidson et al. 2003). In his work on the importance of early experience on school readiness, Guralnick (2013) describes the toll on motivation and self-esteem of early adversity. Good quality child care and education can act as a buffer against adverse experience and Guralnick suggests that readiness for school operates through family mechanisms such as: (1) parent to parent transactions (sensitivity, responsiveness warmth); and (2) family orchestrated child experiences (stimulation, child care, community learning).

Given that children will always arrive at school with different levels of readiness, it is important that learning in the classroom is maximized (Hansen and Jones 2010). Children need the opportunity to develop learning relationships with teachers, experiencing the personal exchange of knowledge, skill acquisition, allowing the child to develop a positive approach, and be active in his or her own learning, which may be a different experience to the one at home. When children are active parties in learning relationships, the child influences the nature of their learning experience. It opens the way for an understanding of the unique proximal and distal factors operating in each child's multi-tiered environment and how they work together in non-linear and non-predictable ways with his/her repertoire of biological, cognitive, emotional and behavioural characteristics, shaping his/her development and learning trajectory, recognizing that development cannot be a uniform process. This approach to learning is more likely to help the child to develop a sense of self-efficacy or also described in terms of the belief in the self capacity to organize and execute actions that are necessary to exert control on future situations (Bandura 1995), helping the child develop traits that promote resilience. For the self-regulated learner, the ability to use metacognitive strategies, such as planning and problem-solving, to enhance performance in a given situation is dependent on the nature of his/her self-efficacy beliefs. The best way to do this is to work within zones of proximal development.

A Different Understanding of Intelligence

In order to maintain engagement and interest in education, school has to be relevant to the skills and interests of young people. The concept of intelligence needs to be expanded beyond Spearman's (1927). Gardner (1993, 1997, 2006a, b) (Fig. 3.2) in an inspiring book called *Frames of Mind* (Gardner 1983) puts forward a pluralistic view of intelligence, arguing that only two types of intelligence, linguistic and logical-mathematical, were being used at school. According to Gardner, there are

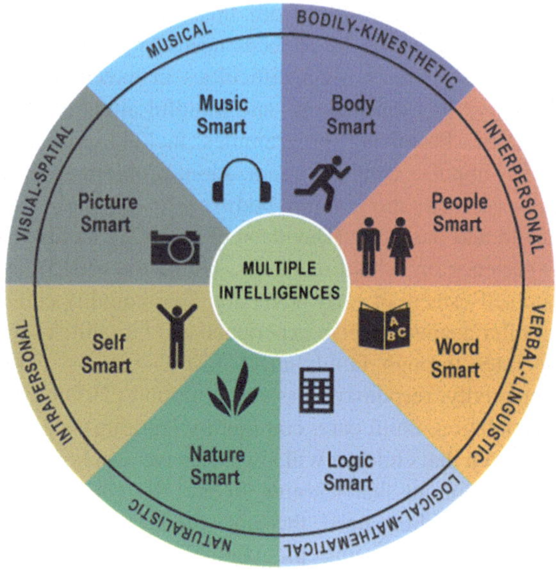

Fig. 3.2 Gardner's model of multiple intelligence

eight forms of intelligence: linguistic, logical-mathematical, musical, spatial, bodily kinaesthetic, interpersonal and intrapersonal, and naturalist intelligence. Gardner maintains that individuals draw on these intelligences, individually and cooperatively, to create products and solve problems that are relevant to the societies in which they live (Gardner 1997; Gardner and Moran 2006). Multiple Intelligence Theory is a departure from traditional twentieth-century conceptions of intelligence, measured today by IQ tests, and is a precursor to the works of Goleman on emotional and social intelligence (Goleman 1995, 2006).

Unlike traditional theories of intelligence that involve debates over the relative importance of nurture and nature (Neisser et al. 1996; Eysenck 1994; Herrnstein and Murray 1994), Multiple Intelligence views intelligence as a combination of heritable potentials and skills that develop in unique ways depending on experience with the environment (Gardner 1983, 1993, 2006a, b). The example given by Gardner is that one individual might be born with a high intellectual potential in the bodily-kinaesthetic sphere that allows him or her to master the intricate steps of a ballet performance with relative ease. For another individual, achieving similar expertise in the domain of ballet requires many additional hours of study and practice. Both individuals can become strong performers—even experts—in a domain that draws on their bodily-kinaesthetic intelligence; however, the pathways along which they travel in order to become strong performers may well differ quantitatively (in terms of speed), and perhaps qualitatively (Ramos-Ford et al. 1988). Gardner's theory fits with Vygotsky's ideas of unique learning pathways for individuals that are shaped and influenced by the ecology of the surrounding context. The theory has implications for curricula and teaching methods. Gardner welcomes and advocates the use of technology to individualize the teaching and assessment methods in schools as much as possible (Vaneema and Gardner 1996). The individuation of teaching then needs to be based on a learner's profile (Normak et al. 2012). Gardner refers to the fact that individualizing tuition has previously been available for the more affluent in society that hire tutors to tailor their pedagogical approach to the learner's needs, and technology may open up more opportunities for this to be made available for all.

Conclusion

The ecological model suggests that an effective education system adopts a holistic development approach, and is rooted in a society that supports parents and provides teachers with the resources to devote time and attention to devote learning relationships with children (Smyth et al. 2010). Schools and parents needs to work in partnership. Parents need to be adequately supported to raise their children and work in partnership with properly trained, respected teachers who have an interest in promoting children's development, as opposed to assessment focused and outcome driven measures (Nomark et al. 2012). Good progress in the early years is associated with an education system that includes differentiation and feedback, adult support for children in talking through conflict situations, and parental partnership centred on developing the educational environment at home (Sharp 2002). An individualized approach to learning—working in the child's zone of proximal development, with the child as an active learner—is more likely to cultivate a sense of self efficacy and mastery, which are character traits associated with better life outcomes—such as employment and well-being— but not necessarily academic performance (Hansen and Jones 2010; Heckman 2011). The goals of education should be to develop a multiplicity of abilities that are nurtured through different types of education (academic, technological, and vocational) (Emig 1997; Özdemir et al. 2006). Education may then be less a source of stress and anxiety and more a source of resilience.

Successful Educational Systems

Putting children at the centre of education entails listening to what they say. In this section, I review some of the information available, on children and young people's experience of school, to see if it matches with what is being written about the system. I will then analyze two successful education systems and understand them in the ecological perspective I have put forward above.

Children and Young People's Views

Riley and Docking (2004) investigated students' perceptions from academic Years 6–10 (6 is the last Year of primary school) and teachers' perceptions of school life. They explored attitudes to rules, discipline, teacher–pupil relationships, parental support, as well as qualitative feedback on schooling. Most pupils valued school, and were supportive of their teachers' efforts to set high standards of behaviour and effort. But, there seemed to be a difference between how positive primary and secondary children were about their experience of school. While Year 6 pupils perceived the schooling experience as satisfactory, secondary pupils—in Year 8 and particularly those in Year 10—reported greater criticism of lessons, disciplinary issues, and student–teacher relations. Schools were seen as having too many rules that were irrelevant to learning. The teachers overestimated the extent to which children enjoyed school and the interest they took in their studies, and underestimated the value pupils placed on completing their school work and the ramifications of bullying.

A more recent study by the Children's Commissioner (2011) also found that children and young people recognized the value of school in supporting their learning and achievement, with three in five enjoying school, and half finding their lessons interesting. Pressure to achieve remained an important theme, with about half worrying about school work and exams, and about a third feeling their school puts too much pressure on them to do well, and a quarter feeling that parents/careers put too much pressure on them to do well at school. The most important priorities for children and young people to improve their school life and education were preventing bullying and having good teachers. Other top priorities focused around the quality of learning opportunities, support to do well in exams, and secondary school admissions. The views of the children suggest that children and young people are experiencing stress in school, and that satisfaction with the school environment decreases with age; a concern, given the social costs when young people lose interest and leave (Robinson and Taylor 2007; Tunnard and Sharp 2009; Robinson and Fielding 2010).

Successful Systems

Finland

Education in Finland is recognized as being one of the best in the world. It is consistently ranked at, or close to, the top in the PISA tables.

Finnish education places the child 'at the heart of the process', and the approach is characterized by co-operation, collaboration, and trust between parents and teachers. Finnish children do not begin school until the age of seven, an age when they are considered developmentally ready. Classes are smaller in Finland—up to

20—and, in primary school, students often have the same teacher for up to six years of their education.

The school day is short, and homework minimal, until they reach adolescence. Students in Finland only have three to four classes a day, and frequent breaks to allow children time to absorb what they have learnt, and to play and exercise in the fresh air. Less time in the classroom is thought to benefit teachers, who use it to think, plan, and create lessons, and this is needed as each school has autonomy over its own curriculum, and students and teachers have a role in educational planning.

Pupils are encouraged to learn through experimentation and interaction, not learning by heart. There are no mandated standardized tests, rankings, comparisons or competition between students, schools, or regions. Teachers get to know their students, their individual needs, and learning styles, with weaker students getting assistance early, and gifted ones being stretched. The Finnish system stresses warmth, collaboration, encouragement, and assessment. Over 90% of Finns graduate from academic or vocational high schools, and 60% go on to higher education.

The teaching profession is a respected and sought-after profession. Candidates have to pass interviews and personality screenings, designed to determine not only their ability to teach but how motivated they are. Teachers must have a Master's degree, and they enjoy a social status equal to other professionals like doctors or lawyers. Teachers are well-trained, and are free to innovate, rather than being subjected to excessive regulation. The culture in Finland is that teachers and parents play an active role and take responsibility for their children's education.

Singapore

The Program for International Student Assessment (PISA) ranking confirms that Singapore has an education system near the top of the international leagues tables which measure student achievement in literacy, numeracy, and science. The country's success has been of interest, especially because the ranking was quite low until 2004.

In 2004, teaching in Singapore became more student-centred, with the introduction of a new educational vision for the country: 'Thinking Schools, Learning Nation'. This focused on the quality of learning rather than the quantity of learning, stressed innovation, creativity and lifelong learning. This is exemplified in two education innovations: the Mastery Method for Mathematics, and the STELLAR approach to English. The Mastery Method for Mathematics enables students to spend time focusing on core principles of mathematics, through a range of activities such as problem-solving exercises, which utilize visual and hands-on aids like blocks, cards, and bar charts. Students are required to become proficient at each step of their learning, and only move on when they have mastered each topic. The STELLAR approach encourages students to improve their language skills through interactive lessons which incorporate drama techniques and role-play, which helps students understand what they have read, evaluate stories and communicate their thoughts; it also makes learners more confident and fluent.

Developing high-quality teachers was an essential aspect of the 'Thinking Schools, Learning Nation' programs. Singapore's educational success is due to the country's ability to develop highly proficient educators by capacity building through selection, training, and professional development. Recruiting high-quality individuals, and providing them with good training and support, has reinforced teaching as a well-regarded occupation, with prospective teachers being selected from the top third of high school graduates. Strong academic ability and a commitment to education are essential for individuals hoping to become teachers. They are well paid and benefit from ongoing professional development; up to 100 h per year. The management of schools is decentralized, and teachers who have the potential to become school leaders are identified early through an initial leadership assessment.

Education is a part of a commitment to equality and meritocracy, encouraging hard work and self-improvement. Confucian ideals are also important to Singaporeans, and these ideals place value on education and diligence. Parents take their children's education seriously and strive to give their children the best possible opportunities, supporting learning with books and tutoring. They have high expectations of their children, which translate into children having high expectations of themselves.

Conclusions

The common features of these educational systems are a focus on the child as a learner, highly trained, valued teachers, and an interactive environment for the child to learn in. Teachers work in partnership with parents in a society where education is seen as essential to self-improvement.

Conclusions and Recommendations

The recent PISA rating of UK education has revealed problems with a system whose focus on outcomes and assessment procedures risks losing sight of the variety of needs of children and young people. The education system reflects deep divisions in society, and a narrow view of what success looks like for children and young people. The UK is notable by how linked educational outcomes are across generations, suggesting limited social mobility. Whilst some children may be prepared to enter the world of schooling, others are less prepared: often children coming from families of a lower social class, with less access to resources and a limited knowledge of the educational system and thus valuing it less (Bourdieu and Passeron 1977). These cultural aspects influence a child's attitude, expectations, and sense of self-efficacy which affect the long-term choices and impact that education will have on a child's life. The lack of funding for early years' provision means that nursery places are in short supply, and that the children who might benefit most from the provision usually do not access it.

The cognitive hypothesis continues to inform education, because, in times of uncertainty. Parents continue to think in simple linear way that training children's cognitive skills will lead to them doing well academically. This may be comforting to parents, teachers and policy holders but does not suit all children (Tough 2014). In practice, it is not proving to be effective either in the state or the private system. Instead, an increasing proportion of young people are becoming disillusioned and/ or stressed. While there is increasing recognition of the importance of social and emotional factors in determining a child's readiness to learn, this is not being translated into practice. In the state system, class size and the young age of children, when they enter the world of formal schooling, means that there is little time and space for children to explore and learn in an age-appropriate fashion. Once in school, the emphasis is on performance, and enhancing outcomes which reflect positively on schools, with children often being denied access to preferred educational pathways because the school is risk-averse in terms of allowing children and young people to choose options which they may not excel at. The narrow definition of success built into the system does not acknowledge that society requires young people with a variety of skills and education needs, and does not prepare them for different roles with good quality technical and vocational training, although there is evidence in recent years that this may be changing.

Educational systems are a product of different cultures and communicate their values. While it is unlikely that the education system is England is likely to change, to become like the Finnish or the Singapore system—whose success is also liked to social and cultural factors—the learning from these systems is: (1) children and an understanding of their development needs to be at the heart of education; (2) children need to be inspired to learn in an interactive process, with good quality well-paid teachers; (3) a successful education system relies on the investment and joint working of all stakeholders (teachers, parents, and policy makers); and (4) successful education systems exist in cultures that value learning for learning's sake and are not driven solely by outcomes that may not be relevant to all. A holistic developmental approach to education is required, for children and young people to succeed; one where schools and their teachers work together with families in a culture that support parents, and prepares and respects teachers to develop a range of skills and competencies.

Going back to the case studies; would a system that promoted working together of families and schools, where children were supported to learn in a way that matched their capacities and interest, be generating the high proportion of difficulties seen in UK schools at the moment? With adequate resources, and a whole system approach where the pupil referral unit was tied into a well-run vocational and apprenticeship schemes and support for families, would so many young people become marginalized and disenfranchised? Would a system built on a holistic vision of a child/young person and their learning, lead to a 16-year-old boy failing their exams after 5 years in a school, or a 12-year-old become so worried about her homework that she started to refuse to attend school. Of course, we don't have the answers to these questions, but asking the questions, suggests the need for a modified and renewed vision for education. It has to put children and young people's learning and development back at the centre of the system, and support teachers and parents to enable children and young people to achieve their aspirations, whatever they may be. This type of education system will help build resilience, and prepare children and young people for a future that matches their strengths and abilities.

References

Amato, P. R. (2000). The consequences of divorce for adults and children. *Journal of Marriage and the Family, 62,* 1269–1287.

Babcock, E. D. (2014). *Using brain science to design new: Pathways out of poverty*. Boston, MA: Crittenton Women's Union.

Bandura, A. (1995). *Self-efficacy in changing societies*. Cambridge: Cambridge University Press.

Barlow, J., & Svanberg, P. O. (2009). *Keeping the baby in mind*. London: Routledge.

Belsky, J. (2005). The developmental and evolutionary psychology of intergenerational transmission of attachment. In C. S. Carter, L. Ahnert, K. E. Grossman, S. B. Hardy, M. E. Lamb, S. W. Porges, & N. Sachser (Eds.), *Attachment and bonding: A new synthesis* (pp. 169–198). Cambridge, MA: The MIT Press.

Belsky, J., & Fearon, R. (2002). Early attachment security, subsequent maternal sensitivity and later child development: Does continuity in development depend upon continuity of care giving? *Attachment and Human Development, 4,* 361–387.

Bernier, A., Carlson, S. M., Deschanes, M., & Matte-Gagne, C. (2012). Social factors in the development of early executive functioning: A closer look at the care giving environment. *Developmental Science, 15*(1), 12–24.

Binet, A., & Simon, T. (1911). *A method of measuring the development of the intelligence of young children*. Lincoln, IL: Courier Company.

Bourdieu, P. (1973). Cultural reproduction and social reproduction. In R. K. Brown (Ed.), *Knowledge Education and Cutura Change*. London, Tavistock.

Bourdieu, P., & Passeron, J. (1977). *Reproduction in education, society and culture*. London: Sage.

Bradbury, B., Corak, M., Waldfogel, J., & Washbrook, E. (2012). Inequality in early child outcomes. In J. Ermisch, M. Jantti, & T. Smeeding (Eds.), *From Parents to Children: The Intergenerational Transmission of Advantage*. New York: The Guilford Press.

Breakspear, S. 2012. The policy impact of PISA: An exploration of the normative effects of international benchmarking in school system performance. *OECD Education Working Papers*. www.search.proquest.com.

Bronfenbrenner, U. (1979). *The ecology of human development: Experiments by nature and design*. Cambridge, MA: Harvard University Press.

Brooks-Gunn, J. (2011). Early childhood education: The likelihood of sustained effects. In E. Zigler, W. S. Gilliam, & W. S. Barnett (Eds.), *The pre-K debates: Current controversies and issues* (pp. 200–205). Baltimor, MD: Brookes.

Brooks-Gunn, J., Berlin, L., & Fulligni, A. (2000). Early childhood intervention programs: What about the family? In J. Shonkoff & J. Meisels (Eds.), *Handbook of early childhood intervention* (pp. 549–577). Cambridge: Cambridge University Press.

Carlivati, J. (2001). *Adolescent attachment, peer relationships, and school success: Predictor, mediator, and moderator relations distinguished majors thesis*. University of Virginia.

Caspi, A., Moffitt, T. E., Wright, B. R. E., & Silva, P. A. (1998). Early failure in the labour market: Childhood and adolescent predictors of unemployment in the transition to adulthood. *American Sociological Review, 63,* 424–451.

Davidson, R. J., Kabat-Zinn, J., Schumacher, J., Rosenkranz, M., Muller, D., Santorelli, S. F., et al. (2003). Alterations in brain and immune function produced by mindfulness meditation. *Psychosomatic Medicine, 65*(4), 564–570.

Deary, I., Strand, S., Smith, P., & Fernandes, C. (2007). Intelligence and educational achievement. *Intelligence, 35,* 13–21.

Duchesne, S., Ratelle, C. F., Poitras, S. C., & Drouin, E. (2009). Early adolescent attachment to parents, emotional problems, and teacher-academic worries about the middle school transition. *The Journal of Early Adolescence, 29*(5), 743–766.

Duncan, G. J., Dowsett, C. J., Claessens, A., Magnuson, K., & Huston, A. C. (2007). School readiness and later achievement. *Developmental Psychology, 43*(6), 1428–1446.

Duncan, G. J., Kalil, A., Mayer, S. E., Tepper, R., & Payne, M. R. (2005). The apple does not fall far from the tree. In S. Bowles, H. Gintis, & M. O. Groves (Eds.), *Unequal chances: Family background and economic success* (pp. 23–79). Princeton, NJ: University Press.

Duncan, G., & Murnance, R. (Eds.). (2011). *Wither opportunity? Rising inequality, schools and children's life chances.* New York: Russell Sage Foundation.

Dweck, C. S. (2008). *Mindset: The new psychology of success.* New York: Ballantine.

Egeland, B., Sroufe, A., Carlson, E., & Collin, A. (2005). *The development of the person: The minnesota study of risk and adaptation from birth to adulthood.* New York: Guilford Press.

Elkind, D. (1996). Early childhood education: What should we expect? *Principal, 75*(5), 11–13.

Elkind, D., & Whithurst, G. J. (2001). Young Einsteins much too early: Much too late. *Education Matters, 1*(2), 8–21.

Elley, W. B. (1992). *How in the world do students read?* The Hague, IEA: IEA Study of Reading Literacy.

Emig, V. B. (1997). A multiple intelligences inventory. *Educational Leadership, 55*(1), 47.

Evans, M., & Schamberg, M. A. (2009). Childhood poverty, chronic stress and adult working memory. *Proceedings of the National Academy of Science, 106*(16), 6545–6549.

Eysenck, H. (1994). *Manual for the Eysenck personality questionnaire (EPQ-R Adult).* San Diego: Educational Industrial Testing Service.

Feinstein, L., & Bynner, J. (2004). The importance of cognitive development in middle childhood for adulthood socioeconomic status, mental health, and problem behaviour. *Child Development, 75*(5), 1329–1339.

Fonagy, P., Gergely, G., Jurist, E., & Target, M. (2004). *Affect regulation, mentalization and the development of self.* London: Karnac.

Gardner, H. (1983). *Frames of mind: The theory of multiple intelligences.* New York: Basic Books.

Gardner, H. (1993). *Frames of mind: The theory of multiple intelligences* (10th ed.). New York, NY: Basic Books.

Gardner, H. (1997). Is there a moral intelligence? In M. Runco (Ed.), *The creativity research handbook.* Cresskill, NJ: Hampton Press.

Gardner, H. (2006a). *Five minds for the future.* Boston, MA: Harvard Business School Press.

Gardner, H. (2006b). *Multiple intelligences: New horizons.* New York: Basic Books.

Gardner, H., & Moran, S. (2006). The science of multiple intelligences theory: A response to Lynn waterhouse. *Educational Psychologist, 41*(4), 227–232.

Gerhardt, S. (2004). *Why love matter: How affection shapes a baby's brain.* Hove, Sussex: Brunner-Routledge.

Goldthorpe, J. H. (2007). Class analysis and the reorientation of class theory: the case of persisting differentials in educational attainment. *British Journal of Sociology, 47*(3), 481–505.

Goleman, D. (1995). *Emotional intelligence.* New York: Bantam Books.

Goleman, D. (2006). *Social intelligence: The new science of human relationships.* New York.

Guralnick, M. J. (2013). Developmental science and preventive interventions for children at environmental risk. *Infants and Young Children, 26*(4), 270–285.

Gutman, L., & Feinstein, L. (n.d.). Children's Well-being in Primary School: Pupil and School Effects. Centre for Research on the Wider Benefits of Learning Research Reports, Bristol, CMDO; 25, Nottingham, DCFS.

Hansen, K., & Jones, E. M. (2010). Cognitive development in England. *Child Indicators Research, 3*(1), 105–126.

Hayes, J. R. (1989). *Cognitive processes in creativity*. In J. A. Glover, R. R. Ronning, C. R.

Heckman, J. (2000). Policies to Foster Human Capital. *Research in Economics, 54*(1), 3–56.

Heckman, J. J. (2011). *The GED in handbook of the economics of education (3)*. In EA Hanusek et al. (Eds.), Oxford: Elsevier.

Herrnstein, R. J., & Murray, C. (1994). *The bell curve: Intelligence and class structure in American life*. New York: Free Press.

Hoerr, T. R. (1992). How our school applied multiple intelligences theory. *Educational Leadership, 50*(2), 67–68.

Hoeve, K., Stams, G. J. J. M., Van de Put, C. E., Dubas, J. S., Van de Laan, P., & Gerris, J. R. M. (2012). A meta-analysis of attachment to parents and delinquency. *Journal of Abnormal Child Psychology, 40*(5), 771–785.

Kalil. (2012). *Promoting early childhood development, addressing the parenting divide to promote early childhood development for disadvantaged children*. The Hamilton Project.

Landry, S. H., Anthony, J. L., Swank, P. R., & Monseque-Bailey, P. (2009). Effectiveness of comprehensive professional development for teachers of at-risk preschoolers. *Journal of Educational Psychology, 101*(2), 448–456.

Luthar, S. S., & Latendress, S. J. (2005). Children of the affluent: Challenges to well-being. *Current Directions in Psychological Science, 14,* 49–53.

Moulin, S., Waldfogel, J., & Washbrook, E. (2014). *Baby bonds parenting, attachment and a secure base for children*. London: The Sutton Trust.

Neisser, U., Boodoo, G., Bouchard, T. J., Jr., Boykin, A. W., Brody, N., Ceci, S. J., et al. (1996). Intelligence: Knowns and unknowns. *American Psychologist, 51*(2), 77.

NICE. (2006). Infant-mother attachment classification: Risk and protection in relation to changing maternal caregiving quality. *Development Psychology, 42*(1), 38–58.

Normak, P., Pata, K., & Kaipainen, M. (2012). An ecological approach to learning dynamics. *Educational Technology and Society, 15*(3), 262–274.

Office of the Children's Commissioner: Children and young people's views of education policy, March 2011.

Owens E, Shaw D (2003) Poverty and early child adjustment. In Luther S (ed) *Resilience and vulnerability: Adaptation in the context of childhood adversities* (pp. 267–292).

Özdemir, P., Güneysu, S., & Tekkaya, C. (2006). Enhancing learning through multiple intelligences. *Journal of Biological Education, 40*(2), 74–78.

Perry, B. D. (1995). Childhood trauma: The neurobiology of adaptation and use-dependent development of the brain. *Journal of Infant Mental Health, 16,* 271–291.

Piaget, J. (1950). *The psychology of intelligence*. London: Routledge & Paul.

Piaget, J. (1952). *The origins of intelligence in children*. New York: International Universities Press.

Price, J. (2010). *Effects of parental time investments: Evidence from natural within family variation*. Mimeo: Brigham Young University.

Ramos-Ford, V., Feldman, D. H., & Gardner, H. (1988). A new look at intelligence through project spectrum. *New Horizons for Learning, 8*(3), 6–15.

Reardon, S. F. (2011). The widening socioeconomic status achievement gap: New evidence and possible explanations. In G. J. Duncan & R. J. Murnane (Eds.), *Wither opportunity? rising inequality and the uncertain life chances of low income children*. New York: Russel Sage Foundation and Spencer Foundation.

Riley, K., & Docking, J. (2004). Voices of disaffecting pupils: Implications for policy and practice. *British Journal of Educational Studies, 52*(2), 166–179.

Robinson, C., & Fielding, M. (2010). Children and their primary schools: pupils voices. In Alexander et al. (Eds.), *The Cambridge primary review research surveys* (pp. 17–48).

Robinson, C., & Taylor, C. (2007). Theorising student voice: Values and perspectives. *Improving Schools, 10*(1), 5–17.
Robson, K. (2010). Changes in Family Structure and the Well-Being of British Children: Evidence from a Fifteen-Year Panel Study. *Child Indicator Research, 3*(1), 65–83.
Sameroff, A. J., Seifer, R., Baldwin, A., & Baldwin, C. (1993). Stability of Intelligence from preschool to adolescent: The influence of social and family risk factors. *Child Development, 64,* 80–97.
Schore, A. (2003). The effect of secure attachment relationship on the right brain development, affect regulations and infant mental health. *Infant Mental Health Journal, 22,* 7–66.
Scott, J. (2004). Family, gender and educational attainments in Britain. *Journal of Comparative Family Studies, 35,* 565–589.
Sharp, C. School starting age: European policy and recent research. In *Paper presented at the LGA Seminar 'When Should Our Children Start School?'*. LGA Conference Centre, Smith Square, London. Nov 1, 2002. www.nfer.ac.uk/publications/44414.
Sharp, C., Hutchison, D., & Keys, W. (2002). Comparing school systems to explain enduring birth date effects: a response to Mcdonald (2001). *Compare: A Journal of Comparative and International Education, 32*(2), 239–241.
Sheridan, M. A., & McLaughlin, K. A. (2016). Neurobiological models of the impact of adversity on education. *Current Opinion in Behavioral Sciences, 10,* 108–113.
Shonkoff, J. P. (2012). Leveraging the biology of adversity to address the roots of disparity in health and development. *Proceedings of the National Academy of Sciences of the United States of America, 109*(2), 17302–17307.
Shonkoff, J. P., & Garner, A. S. (2012). The lifelong effects of early childhood adversity and toxic stress. *Peadiatrics, 129*(1), 232–246.
Siegel, D. J., & Hartzell, M. (2003). *Parenting from the inside out: How a deeper understanding can help you raise children who thrive*. New York: Penguin Books.
Smyth, E., Whelan, C. T., McCoy, S., Quail, A., & Dole, E. (2010). Understanding parental influence on educational outcomes among 9 year olds in Ireland: The mediating role of resources, attitudes and children's own perspective. *Child Indicators Research, 3*(1), 85–104.
Spearman, C. (1927). *The abilities of man*. London, UK: Macmillan.
Toth, S. L., Rogosch, F. A., Manly, J. T., & Cicchetti, D. (2006). The efficacy of toddler-parent psychotherapy to reorganize attachment in the young offspring of mothers with major depressive disorder: A randomized preventive trial. *Journal of Consulting and Clinical Psychology, 74*(6), 1006–1016.
Tough, T. (2014). *How children succeed*. London: Arrow Books.
Tunnard, S., & Sharp, J. (2009). Children's views of collaborative learning. *Education 3–13, 37* (2), 159–164.
Vaneema, S., & Gardner, H. (1996). Multi-media multiple intelligence. *American Prospect*, 26.
Villena-Rodan, B., Rios-Aguilar, C. (2011). Causal effects of maternal time-investment on children's cognitive outcomes. In *Working Paper 285, Centro de EconomiaAplicada*. Santiago: Universidad de Chile.
Vygotsky, L. S. (1978). *Mind in society*. Cambridge, MA: Harvard University Press.
Waldfogel, J., & Washbrook, E. (2010). *Low income and cognitive development in the UK: A report for the Sutton Trust*. London: The Sutton Trust.

Electronic Resources

Binet, A., & Simon, T. (1916). *The development of intelligence in children*. Baltimore, Williams & Wilkins. (Reprinted 1973, New York: Arno Press; 1983, Salem, NH: Ayer Company).
Every Child Matters www.gov.uk/government/publications/every-child-matters.
Gutman, L., & Feinstein, L. (2007). Wider beneftis of Learning report 22. www.learningbenefits.net.

Hansen, K., & Vignoles, A. (2005). The United Kingdom education system in comparative context. https://www.cls.ioe.ac.uk/library.

Hanson et al. (2013). Family poverty affects the rate of human infant brain growth. *PLOS* 8, 12. www.plos.org.

Joseph Rowntree Foundation. www.Jrht.org.uk.

Machin, S., & Vignole, A. (2006). Education policy in the UK. cee.lse.ac.uk/ceedps/ceedp57.pdf.

National Scientific Council on the Developing Child. (2005/2014). *Excessive stress disrupts the architecture of the developing brain: Working paper 3*. Updated Edition. http://www.developingchild.harvard.edu.

No Child Left Behind www.nochildleftbehind.co.uk.

Stivaros, H. (2007). *An ecological perspective of children's school experiences and educational outcome*. Doctoral thesis, University of Huddersfield.

This version is available at http://eprints.hud.ac.uk/959/.

Tait Telegraph (2015, June 4). www.journalisted.com/peter-tait?allarticles.

United Nations (1989). *Convention on the rights of the child*. General Assembly Resolution 44/25, 20th Nov 1989. U.N Doc. A/RES/44/25.

Young Minds (2017). *Children and adolescent mental health*. https://youngminds.org.uk.

Chapter 4
Understanding and Supporting Student Motivation for Learning

Linda Gilmore

Abstract This chapter highlights the importance of motivation for children's learning, and describes the ways in which motivation may be strengthened. We begin by discussing the construct of motivation and the various theories that have attempted to explain why some students are more highly motivated than others. Drawing on the framework of mastery motivation, we describe developmental aspects of the drive for mastery, highlighting the ways in which this drive increasingly becomes differentiated and affected by the interplay of individual child characteristics, such as self-efficacy and self-regulation, and contextual factors, such as cognitively stimulating environments, optimal challenge, and support for autonomy. The contexts in which children live and learn have important implications for motivation. We discuss motivation in children with learning and developmental disabilities, considering the experiences that potentially undermine their engagement with learning. The final part of the chapter focuses on strategies for promoting and sustaining motivation. In particular, we emphasize the importance of providing optimal challenge, experiences of success, and support for autonomy, as well as the benefits of positive strategies for developing self-regulatory skills.

Keywords Student · Motivation · Learning · Developmental disabilities
Self-efficacy · Self-regulation

Introduction

Motivation is critical for effective learning. Highly motivated students are enthusiastic about learning, and committed to working towards goals. They make use of effective strategies to achieve their goals, hold positive beliefs about the value of learning, and display confidence in their own ability. Poorly motivated students, on the other hand, tend to be disengaged, displaying a reluctance to attempt or persist

L. Gilmore (✉)
Queensland University of Technology, Brisbane, Australia
e-mail: l.gilmore@qut.edu.au

S. Deb (ed.), *Positive Schooling and Child Development*,
https://doi.org/10.1007/978-981-13-0077-6_4

with tasks, and appearing uninterested in learning. Not surprisingly, reduced levels of motivation are associated with lower academic achievement.

Teachers naturally want children to be keen to learn. Ideally, they want them to be *intrinsically* motivated; that is, they want them to be motivated to learn because they perceive the material to be inherently interesting and they recognize its value. Students who are intrinsically motivated are keen to acquire knowledge and skills; their goal is to achieve mastery of, or competence in, a particular area. By contrast, children who are extrinsically motivated are driven by external factors, such as the desire to achieve passing grades or to impress others. Realistically, although individuals may be intrinsically motivated by some topics or areas, much learning is not inherently interesting. Students may struggle to see the relevance of required learning for later goals, leading them to be more extrinsically motivated.

This chapter focuses on evidence from research studies that have attempted to answer some of the key questions teachers have about student motivation: What motivates children to learn and achieve? Why are some children more motivated than others? How can teachers encourage children to be more engaged with learning?

Drawing on a considerable body of research from the area of educational psychology, the chapter begins with an overview of various theoretical perspectives on motivation, before considering the child and contextual factors that are associated with higher motivation for learning. The final section of the chapter describes positive strategies for promoting and sustaining children's engagement with learning.

Definitions and Theoretical Perspectives on Motivation

Motivation has been defined as the force that energizes, directs, and sustains goal-directed behaviour (Morgan et al. 1990; Schunk et al. 2014). White (1959) argued that all individuals are born with an inherent drive to master their environments. This drive provides the energy for individuals to work towards goals; it directs their behaviour towards those goals, and sustains the necessary effort for achieving them. Stipek (1997) described motivated students as "willingly engaged in the learning process, self-confident in their ability to learn and to complete school tasks, persistent in the face of difficulty, oriented towards developing, understanding and mastering skills, enthusiastic and optimistic about learning, and proud of their accomplishments" (1997, 77). This definition illustrates the behaviours, emotions, and cognitions that are associated with the concept of motivation. We infer motivation from behaviours such as the willingness to engage and persist with challenging tasks, and from emotional responses, such as enthusiasm for tasks, and pride following achievement. Cognitive influences on motivation include beliefs about one's own competence and the attributions one makes for successes and failures. Such cognitions affect the ways in which students approach learning, including their levels of persistence and their responses to failure. Cognitive aspects of motivation also include self-regulation skills such as goal-setting, planning, monitoring progress, and resisting distractions.

Various theoretical perspectives emphasize specific cognitive, emotional, and behavioural components of motivation. For example, social cognitive theory (Bandura 1986) stresses the importance of self-efficacy - that is, cognitive beliefs about one's own competence. Self-worth theory (Covington 1992) focuses on emotional self-evaluations and self-acceptance. Expectancy-value theory (Wigfield and Eccles 2000) proposes that students' motivation for achievement depends on their expectations about future success with a particular task, as well as their perceptions of the task's intrinsic value. Goal theory (Maehr and Zusho 2009) has contributed to our understanding of motivation by distinguishing mastery, with its focus on *developing* competence, from performance recognition, which is the *demonstration* of competence. Mastery goals are associated with more positive academic outcomes than performance goals. The impact on motivation of the ways in which we reason about the causes of our successes and failures is the focus of attribution theory (Weiner 1985), while operant theory (Skinner 1953) emphasizes the motivational effects of reinforcement or punishment.

According to self-determination theory (Ryan and Deci 2000), motivated behaviour is driven by the basic human needs for autonomy, competence, and social relatedness. People need to feel a sense of volition and control over their own actions, they need to feel effective in their interactions with the environment, and they need to feel connected to others. Self-determination theory proposes a motivation continuum of autonomy versus control. Between the opposite end points of intrinsic motivation (high autonomy) and amotivation (unmotivated, uninterested) there exist four different subtypes of extrinsic motivation that differ according to the degree of autonomy or self-determination that is involved (Ryan and Deci 2000). In the two higher levels, individuals are motivated for activities they value (identified motivation) or by ones that are consistent with their personal values (integrated motivation). By contrast, lower levels of self-determination characterize introjected motivation in which individuals seek to feel satisfaction or pride, and to avoid feelings of shame and guilt. The least self-determined level of motivation is external motivation where actions are driven purely by the need to obtain rewards and avoid punishment. There is evidence that these subtypes of extrinsic motivation also apply to individuals who are developing atypically (Frielink et al. 2017).

Better outcomes are associated with autonomous than controlled motivation (Deci and Ryan 2002). Intrinsic motivation is related to higher academic achievement and self-efficacy (Froiland and Oros 2014; Gottfried 1990; Lepper et al. 2005). In this most autonomous and self-determined level of motivation, individuals engage in an activity of their choosing for its own sake, displaying high levels of enthusiasm, absorption, concentration, and enjoyment of the activity. Those who are deeply immersed in an intrinsically rewarding activity may experience a state of flow in which there is no longer any awareness of time, place, and even self (Csikszentmihalyi 1990). An important characteristic of flow is the notion of optimal challenge that represents a perfect balance between the inherent challenge of a task and the individual's ability. Csikszentmihalyi (1975) argued that when task difficulty exceeds an individual's capabilities, anxiety results. But when a task is perceived as not sufficiently challenging, boredom is likely to follow. Although flow may not be experienced commonly in school settings (Shernoff and Csikszentmihalyi 2009), the concept provides a worthy goal for teachers. Ideal engagement in learning can be viewed as deep engrossment in tasks that are inherently interesting, optimally challenging, and personally satisfying. Of particular note is that either anxiety or boredom may result if learning tasks are not appropriate for individual ability.

The construct of mastery motivation offers a framework for considering the developmental nature of motivation. It is presumed that all infants have an instinctive and undifferentiated drive to explore and master their environments (White 1959). Over time, experiences of success and failure influence motivation, and children become more motivated to engage in activities they enjoy and feel competent with (Guay et al. 2010; Harter 1978). Thus, mastery motivation becomes increasingly differentiated and focused with age. Older children and adults naturally display greater motivation to master activities that are within their realm of interest and aptitude, whereas they are less likely to be motivated in areas that they perceive to be difficult or uninteresting, or in which they have experienced constant failure.

Numerous studies have found that early motivation predicts later competence and academic success (Gilmore et al. 2003a, b; Hustinx et al. 2009; Turner and Johnson 2003). The importance of mastery motivation has been demonstrated also in atypical populations. In a sample with Down syndrome, motivation in early childhood predicted academic success in adolescence (Gilmore and Cuskelly 2009) and adaptive functioning in young adulthood (Gilmore and Cuskelly 2017). Hauser-Cram et al. (2014) also reported associations of early childhood motivation with executive functioning 20 years later, in a group of individuals with developmental disabilities. The importance of mastery motivation has also been demonstrated for individuals with neurodevelopmental disorders such as cerebral palsy (Warschausky et al. 2017).

Over time, children become more susceptible to the reactions of others, such as parents, teachers, and peers, and these reactions influence their continuing motivation. Social acknowledgement of mastery attempts and achievements may become more important than intrinsic feelings of satisfaction associated with success. According to the construct of achievement motivation, children with a performance orientation focus on demonstrating their competence to others, while those with a mastery orientation are more focused on the development of competence (Senko et al. 2008).

For older children and adults, preference for challenge or novelty is often viewed as an indicator of motivation, along with persistence, curiosity, and inherent pleasure in learning. Although the construct of mastery motivation has sometimes been used in motivation studies with older children and adults (Gilmore et al. 2017), it is more common for research with older samples to draw on the broader construct of achievement motivation that includes beliefs and expectations about performance, as well as self-perceptions of competence and the value placed on learning.

Developmentally, declines in intrinsic motivation with age are frequently documented, especially at the time of school entry and in the transition from elementary to high school (Gottfried et al. 2009; Lepper et al. 1997; Otis et al. 2005). There are numerous possible explanations for such declines, including an increasing focus on performance instead of mastery outcomes, greater social comparisons against the achievement of peers, boredom associated with lack of meaning or relevance of learning tasks, and less perceived control over learning in adolescence, a developmental phase in which autonomy becomes increasingly important.

Each of the theoretical perspectives and motivational constructs discussed above offers potentially useful insights that help us to make sense of individual differences in motivation. Children vary hugely with respect to their self-concepts, attributions, expectancies of success, persistence, and interest in different areas of learning. In addition, individuals rarely display similar levels of motivation across all learning domains, and they are likely to display different motivational profiles or patterns in different contexts (for example, home, school, sporting arena) and at different times. Thus, we need a range of theoretical perspectives to draw upon when attempting to understand and respond to motivational issues.

Research with Typically Developing Children

Research with typically developing children has focused on two main aspects of motivation: Why are some children more motivated than others? And, how can motivation be improved? We first need to understand individual differences in motivation in order to recommend particular teaching practices or interventions that will improve children's motivation for learning. We focus first here on individual child characteristics that affect motivation, then on environmental factors, although child and environmental factors are inevitably interconnected and reciprocally influencing.

Individual Child Characteristics

Many child characteristics are associated with motivation for learning. The most basic, yet often overlooked, reasons for low motivation are those associated with physical health, sensory difficulties, and motor skills. Children who have difficulties in these areas are likely to have reduced interest in learning because of problems such as inadequate hearing, pain, lack of sleep, or low energy levels. For example, the child who does not have a good night's sleep because of pain from an ear infection, or breathing difficulties due to asthma, or disturbances by parents arguing, is unlikely to display highly motivated behaviour at school the following day. Numerous other factors, such as medication side-effects, substance misuse, anxiety, and depression, may influence student engagement in the classroom.

Some of the theories of motivation discussed earlier help us to understand how children's cognitions can undermine their motivation for learning. The ways they think about their ability are particularly relevant. Students who have low levels of belief in their own competence and a low expectancy of success will tend to avoid challenge and not persist after failure. The attributions they make for successes and failures can have critical impacts on motivation. Children who view their failures as due to low ability, or simply luck, will see learning as uncontrollable and believe persistence is pointless. On the other hand, those who explain failure as the result of insufficient effort may be more motivated to try harder in order to avoid repeated failure. As discussed later in this chapter, students' attributions are likely to be influenced by the direct and indirect messages they receive from teachers and other significant people.

Children whose individual learning goals are directed towards mastery tend to display greater persistence and higher self-efficacy than those whose learning is overshadowed by the need to demonstrate their achievements to others or to compete with peers. The latter group is more likely to avoid challenge and to demonstrate a learned helpless pattern of motivation. Another individual characteristic that influences motivation is the capacity for self-regulation. Motivated behaviour requires the ability to resist distractions, monitor and evaluate progress with a task, change approaches if necessary, cope adaptively with frustration and other emotional responses, and ask for help when necessary. Children vary in their ability to use these self-regulation skills, with some groups such as those with attention-hyperactivity disorders (Barkley 2011) or intellectual impairment (Cuskelly et al. 2013) having more difficulty than others.

Although some of these individual characteristics are intrinsic to the child, most are influenced by environmental factors, or can be modified by appropriate interventions. The environments within which children live and learn have important implications for their motivation.

Children's Environments

Motivation is likely to be impacted by a range of factors within children's family, school, community, and cultural contexts. Research evidence shows that environments which provide cognitive stimulation and challenge, opportunities for success, support for autonomy, and positive reinforcement, are optimal for promoting and sustaining children's motivation for learning.

Numerous studies have demonstrated associations between cognitively stimulating environments and children's motivation and achievement (see Gottfried et al. 1998; Wang et al. 2011). Gottfried et al. (2016) found that 8-year-old children, whose parents provided cognitively stimulating activities, went on to display higher academic intrinsic motivation and achievement in science at high school. Students who are intrinsically motivated prefer challenging activities (Deci and Ryan 1985). Optimally challenging tasks are neither too easy nor too difficult, but rather are within a child's zone of proximal development (Vygotsky 1986). Not only are such activities more cognitively stimulating, but they are also more likely to produce feelings of satisfaction following success and to reinforce a child's feelings of self-efficacy.

The ways in which teachers respond to students' efforts in the classroom are likely to influence their motivation for further attempts. Clear, informative feedback, that focuses on effort rather than ability, is most useful for promoting mastery goals (Mueller and Dweck 1998). There is extensive evidence for the effectiveness of positive reinforcement for shaping children's behaviour, provided it is used judiciously. Commonly used reinforcers include praise, rewards, and treats or privileges of different kinds. Some studies have demonstrated the potentially adverse effects of reinforcers for children's motivation. Referred to as the "overjustification effect", it seems that offering external incentives for activities that are intrinsically interesting may reduce motivation, although this effect may not be observed when rewards are unexpected (Lepper et al. 1973). Reinforcement in the form of praise can positively impact intrinsic motivation when the focus is on mastery rather than social comparisons (Henderlong Corpus et al. 2006). Later in this chapter, we will consider the ways in which praise can most effectively be used for promoting children's motivation.

Various teacher characteristics potentially influence children's motivation for learning. Students tend to be more highly motivated when teachers display their own high levels of motivation and enthusiasm for learning (Patrick et al. 2000). Teacher passion tends to be contagious and to increase student engagement (Keller et al. 2013). Not surprisingly, teachers themselves report more enjoyment and greater confidence in the classroom when their students are highly motivated to learn and oriented towards mastery (Martin 2006).

High levels of teacher stress can have adverse consequences, not only for teachers' well-being, but also for children's motivation for learning (Pakarinen et al. 2010). Stressed teachers are likely to be less engaged with their students and to provide less effective instruction. In a large sample of high school students, Shen and colleagues (2015) found negative relationships of teacher burnout with students' motivation and their perceptions of the extent to which teachers supported their autonomy.

Many studies have demonstrated links of student motivation with supportive teacher behaviours such as respect and empathy (Patrick et al. 2007; Skinner et al. 2008). One of the most important ways in which teachers can support their students is by encouraging their autonomy. A considerable body of research has demonstrated the associations of autonomy support with children's social, emotional, cognitive, and motivational outcomes (Jang et al. 2010; Reeve 2009; Ruzek et al. 2016; Taylor and Ntoumanis 2007; van der Kaap-Deeder et al. 2017; Vasquez et al. 2016). Similar relationships have been documented for children with learning disabilities (Deci et al. 1992), intellectual disability (Emond Pelletier and Joussemet 2016; Gilmore et al. 2009) and behavioural disorders (Savard et al. 2013). Autonomy supportive behaviours include involving children in decision-making, acknowledging their feelings and respecting their views, minimizing directives and demands, encouraging children to take the initiative, and offering choices. By contrast, directive adults tend to be controlling and intrusive, ignoring children's perspectives, and giving them few if any opportunities for autonomous behaviour.

Collaborative environments in which groups of students work towards common goals can contribute to motivation. Self-determination theory stresses the importance of human connectedness. Even young children appear to have an innate drive to cooperate with others (Warneken and Tomasello 2007) and opportunities for collaboration enhance persistence and task enjoyment (Butler and Walton 2013). Turner (1995) found that Grade One students who had opportunities to work on interesting and challenging tasks, in collaborative settings in which they perceived some control, displayed the highest levels of motivation for literacy. However, students may benefit most when they feel that they are part of the group and also that they stand out as individuals. In a recent study of high school students, Gray (2017) found that academic motivation was strongest for those who felt not only that they belonged within their peer group but also that their unique contributions were valued by the group. Developmentally, adolescence is a time when, somewhat paradoxically, young people strive both for conformity to peer norms and for the establishment of a unique individual identity. Thus, they are seeking simultaneously to 'fit in' and to 'stand out'. Satisfying both of these needs is associated with achievement motivation and well-being.

Cultural Contexts

The overwhelming majority of research studies published in international journals report data collected in western countries, predominantly the United States. Cultural influences have generally been overlooked in motivation research (King and McInerney 2014) and, when culture is considered, comparisons often tend to be made between children in western countries and immigrants from non-western countries who are now living in western countries. There is a scarcity of research conducted in less-developed countries and published in journals that are accessible for international audiences. Yet, we cannot presume that the findings of motivation research in western countries always apply in non-western contexts, especially collectivist cultures.

Cross-culturally, there appear to be both similarities and differences in motivational processes. A generally universal finding is the decline in motivation at school entry and the further decline around the transition from primary to secondary school; in addition, girls are commonly found to be more highly motivated than boys (Lam et al. 2016). Many studies have described common motivation profiles across different cultural groups. De Castella et al. (2013) reported similar patterns of motivation for high school students in Australia and Japan and, in a study of mastery motivation of university students in four different cultural contexts—Australia, Hungary, Bangladesh, and Iran—there were no significant differences in self-reported motivation (Gilmore et al. 2017). However, some motivation theories may not be supported in non-western cultures, and motivation concepts may have different meaning or salience in different cultural contexts (King and McInerney 2014; Täht et al. 2014). In particular, the fact that western countries tend to emphasize individual goals and autonomy, whereas collectivist cultures generally focus more on group goals and relatedness, suggests that academic achievement in individualistic cultures is more likely to be driven by mastery, while in collectivist societies performance or social goals may be more important (Dekker and Fischer 2008; King et al. 2014). Self-determination theory proposes, however, that the needs for autonomy, competence, and relatedness are universal, even though collectivist cultures may not necessarily value autonomy to the same extent as western countries. Indeed, there is evidence that autonomy-supportive teaching has similarly positive benefits for motivation of children in China (Zhou et al. 2009).

Children with Learning or Developmental Difficulties

Children with learning or developmental difficulties may have physical health and sensory impairments, cognitive impairments, difficulties with motor skills, problems with social interaction, and limitations with language and communication. At school, these children are likely to experience not only difficulties with learning, but also experiences of failure, discouraging feedback from others, negative self-evaluations, and social exclusion. All of these experiences potentially undermine their motivation for learning.

Students with learning disabilities may display problems with motivation, such as poor task persistence, avoidance of challenge, low academic self-efficacy, and negative affect (Ayers et al. 1990; Baird et al. 2009; Meltzer et al. 2004; Poskiparta et al. 2003; Sideridis 2006). This is not surprising, given their difficulties with learning and the greater number of failures they are likely to experience. But learning disabilities are not always easily recognized. Children may be presumed to be poorly motivated - in other words, simply lazy. Gilmore and Boulton-Lewis (2009) demonstrated this presumption powerfully in a study of 20 children who, according to their teachers, could be successful at school if only they made greater effort and applied themselves more. The researchers hypothesized that specific difficulties might underlie the presumed laziness of these children, and indeed the results of comprehensive psycho-educational assessments supported this hypothesis. Of the 20 children in the sample, 17 had diagnosable, but previously unrecognized, learning disabilities or attention disorders. These findings highlight the importance of considering individual child characteristics if we are trying to understand motivation for learning.

Several studies have demonstrated the ways in which the environments of students with learning disabilities may impact their motivation. Teachers may inadvertently convey the message that children with learning disabilities have low levels of ability and thus should expect failure (Georgiou et al. 2002; Woodcock and Vialle 2016). Woodcock and Vialle (2011) reported that pre-service teachers had lower expectations of students with learning disabilities, and conveyed negative attributions that had the potential to undermine students' beliefs about the level of achievement they might expect to attain. Children with learning disabilities are more likely to attribute their successes to external factors such as luck, and their failures to low ability (Waheeda and Grainger 2002).

Students who experience constant failure and negative feedback may come to believe that they do not have the necessary ability or that they have little control over learning outcomes (Kunnen and Steenbeek 1999). In the former case (low perceptions of competence), students may seek to avoid failure, whereas in the latter case (low perceptions of control) they may feel helpless (Craske 1988). Children with learning disabilities are more vulnerable to developing learned helplessness than others (Sideridis 2003). Learned helplessness is associated with low self-esteem, low self-perceptions of ability, and low expectations about future success. Dweck and Sorich (1999) reported that some children as young as, or even younger than, 8 years of age displayed signs of helplessness such as poor task persistence, ineffective learning strategies, self-blame for failure, and the belief that increased effort would not make a difference.

There is a relative scarcity of research about motivation in children with developmental disabilities. Most of the available research is quite dated (Jacobs 1972; Switzky 1997; Wong 1980) and overwhelmingly comes from western countries, mainly the United States. One of the earliest studies concluded that children and adolescents with intellectual disability had lower levels of motivation than those who were developing typically (Harter and Zigler 1974). At this time, however, individuals with developmental disabilities experienced exclusion and discrimination that limited their opportunities for engagement and success with learning (Gilmore and Cuskelly 2014). Nevertheless, the view that individuals with intellectual disability have deficits in motivation has tended to persist (Deci 2003; Emond Pelletier and Joussemet 2016; Greenspan 2006). This is despite evidence from more recent studies that have found no differences in task persistence when children with intellectual disability are compared to others of the same mental age (Gilmore and Cuskelly 2011; Gilmore et al. 2003a, b; Glenn et al. 2001; Nader-Grosbois and Lefévre 2011; Nader-Grosbois and Vieillevoye 2012). At times, however, subtle differences have been identified, such as with respect to sustained task engagement (Ruskin et al. 1994), and parents or teachers generally rate children with intellectual disability as less persistent (Gilmore and Cuskelly 2011; Zigler et al. 2002), possibly because they make comparisons to peers of the same chronological, rather than mental, age. Some researchers have argued that motivational deficits are part of the learning and behavioural profile of specific disabilities, such as Down syndrome (Fidler 2006), although others have challenged this view (Gilmore et al. 2015).

Positive Strategies for Promoting Motivation

The evidence from research studies reviewed above provides a strong foundation for the development of a range of positive strategies that teachers can use to promote and sustain children's motivation for learning.

Consider Possible Underlying Issues

As mentioned earlier, there may be specific reasons for a child's lack of engagement with learning. Teachers need to be aware of the range of difficulties that undermine motivation, and watch for possible indicators of problems. For example, the child who appears inattentive to instructions may have undiagnosed difficulties with hearing or auditory processing or speech and language. The student who seems to be daydreaming and staring into space as if uninterested in learning, could potentially be experiencing absence seizures, sleep deprivation, anxiety, or attention deficit disorder. Children who have unrecognized learning disabilities may present as 'lazy' and unmotivated, because their learning needs have not been recognized. At times, teachers may misinterpret certain child behaviours, such as slowness and passivity, as being reflective of low levels of motivation. But some children, especially those with intellectual disability, require more time for processing and formulating responses. These children may also need time-out breaks from concentration if learning is particularly effortful; during such breaks, they may appear passive and uninterested in their surroundings, but it is not appropriate to conclude automatically that these behaviours imply low levels of motivation. Research about flow experiences suggests that individuals with low levels of ability who are given tasks that are low in challenge may become passive or apathetic about learning. Even children with intellectual disability need to be offered tasks that are challenging for them. Yet this does not necessarily happen in classrooms, as illustrated in the following example. An 11-year-old boy with a mild intellectual disability was asked: "What do you do if the teacher gives you some work and it's too hard for you?"; he replied: "I tell her it's too hard and then she just gives me colouring in to do."

It is clearly important to consider possible issues that underlie what, on the surface, appear to be problems with motivation. When teachers believe a student is poorly motivated, they tend to respond with less involvement, less structure, and less autonomy support than they provide to students who they perceive to be highly motivated. Such responses will undermine the children's inherent interest and engagement in learning activities, and consequently limit their achievement. If they are aware of the range of difficulties that can potentially underlie apparent motivational problems, teachers can respond more sensitively, referring students to school psychologists or counsellors for proper evaluation if necessary.

Identify and Modify Children's Self-efficacy Beliefs and Attributions

Earlier, we discussed the critical influences of self-efficacy, expectations, and attributions on children's motivation. Teachers can identify, challenge, and modify the beliefs students have about their own competence, the expectations they have about future achievement, and the attributions they make for their successes and failures. Of course, teachers also need to be aware of their own expectations about the level of achievement a child may attain, as well as the attributions they make for a student's successful and unsuccessful attempts. It is important to have realistic, but optimistic, expectations of children, neither unnecessarily low nor unrealistically high. When teachers have low expectations, they are more likely to attribute a child's failures to low ability, and their successes to luck. These teacher expectations and attributions, if conveyed directly or indirectly to students, can undermine their motivation.

In order to strengthen self-efficacy, self-competence beliefs, and expectations, children need opportunities to experience success. Learning activities can be structured so that some degree of success is achievable and a child's particular strengths, interests, curiosities, and talents may be identified, incorporated, and nurtured (Cuskelly and Gilmore 2014). Self-efficacy contributes not only to motivation and academic achievement, but also to psychosocial well-being (Erikson 1963) and a host of other positive developmental outcomes, such as self-regulation and resilience (Benight and Bandura 2004).

Identifying and modifying the attributions students make about their own performance can be a powerful strategy for enhancing motivation. Children who make comments such as "I'm just a dumb kid" are likely to be attributing their failures to low ability and, if failure is common, they may develop a pattern of learned helplessness in which effort is seen as useless, because failure is believed to be inevitable. For these children, there is a sense of hopelessness as well as helplessness. They are pessimistic about the possibility of succeeding, and tend to either give up quickly or not try at all. It is important to identify maladaptive attributions early before they become deeply entrenched. In order to modify those attributions, teachers can provide opportunities for success, modifying tasks if necessary, and giving students strategies such as mnemonics, to increase their sense of control and likelihood of success. Offer feedback which emphasizes that successes are due to effort, and failures are due to lack of effort, but beware of attributing failure to lack of effort if a child does not have the necessary ability or strategies for success. Some children may try very hard, but their efforts still do not result in success. This may be because of a learning disability or speech and language disorder or some other problem that has not been recognized, so considering the possibility of such underlying issues is critical when a child's progress is slow or inconsistent.

Attribution-retraining programmes commonly use cognitive-behavioural techniques to challenge existing attributions. Many studies have reported on positive improvements in student motivation (Dresel and Haugwitz 2008; Sinnott and

Biddle 1998) including for children with learning disabilities (Okolo 1992; Toland and Boyle 2008). Toland and Boyle (2008) showed that it was possible to modify children's attributions, with subsequent benefits for their motivation, self-esteem, and academic performance. Using strategies based on cognitive behaviour therapy and a range of activities that included role plays, modelling, verbal rehearsal, peer support, the intervention encouraged children to think more positively about learning, to see success as a result of their own efforts, and to use positive self-talk to dispute negative thoughts.

Use Positive Teaching Strategies

Positive teaching strategies that promote students' motivation include the provision of well-structured and well-scaffolded lessons. Breaking down complex tasks into smaller integrated steps with short-term goals not only makes learning more manageable, but also gives children opportunities to experience success at each step, as well as opportunities to practice dealing appropriately with failure if it occurs. Success contributes to feelings of self-efficacy and well-being. Although constant failure is likely to undermine motivation, this does not mean that learning should be organized so that failure is avoided. Children need to understand that failure is an inevitable part of life and view failure experiences as opportunities for learning. They can be helped to recognize, understand, and manage responses such as frustration and disappointment.

In addition to the regulation of emotions, other self-regulatory strategies can be incorporated in positive teaching practices. Direct teaching of skills such as goal-setting, self-management of attention, and inhibition of impulsive responding can be useful for many students. Self-talk is a valuable strategy for regulating thinking and behaviour. Encourage positive self-talk such as "I can do it, yes I can" or "Try, try again" to replace pessimistic thoughts such as "This is too hard for me, I can't do it". Help-seeking is another adaptive self-regulatory strategy. Children need to feel that it is OK to request help but some may be reluctant for fear of being ridiculed by their peers. Help them to know when it is appropriate to seek help and how to ask for it, perhaps by practicing ways of asking for help using role-plays or self-talk.

As an example of a self-regulation intervention, the Self-Regulated Strategy Development programme (SRSD; Harris and Graham 1996; Harris et al. 2008) was developed specifically to address children's writing skills. Writing demands multiple self-regulatory strategies such as planning, monitoring, evaluation, and self-reinforcement. The SRSD programme includes both scaffolded instruction about writing processes and the development of appropriate self-regulatory strategies. Through its focus on enhancing feelings of writing self-efficacy, and encouraging attributions to effort and strategy use, the intervention has been shown to be effective for improving motivation and achievement in writing, including for students with learning disabilities (for a meta-analysis of the evidence, see Graham et al. 2013).

Students will more likely be engaged with learning when they find the material interesting, when they see it as relevant, and when their teacher is enthusiastic about the subject matter. Highlighting the value and relevance of new learning can potentially promote students' motivation. Hulleman and Harackiewicz (2009) developed and evaluated an intervention that encouraged students to see the relevance of science learning to their own lives. High school pupils were randomly allocated to either an experimental group, in which they were asked to write essays about the perceived usefulness of science in their own lives, or a control group that simply wrote summaries of science classes. At the end of the semester, students in the experimental group who reported low expectancies of success in science at the beginning of the study displayed more interest in science and higher achievement than those in the control group. There were no differences for pupils whose expectancies of success had initially been high. These results show that encouraging students' awareness of the relevance of new learning can improve their motivation and achievement.

Another key teaching strategy for promoting intrinsic motivation is the provision of optimal challenge matched to an individual child's skills. Optimally challenging and intrinsically interesting activities with clear goals are more likely to produce intense absorption and a state of flow. Students who experience flow feel in control of their own learning and derive great satisfaction, even exhilaration, from the experience. Encouraging children's curiosity and autonomy can also foster their intrinsic motivation for learning.

One of the most important influences teachers have on children's motivation and learning is through the feedback they provide. Most valuable is clear and informative feedback that highlights improvement and mastery. Specific feedback with a focus on effort and the processes involved in learning, not merely on successful completion, is more effective (Cimpian 2010; Zentall and Morris 2010). But praise should be used judiciously - not too often and not too lavishly. Social comparisons can be motivating for high-achieving students, especially boys, but may be harmful for other children, especially those with learning or developmental disabilities. For promoting intrinsic motivation, feedback that is focused on individual progress, skill development, personal strengths, and mastery is likely to be more effective than social comparisons (Henderlong Corpus et al. 2006).

Praise is a form of positive reinforcement that provides more than informational feedback because it contains teacher approval and sometimes an emotional quality. Effective praise is sincere, specific, and contingent, rather than excessively effusive, haphazard, or ambiguous. But, at times, praise may inadvertently convey the wrong messages to students. Especially in early childhood classrooms, it seems to be relatively common to praise children with comments such as "good boy" or "good girl" and "You're so clever", which convey messages about goodness and ability, rather than effort (for example, "You tried so hard") or achievement ("You did it!"). Some forms of praise are likely to be more effective than others for enhancing intrinsic motivation. For instance, the feedback "I'm so proud of you for doing well on this test" conveys the teacher's pleasure; by contrast, "You must feel so proud of yourself for doing well on this test" implies that the child has achieved, not for the teacher's praise, but for his or her own satisfaction. Subtle messages may also sometimes be conveyed through nonverbal feedback. For instance, when a teacher gives a small sigh following a child's efforts with a task, this could be taken to suggest that her expectations of the child's low ability have just been confirmed.

It is not necessary to praise every single success and it is not appropriate to praise successful completion of very easy tasks. Children usually know when their efforts have been praiseworthy, and praise for success with tasks that were not particularly difficult or challenging suggests that teachers have low expectations of the child. Constant praise may lead to children becoming dependent on adult reinforcement and unwilling to persist without it. As an example, a young child was completing a series of moderately challenging puzzle tasks in a research study, with his mother present but not assisting. When her son completed the first puzzle, she applauded enthusiastically. Because the researcher did not join in, she said, "You have to clap, otherwise he won't do any more"; indeed, she was right, for the child refused to continue when the researcher did not applaud.

In some situations, rewards such as treats or free time can be motivating provided they are valued by students. However, as discussed earlier, rewards may potentially undermine intrinsic motivation when interest and enjoyment of an activity are high. For children who need encouragement to persist, rewards linked to progress can be useful, whereas rewarding task completion or time spent on a task, irrespective of the quality of work, are not helpful. Rewards may also have some value when the tasks that students are required to undertake are not inherently interesting, but nevertheless are important building blocks for later learning (for example, memorizing multiplication tables). For such tasks that students consider boring or irrelevant, rewards may be useful for encouraging effort.

Create a Supportive Classroom Environment

Motivation for learning is nurtured within warm classroom environments where children are accepted and respected, where they are encouraged to express their opinions, and where their views are accepted and valued. Bempechat and Shernoff (2012) said that "expressions of warmth and care are critical to well-being and essential in students' motivation to learn" (2012, 334). Supportive environments promote a sense of belonging and relatedness, and minimize social comparisons, encouraging cooperation rather than competition.

Collaboration has a range of positive outcomes for motivation and achievement. Opportunities to work with others may make learning tasks more enjoyable, and increase the likelihood of sustained effort with a task and shared pleasure upon success. At the same time, identifying and valuing individual strengths and talents is important, especially for adolescents (Gray 2017). Students need to feel that they are part of the group, and also that their unique contributions are valued by their peers. Ideally, teachers need skills in facilitating groups, especially when the class includes students with a range of individual differences in abilities/disabilities and cultural identities.

Supporting children's autonomy is one of the most important ways for promoting and sustaining motivation. External control reduces autonomy, so students need opportunities for self-initiation, involvement in decision-making, choice, and control. Autonomy-supportive teachers explain reasons for requests and rules instead of just giving directions, avoid using controlling language of techniques, and genuinely value students' perspectives and input.

Choice is an important element of autonomy support. Children are more likely to persist with a task if they have chosen it themselves from a range of appealing alternatives. Choice enhances effort, performance, and feelings of competence (Patall et al. 2008) although this is not always the case (Flowerday and Schraw 2003). Merely offering choice is not necessarily motivating, and indeed may even reduce motivation (Katz and Assor 2007). Ideally, choices on offer need to be relevant and meaningful in order to satisfy children's needs for autonomy, competence, and relatedness. Offering high school students choices about the type and amount of homework they do has been shown to have positive influences on motivation (Akioka and Gilmore 2013; Patall et al. 2010). But there is a cognitive load involved in making choices: if there are too many options, students may feel stressed and overwhelmed. Children with intellectual disability need a limited number of choices (ideally only 2 or 3) and help to consider each option. Of course, the choices on offer should be appropriate for the children's ages and ability levels, as well as being alternatives that they are likely to value, and that the teacher finds acceptable. Choices of topics, methods of learning, and styles of presentation can be offered. Supporting the autonomy of students with intellectual disability can be more demanding because of the need to wait for a child's independent attempts without intervening, and to be sensitive to child cues that indicate the need for teacher prompts or assistance, in order to avoid frustration or task refusal.

One final way in which teachers can encourage children's persistence is through case examples of both real and fictional characters. Arguably, one of the very best models of persistence that children will easily relate to is J. K. Rowling, whose first Harry Potter book was rejected by 12 major publishers before it was finally accepted. Discussions with students could focus on the discouraging effects of rejection, and the need to believe in oneself and persist nevertheless. What would have happened if J. K. Rowling had given up after the third, eighth or twelfth rejection? Many millions of children and adults would never have had the opportunity to enjoy these wonderful books! There are numerous other examples of persistent individuals, such as Michael Jordon, who was told at high school that he would never be a good basketball player, and Thomas Edison, who reportedly had to make around 1,000 attempts before eventually creating a light bulb that worked.

Fictional characters can also be introduced to illustrate the importance of persistence. For young children, the classic "The Little Engine That Could" (Piper 2011) provides the catchy line "I think I can, I think I can" that children could incorporate as self-talk, to remind themselves of the importance of not giving up. The picture book "Stickley Sticks to It" (Miles and Mack 2015) tells of a frog named Stickley with a special gift called "stick-to-it-ness", which refers not only to his sticky suction toes, but also to his highly persistent attitude towards getting things done. In Stickley's own words, this means "taking chances and believing in yourself–even when you're not sure what will happen". The book ends with notes for parents and teachers, including suggestions for promoting persistence, such as taking breaks for recharging, thinking about the problem in a different way, and asking for help when necessary.

Another motivational picture book suitable for young readers is "The Most Magnificent Thing" by Spires (2017). This engaging story is about a young girl who tries and tries to create the "most magnificent thing" in the world with the help of her canine assistant. But it turns out to be more difficult than she expected. There are many important messages in this book about planning, overcoming failure and frustration, and never giving up; all of these messages are conveyed with the use of interesting vocabulary and delightful illustrations. And for older students, "Alexander Conquers the World" by Lehn (2014) tells about a teenage boy who is very poorly motivated at school, until he meets a mysterious stranger who stimulates his interest in learning using a range of assignments and special missions.

It seems that even robots can make good models of persistence for children. Research being conducted at the Massachusetts Institute of Technology is demonstrating that children's approaches to learning can be improved with assistance from robots (New Scientist 25 February 2017). Children who completed a puzzle in collaboration with a robot that displayed persistent and positive approaches to learning, learnt to be more persistent and dealt better with failure, compared with children whose robot companion behaved in ways that were more neutral.

Conclusions

In this chapter, we have considered the various theoretical perspectives on motivation, reviewed research evidence about individual differences in motivation, and described the ways in which children's environments can potentially impact their motivation for learning. Drawing on theory and empirical evidence, we identified a range of positive strategies teachers can use to promote and sustain children's motivation. These strategies include considering issues that may underlie low motivation, identifying and modifying children's self-efficacy beliefs and attributions, using positive teaching strategies, and creating supportive classroom environments. Fostering children's motivation for learning is likely to promote higher levels of academic achievement, as well as positive psychological well-being and future successes throughout the lifespan.

References

Akioka, E., & Gilmore, L. (2013). An intervention to improve motivation for homework. *Australian Journal of Guidance and Counselling, 23,* 34–48. https://doi.org/10.1017/jgc.2013.2.

Ayers, R., Cooley, E., & Dunn, C. (1990). Self-concept, attribution, and persistence in learning-disabled students. *Journal of School Psychology, 28,* 153–163.

Baird, G. L., Scott, W. D., Dearing, E., & Hamill, S. K. (2009). Cognitive self-regulation in youth with and without learning disabilities: Academic self-efficacy, theories of intelligence, learning versus performance goal preferences, and effort attributions. *Journal of Social and Clinical Psychology, 28,* 881–908. https://doi.org/10.1521/jscp.2009.28.7.881.

Bandura, A. (1986). *Social foundations of thought and action: A social cognitive theory.* Englewoods Cliffs, NJ: Prentice Hall.

Barkley, R. A. (2011). *Handbook of self-regulation: Research, theory and applications* (2nd ed.). New York: Guilford Press.

Bempechat, J., & Shernoff, D. J. (2012). Parental influences on achievement motivation and student engagement. In S. L. Christenson, A. L. Reschly, & C. Wylie (Eds.), *Handbook of research on student engagement* (pp. 315–342). New York: Springer.

Benight, C. C., & Bandura, A. (2004). Social cognitive theory of posttraumatic recovery: The role of perceived self-efficacy. *Behavior Research and Therapy, 42,* 1129–1148. https://doi.org/10.1016/j.brat.2003.08.008.

Butler, L. P., & Walton, G. M. (2013). The opportunity to collaborate increases preschoolers' motivation for challenging tasks. *Journal of Experimental Child Psychology, 116,* 953–961. https://doi.org/10.1016/j.jecp.2013.06.007.

Cimpian, A. (2010). The impact of generic language about ability onchildren's achievement motivation. *Developmental Psychology, 46,* 1333–1340. https://doi.org/10.1037/a0019665.

Covington, M. V. (1992). *Making the grade: A self-worth perspective on motivation and school reform.* New York: Cambridge University Press.

Craske, M. L. (1988). Learned helplessness, self-worth motivation and attribution retraining for primary school children. *British Journal of Educational Psychology, 58,* 152–164. https://doi.org/10.1111/j.2044-8279.1988.tb00888.x.

Csikszentmihalyi, M. (1975). *Beyond boredom and anxiety.* San Francisco: Jossey-Bass.

Csikszentmihalyi, M. (1990). *Flow: The psychology of optimal experience.* New York: Harper Perennial.

Cuskelly, M., & Gilmore, L. (2014). Motivation for learning in children with intellectual disabilities. *Research and Practice in Intellectual and Developmental Disabilities, 1,* 51–59. https://doi.org/10.1080/23297018.2014.906051.

Cuskelly, M., Gilmore, L., & Carroll, A. (2013). Self-regulation and mastery motivation in individuals with developmental disabilities: Barriers, supports, and strategies. In K. C. Barrett, N. A. Fox, G. A. Morgan, D. J. Fidler, & L. A. Daunhauer (Eds.), *Handbook of self-regulatory processes in development: New directions and international perspectives* (pp. 381–402). New York: Taylor & Francis.

De Castella, K., Byrne, D., & Covington, M. (2013). Unmotivated or motivated to fail? A cross-cultural study of achievement motivation, fear of failure, and student disengagement. *Journal of Educational Psychology, 105,* 861–880. https://doi.org/10.1037/a0032464.

Deci, E. L. (2003). Promoting intrinsic motivation and self-determination in people with mental retardation. In H. N. Switzky (Ed.), *Personality and motivational systems in mental retardation* (pp. 1–20). San Diego, CA: Elsevier Academic Press.

Deci, E. L., Hodges, R., Pierson, L., & Tomassone, J. (1992). Autonomy and competence as motivational factors in students with learning disabilities and emotional handicaps. *Journal of Learning Disabilities, 25,* 457–471. https://doi.org/10.1177/002221949202500706.

Deci, E. L., & Ryan, R. M. (1985). *Intrinsic motivation and self-determination in human behaviour.* New York: Academic Press.

Deci, E. L., & Ryan, R. M. (2002). *Handbook of self-determination research*. Rochester: University of Rochester Press.

Dekker, S., & Fischer, R. (2008). Cultural differences in academic motivation goals: A meta-analysis across 13 societies. *Journal of Educational Research, 102,* 99–110. https://doi.org/10.3200/JOER.102.2.99-110.

Dresel, M., & Haugwitz, M. (2008). A computer-based approach to fostering motivation and self-regulated learning. *Journal of Experimental Education, 77,* 3–18. https://doi.org/10.3200/JEXE.77.1.3-20.

Dweck, C. S., & Sorich, L. A. (1999). Mastery-oriented thinking. In C. R. Snyder (Ed.), *Coping: The psychology of what works*. New York: Oxford University Press.

Emond Pelletier, J., & Joussemet, M. (2016). The benefits of supporting the autonomy of individuals with mild intellectual disabilities: An experimental study. *Journal of Applied Research in Intellectual Disabilities*. https://doi.org/10.1111/jar.12274.

Erikson, E. H. (1963). *Childhood and society*. New York: Norton.

Fidler, D. J. (2006). The emergence of a syndrome-specific personality profile in young children with Down syndrome. *Down Syndrome Research and Practice, 10,* 53–60. https://doi.org/10.3104/reprints.305.

Flowerday, T., & Schraw, G. (2003). Effect of choice on cognitive and affective engagement. *Journal of Educational Research, 96,* 207–215. https://doi.org/10.1080/00220670309598810.

Frielink, N., Schuengel, C., & Embregts, P. (2017). Distinguishing subtypes of extrinsic motivation among people with mild o borderline intellectual disability. *Journal of Intellectual Disability Research, 61,* 625–636. https://doi.org/10.1111/jir.12363.

Froiland, J. M., & Oros, E. (2014). Intrinsic motivation, perceived competence and classroom engagement as longitudinal predictors of adolescent reading achievement. *Educational Psychology, 34,* 119–132. https://doi.org/10.1080/01443410.2013.822964.

Georgiou, S., Christou, C., Stavrinides, P., & Panoura, G. (2002). Teacher attributions of student failure and teacher behaviour toward the failing student. *Psychology in the Schools, 39,* 583–595. https://doi.org/10.1002/pits.10049.

Gilmore, L., & Boulton-Lewis, G. (2009). Just try harder and you will shine: A study of 20 lazy children. *Australian Journal of Guidance and Counselling, 19,* 95–103. https://doi.org/10.1375/ajgc.19.2.95.

Gilmore, L., & Cuskelly, M. (2009). A longitudinal study of motivation and competence in children with Down syndrome: Early childhood to early adolescence. *Journal of Intellectual Disability Research, 53,* 484–492. https://doi.org/10.1111/j.1365-2788.2009.01166.x.

Gilmore, L., & Cuskelly, M. (2011). Observational assessment and maternal reports of motivation in children and adolescents with Down syndrome. *American Journal on Intellectual and Developmental Disabilities, 116,* 153–164. https://doi.org/10.1352/1944-7558-116.2.153.

Gilmore, L., & Cuskelly, M. (2014). Mastery motivation in children with Down syndrome: Promoting and sustaining interest in learning. In R. Faragher & B. Clarke (Eds.), *Educating learners with Down syndrome: Research, theory, and practice with children and adolescents*. New York: Routledge/Taylor & Francis.

Gilmore, L., & Cuskelly, M. (2017). Associations of child and adolescent mastery motivation and self-regulation with adult outcomes: A longitudinal study7 of individuals with Down syndrome. *American Journal on Intellectual and Developmental Disabilities, 122,* 235–246. https://doi.org/10.1352/1944-7558-122.3.235.

Gilmore, L., Cuskelly, M., & Browning, M. (2015). Mastery motivation in children with intellectual disability: Is there evidence for a Down syndrome behavioural phenotype? *International Journal of Disability, Development and Education, 62,* 265–275. https://doi.org/10.1080/1034912X.2015.1020923.

Gilmore, L., Cuskelly, M., & Hayes, A. (2003a). A comparative study of mastery motivation in young children with Down syndrome: Similar outcomes, different processes? *Journal of Intellectual Disability Research, 47,* 181–190. https://doi.org/10.1046/j.1365-2788.2003.00460.x.

Gilmore, L., Cuskelly, M., & Purdie, N. (2003b). Mastery motivation: Stability and predictive validity from ages two to eight. *Early Education and Development, 14,* 411–424. https://doi.org/10.1207/s15566935eed1404_2.

Gilmore, L., Cuskelly, M., Jobling, A., & Hayes, A. (2009). Maternal support for autonomy: Relationships with persistence for children with Down syndrome and typically developing children. *Research in Developmental Disabilities, 30,* 1023–1033. https://doi.org/10.1016/j.ridd.2009.02.005.

Gilmore, L., Islam, S., Younesian, S., Bús, E., & Józsa, K. (2017). Mastery motivation of university students in Australia, Hungary, Bangladesh and Iran. *Hungarian Educational Research Journal, 7,* 180–193. https://doi.org/10.14413/herj.2017.02.11.

Glenn, S., Dayus, B., Cunningham, C., & Horgan, M. (2001). Mastery motivation in children with Down syndrome. *Down Syndrome Research and Practice, 7,* 52–59. https://doi.org/10.3104/reports.114.

Gottfried, A. E. (1990). Academic intrinsic motivation in young elementary school children. *Journal of Educational Psychology, 82,* 525–538. https://doi.org/10.1037/0022-06663.82.3.525.

Gottfried, A. E., Fleming, J. S., & Gottfried, A. W. (1998). Role of cognitively stimulating home environment in children's academic intrinsic motivation: A longitudinal study. *Child Development, 69,* 1448–1460. https://doi.org/10.2307/1132277.

Gottfried, A. E., Marcoulides, G. A., Gottfried, A. W., & Oliver, P. H. (2009). A latent curve model of parental motivational practices and developmental decline in math and science academic intrinsic motivation. *Journal of Educational Psychology, 101,* 729–739. https://doi.org/10.1037/a0015084.

Gottfried, A. E., Preston, K. S. J., Gottfried, A. W., Oliver, P. H., Delany, D. E., & Ibrahim, S. M. (2016). Pathways from parental stimulation of children's curiosity to high school science course accomplishments and science career interest and skill. *International Journal of Science Education, 38,* 1972–1995. https://doi.org/10.1080/09500693.2016.1220690.

Graham, S., Harris, K. R., & McKeown, D. (2013). The writing of students with LD and a meta-analysis of SRSD writing intervention studies. In I. Swanson, K. R. Harris, & S. Graham (Eds.), *Handbook of learning disabilities* (2nd ed., pp. 405–438). New York: Guilford Press.

Gray, D. L. (2017). Is psychological membership in the classroom a function of standing out while fitting in? Implications for achievement motivation and emotions. *Journal of School Psychology, 61,* 103–121. https://doi.org/10.1016/j.jsp.2017.02.001.

Greenspan, S. (2006). Functional concepts in mental retardation: Finding the natural essence of an artificial category. *Exceptionality, 14,* 205–224. https://doi.org/10.1207/s15327035ex1404_3.

Guay, F., Chanal, J., Ratelle, C. F., Marsh, H. W., Larose, S., & Boivin, M. (2010). Intrinsic, identified, and controlled types of motivation for school subjects in young elementary school children. *Journal of Educational Psychology, 80,* 711–735. https://doi.org/10.1348/000709910X499084.

Harris, K., & Graham, S. (1996). *Making the writing process work: Strategies for composition and self-regulation* (2nd ed.). Cambridge, MA: Brookline Books.

Harris, K., Graham, S., Mason, L., & Friedlander, B. (2008). *Powerful writing strategies for all students.* Baltimore: Paul H. Brookes.

Harter, S. (1978). Effectance motivation reconsidered: Toward a developmental model. *Human Development, 21,* 34–64. https://doi.org/10.1159/000271574.

Harter, S., & Zigler, E. (1974). The assessment of effectance motivation in normal and retarded children. *Developmental Psychology, 10,* 169–180. https://doi.org/10.1037/h0036049.

Hauser-Cram, P., Woodman, A. C., & Heyman, M. (2014). Early mastery motivation as a predictor of executive function in young adults with developmental disabilities. *American Journal on Intellectual and Developmental Disabilities, 119,* 536–551. https://doi.org/10.1352/1944-7588-119.6.536.

Henderlong Corpus, J., Ogle, C. M., & Love-Geiger, K. E. (2006). The effects of social-comparison versus mastery praise on children's intrinsic motivation. *Motivation and Emotion, 30,* 335–345. https://doi.org/10.1007/s11031-006-9039-4.

Hulleman, C. S., & Harackiewicz, J. M. (2009). Promoting interest and performance in high school science classes. *Science, 326,* 1410–1412. https://doi.org/10.1126/science.1178712.

Hustinx, P. W. J., Kuyper, H., & van der Werf, M. P. C. (2009). Achievement motivation revisited: New longitudinal data to demonstrate its predictive power. *Educational Psychology, 29,* 561–582. https://doi.org/10.1080/01443410903132128.

Jacobs, S. U. (1972). Acquisition of achievement motive among mentally retarded boys. *Sociology of Education, 45,* 223–232. https://doi.org/10.2307/2112009.

Jang, H., Deci, E. L., & Reeve, J. (2010). Engaging students in learning activities: It is not autonomy support or structure but autonomy support and structure. *Journal of Educational Psychology, 102,* 588–600. https://doi.org/10.1037/a0019682.

Katz, I., & Assor, A. (2007). When choice motivates and when it does not. *Educational Psychology Review, 19,* 429–442. https://doi.org/10.1007/s10648-006-9027-y.

Keller, M., Neumann, K., & Fischer, H. E. (2013). Teacher enthusiasm and student learning. In J. Hattie & E. M. Anderman (Eds.), *International guide to student achievement* (pp. 247–249). New York: Routledge.

King, R. B., Ganotice, F. A., & Watkins, D. A. (2014). A cross-cultural analysis of achievement and social goals among Chinese and Filipino students. *Social Psychology of Education, 17,* 439–455. https://doi.org/10.1007/s11218-014-9251-0.

King, R. B., & McInerney, D. M. (2014). Culture's consequences on student motivation: Capturing cross-cultural universality and variability through personal investment theory. *Educational Psychologist, 49,* 175–198. https://doi.org/10.1080/00461520.2014.926813.

Kunnen, E. S., & Steenbeek, H. W. (1999). Differences in problems of motivation in different special groups. *Child: Care Health and Development, 25,* 429–446. https://doi.org/10.1046/j.1365-2214.1999.00106.x.

Lam, S.-F., Jimerson, S., Shin, H., Cefai, C., Veiga, F. H., Hatzichristou, C., et al. (2016). Cultural universality and specificity of student engagement in school: The results of an international study from 12 countries. *British Journal of Educational Psychology, 86,* 137–153. https://doi.org/10.1111/bjep.12079.

Lehn, M. (2014). *Alexander conquers the world: A story about learning and motivation.* USA: Createspace.

Lepper, M. R., Greene, D., & Nisbett, R. E. (1973). Undermining children's intrinsic interest with extrinsic reward: A test of the "overjustification" hypothesis. *Journal of Personality and Social Psychology, 28,* 129–137. https://doi.org/10.1037/h0035519.

Lepper, M. R., Henderlong Corpus, J., & Iyengar, S. S. (2005). Intrinsic and extrinsic motivational orientations in the classroom: Age differences and academic correlates. *Journal of Educational Psychology, 97,* 184–196. https://doi.org/10.1037/0022-0663.97.2.184.

Lepper, M. R., Sethi, S., Dialdin, D., & Drake, M. (1997). Intrinsic and extrinsic motivation: A developmental perspective. In S. S. Luthar, J. A. Burack, D. Cicchetti, & J. R. Weisz (Eds.), *Developmental psychopathology: Perspectives on adjustment, risk, and disorder* (pp. 23–50). New York: Cambridge University Press.

Maehr, M. L., & Zusho, A. (2009). Achievement goal theory: The past, present, and future. In K. Wentzel & A. Wigfield (Eds.), *Handbook of motivation at school* (pp. 77–104). New York: Routledge.

Martin, A. J. (2006). The relationship between teachers' perceptions of student motivation and engagement and teachers' enjoyment of and confidence in teaching. *Asia-Pacific Journal of Teacher Education, 34,* 73–93. https://doi.org/10.1080/13598660500480100.

Meltzer, L., Katzir, T., Miller, L., Reddy, R., & Roditi, B. (2004). Academic self-perceptions, effort, and strategy use in students with learning disabilities: Changes over time. *Learning Disabilities Research and Practice, 19,* 99–108. https://doi.org/10.1111/j.1540-5826.2004.00093.x.

Miles, B. S., & Mack, S. (2015). *Stickley sticks to it! A frog's guide to getting things done.* Washington, DC: Magination Press, American Psychological Association.

Morgan, G. A., Harmon, R. J., & Maslin-Cole, C. A. (1990). Mastery motivation: Definition and measurement. *Early Education and Development, 1,* 318–339.

Mueller, C. M., & Dweck, C. S. (1998). Praise for intelligence can undermine children's motivation and performance. *Journal of Personality and Social Psychology, 75,* 33–52. https://doi.org/10.1037/0022-3514.75.1.33.

Nader-Grosbois, N., & Lefévre, N. (2011). Self-regulation and performance in problem-solving using physical materials or computers in children with intellectual disability. *Research in Developmental Disabilities, 32,* 1492–1505. https://doi.org/10.1016/j.ridd.2011.01.020.

Nader-Grosbois, N., & Vieillevoye, S. (2012). Variability of self-regulatory strategies in children with intellectual disability and typically developing children in pretend play situations. *Journal of Intellectual Disability Research, 56,* 140–156. https://doi.org/10.1111/j.1365-2788.2011.01443.x.

Okolo, C. M. (1992). The effects of computer-based attribution retraining on the attributions, persistence, and mathematics computation of students with learning disabilities. *Journal of Learning Disabilities, 25,* 327–334. https://doi.org/10.1177/002221949202500507.

Otis, N., Grouzet, F. M. E., & Pelletier, L. G. (2005). Latent motivational change in an academic setting: A 3-year longitudinal study. *Journal of Educational Psychology, 97,* 170–183. https://doi.org/10.1037/0022-0663.97.2.170.

Pakarinen, E., Kiuru, N., Lerkkanen, M.-K., Poikkeus, A.-M., Siekkinen, M., & Nurmi, J.-E. (2010). Classroom organization and teacher stress predict learning motivation in kindergarten children. *European Journal of Psychology of Education, 25,* 281–300. https://doi.org/10.1007/s10212-010-0025-6.

Patall, E. A., Cooper, H., & Robinson, J. C. (2008). The effects of choice on intrinsic motivation and related outcomes: A meta-analysis of research findings. *Psychological Bulletin, 134,* 270–300. https://doi.org/10.1037/0033-2909.134.2.270.

Patall, E. A., Cooper, H., & Wynn, S. R. (2010). The effectiveness and relative importance of choice in the classroom. *Journal of Educational Psychology, 102,* 896–915. https://doi.org/10.1037/a0019545.

Patrick, B. C., Hisley, J., & Kempler, T. (2000). What's everybody so excited about?: The effects of teacher enthusiasm on student intrinsic motivation and vitality. *Journal of Experimental Education, 68,* 217–236. https://doi.org/10.1080/00220970009600093.

Patrick, H., Ryan, A. M., & Kaplan, A. (2007). Early adolescents' perceptions of the classroom social environment, motivational beliefs, and engagement. *Journal of Educational Psychology, 99,* 83–98. https://doi.org/10.1037/0022-0663.99.1.83.

Piper, W. (2011). *The little engine that could.* New York: Penguin Putnam.

Poskiparta, E., Niemi, P., Lepola, J., Ahtola, A., & Laine, P. (2003). Motivational-emotional vulnerability and difficulties in learning to read and spell. *British Journal of Educational Psychology, 73,* 187–206. https://doi.org/10.1348/00070990360626930.

Reeve, J. (2009). Why teachers adopt a controlling motivating style towards students and how they can become more autonomy supportive. *Educational Psychologist, 44,* 159–175. https://doi.org/10.1080/00461520903028990.

Ruskin, E. M., Mundy, P., Kasari, C., & Sigman, M. (1994). Object mastery motivation of children with Down syndrome. *American Journal on Mental Retardation, 98,* 499–509.

Ruzek, E. A., Hafen, C. A., Allen, J. P., Gregory, A., Mikami, A. Y., & Pianta, R. C. (2016). How teacher emotional support motivates students: The mediating roles of perceived peer relatedness, autonomy support, and competence. *Learning and Instruction, 42,* 95–103. https://doi.org/10.1016/j.learninstruc.2016.01.004.

Ryan, R., & Deci, E. L. (2000). Self-determination theory and the facilitation of intrinsic motivation, social development, and well-being. *American Psychologist, 55,* 68–78. https://doi.org/10.1037/0003-066X.55.1.68.

Savard, A., Joussemet, M., Emond Pelletier, J., & Mageau, G. (2013). The benefits of autonomy support for adolescents with severe emotional and behavioural problems. *Motivation and Emotion, 37,* 688–700. https://doi.org/10.1007/s11031-013-9351-8.

Schunk, D. H., Meece, J. L., & Pintrich, P. R. (2014). *Motivation in education: Theory, research, and applications* (4th ed.). Upper Saddle River, NJ: Pearson Education.

Senko, C., Durik, A., & Harackiewicz, J. (2008). Historical perspectives and new directions in achievement goal theory. In J. Shah & W. Gardner (Eds.), *Handbook of motivation science* (pp. 100–113). New York: Guilford Press.
Shen, B., McCaughtry, N., Martin, J., Garn, A., Kulik, N., & Fahlman, M. (2015). The relationship between teacher burnout and student motivation. *British Journal of Educational Psychology, 85,* 519–532. https://doi.org/10.1111/bjep.12089.
Shernoff, D. J., & Csikszentmihalyi, M. (2009). Flow in schools: Cultivating engaged learners and optimal learning environments. In R. C. Gilman, E. S. Heubner, & M. J. Furlong (Eds.), *Handbook of positive psychology in schools* (pp. 131–145). New York: Routledge.
Sideridis, G. D. (2003). On the origins of helpless behaviour of students with learning disabilities: Avoidance motivation? *International Journal of Educational Research, 39,* 497–517.
Sideridis, G. D. (2006). Achievement goal orientations, "oughts", and self-regulation in students with and without learning disabilities. *Learning Disability Quarterly, 29,* 3–18. https://doi.org/10.2307/30035528.
Sinnott, K., & Biddle, S. (1998). Changes in attributions, perceptions of success and intrinsic motivation after attribution retraining in children's sport. *International Journal of Adolescence and Youth, 7,* 137–144. https://doi.org/10.1080/02673843.1998.9747818.
Skinner, B. F. (1953). *Science and human behaviour*. New York: Free Press.
Skinner, E. A., Furrer, C., Marchand, G., & Kindermann, T. (2008). Engagement and disaffection in the classroom: Part of a larger motivational dynamic? *Journal of Educational Psychology, 100,* 765–781. https://doi.org/10.1037/a0012840.
Spires, A. (2017). *The most magnificent thing*. Toronto, Canada: Kids Can Press.
Stipek, D. J. (1997). Success in school—for a head start in life. In S. S. Luthar, J. A. Burack, D. Cicchetti, & J. R. Weisz (Eds.), *Developmental psychopathology: Perspectives on adjustment, risk, and disorder* (pp. 75–92). Cambridge: Cambridge University Press.
Switzky, H. N. (1997). The educational meaning of mental retardation: Toward a more helpful construct. Mental retardation and the neglected construct of motivation. In *Paper presented at the Annual Convention of the Council for Exceptional Children*, Salt Lake City, UT.
Täht, K., Must, O., Peets, K., & Kattel, R. (2014). Learning motivation from a cross-cultural perspective: A moving target? *Educational Research and Evaluation, 20,* 255–274. https://doi.org/10.1080/13803611.2014.929009.
Taylor, I. M., & Ntoumanis, N. (2007). Teacher motivational strategies and student self-determination in physical education. *Journal of Educational Psychology, 99,* 747–760. https://doi.org/10.1037/0022-0663.99.4.747.
Toland, J., & Boyle, C. (2008). Applying cognitive behavioural methods to retrain children's attributions for success and failure in learning. *School Psychology International, 29,* 286–302. https://doi.org/10.1177/0143034308093674.
Turner, J. C. (1995). The influence of classroom contexts on young children's motivation for literacy. *Reading Research Quarterly, 30,* 410–441. https://doi.org/10.2307/747624.
Turner, L. A., & Johnson, B. (2003). A model of mastery motivation for at-risk pre-schoolers. *Journal of Educational Psychology, 95,* 495–505. https://doi.org/10.1037/0022-0663.95.3.495.
van der Kaap-Deeder, J., Vansteenkiste, M., Soenens, B., & Mabbe, E. (2017). Children's daily well-being: The role of mothers', teachers', and siblings' autonomy support and psychological control. *Developmental Psychology, 53,* 237–251. https://doi.org/10.1037/dev0000218.
Vasquez, A. C., Patall, E. A., Fong, C. J., Corrigan, A. S., & Pine, L. (2016). Parent autonomy support, academic achievement, and psychosocial functioning: A meta-analysis of research. *Educational Psychology Review, 28,* 605–644. https://doi.org/10.1007/s10648-015-9329-z.
Vygotsky, L. S. (1986). *Thoughts and language*. Cambridge, MA: MIT Press.
Waheeda, T., & Grainger, J. (2002). Self-concept, attributional style and self-efficacy beliefs of students with learning disabilities with and without attention deficit hyperactivity disorder. *Learning Disability Quarterly, 25,* 141–151. https://doi.org/10.2307/1511280.
Wang, P.-J., Hwang, A.-W., Liao, H.-F., Chen, P.-C., & Hsieh, W.-S. (2011). The stability of mastery motivation and its relationship with home environment in infants and toddlers. *Infant Behavior and Development, 34,* 434–442. https://doi.org/10.1016/j.infbeh.2011.04.005.

Warneken, F., & Tomasello, M. (2007). Helping and cooperation at 14 months of age. *Infancy, 11,* 271–294. https://doi.org/10.1111/j.1532-7078.2007.tb00227.x.
Warschausky, S., Kaufman, J. N., Evitts, M., Schutt, W., & Hurvitz, E. A. (2017). Mastery motivation and executive functions as predictors of adaptive behaviour in adolescents and young adults with cerebral palsy or myelomeningocele. *Rehabilitation Psychology, 62,* 258–267. https://doi.org/10.1037/rep0000151.
Weiner, B. (1985). An attributional theory of achievement motivation and emotion. *Psychological Review, 92,* 548–573.
White, R. W. (1959). Motivation reconsidered: The concept of competence. *Psychological Review, 66,* 297–333.
Wigfield, A., & Eccles, J. S. (2000). Expectancy-value theory of achievement motivation. *Contemporary Educational Psychology, 25,* 68–81. https://doi.org/10.1006/ceps.1999.1015.
Wong, B. Y. (1980). Motivation for learning in mildly handicapped adolescents and young adults: A review of related theories. *Exceptional Education Quarterly, 1,* 37–45.
Woodcock, S., & Vialle, W. (2011). Are we exacerbating students' learning disabilities? An investigation of preservice teachers' attributions of the educational outcomes of students with learning disabilities. *Annals of Dyslexia, 61,* 223–241. https://doi.org/10.1007/s11881-011-0058-9.
Woodcock, S., & Vialle, W. (2016). An examination of pre-service teachers' attributions for students with specific learning difficulties. *Learning and Individual Differences, 45,* 252–259. https://doi.org/10.1016/j.lindif.2015.12.021.
Zentall, S. R., & Morris, B. J. (2010). Good job, you're so smart: The effects of inconsistency of praise type on young children's motivation. *Journal of Experimental Child Psychology, 107,* 155–163. https://doi.org/10.1016/j.jecp.2010.04.015.
Zhou, M., Ma, W. J., & Deci, E. L. (2009). The importance of autonomy for rural Chinese children's motivation for learning. *Learning and Individual Differences, 19,* 492–498. https://doi.org/10.1016/j.lindif.2009.05.003.
Zigler, E., Bennett-Gates, D., Hodapp, R., & Henrich, C. C. (2002). Assessing personality traits of individuals with mental retardation. *American Journal on Mental Retardation, 107,* 181–193.

Chapter 5
Culturally Responsive Positive Behavioural Interventions and Supports

Amity Noltemeyer, Erin A. Harper and Anthony G. James

Abstract Positive Behavioural Interventions and Supports (PBIS) is a prevention-oriented, data-driven, multi-tiered framework for providing a continuum of behavioural supports to enhance student and school outcomes. PBIS involves the application of increasingly intense tiers of support, based on student need. At Tier 1, a school identifies 3–5 positively worded behavioural expectations that are taught, modelled, practiced, reinforced, and prompted consistently school-wide with all students. At Tier 2, students at risk, or experiencing minimal behavioural concerns, are provided with low-intensity interventions (for example, small group support, mentoring) and their progress is monitored. Finally, at Tier 3, students who are exhibiting significant behavioural concerns, and those who have not sufficiently responded to Tier 1 and Tier 2 services, are provided with intensive supports, often including a functional behaviour assessment and individualized behaviour intervention plan. Research has shown PBIS to improve pro-social behaviour, school climate, and academic achievement, while also reducing discipline referrals, problem behaviour, and school exclusion. However, the effectiveness of PBIS across cultural settings depends on the degree to which PBIS is planned for and implemented in a culturally responsive manner. Although culturally responsive practices have certainly been included within the PBIS discourse, we argue that increased attention to this critical feature of PBIS is warranted. For example, it is important for schools to ensure that the Tier 1 PBIS expectations are developed with the local cultural context in mind, and are taught and reinforced in a culturally congruent way. Furthermore, schools should disaggregate their PBIS student data by student subgroups (such as, racial/ethnic, gender, economic), and analyze and address the causes of any disparities in outcomes. The chapter aims to: (a) describe the key features of PBIS, provide a rationale for its use in schools, and review

A. Noltemeyer (✉) · E. A. Harper
Department of Educational Psychology, Miami University, Oxford, OH, USA
e-mail: anoltemeyer@miamioh.edu

A. G. James
Department of Family Science and Social Work, Miami University, Oxford, OH, USA

S. Deb (ed.), *Positive Schooling and Child Development*,
https://doi.org/10.1007/978-981-13-0077-6_5

research on its effectiveness, (b) highlight the importance of, and key considerations for, ensuring that PBIS is culturally-responsive, and (c) provide recommendations for implementing and evaluating a comprehensive and culturally-responsive PBIS framework.

Keywords Students · School · Positive behavioural interventions
Supports

Introduction

Promoting positive student behaviour and school climate is a goal shared by many educators worldwide. One framework that can be harnessed in pursuit of this goal is Positive Behavioural Interventions and Supports (PBIS). PBIS is a prevention-oriented, data-driven, multi-tiered framework for providing a continuum of behavioural supports to enhance student and school outcomes. Research has shown PBIS to improve prosocial behaviour, school climate, and academic achievement, while also reducing discipline referrals, problem behaviour, and school exclusion. However, we argue that the effectiveness of PBIS across cultural settings depends on the degree to which PBIS is planned for and implemented in a culturally responsive manner. With this context in mind, this chapter: (a) describes the key features of PBIS, provides a rationale for its use in schools, and reviews research on its effectiveness, (b) highlights the importance of, and key considerations for, ensuring that PBIS is culturally-responsive, and (c) provides recommendations for implementing and evaluating a comprehensive and culturally-responsive PBIS framework.

School-Wide PBIS: Description and Key Features

As mentioned, PBIS is a school-wide initiative that involves the application of increasingly intense tiers of behavioural support, based on students' needs (see Fig. 5.1). At Tier 1, a school identifies 3–5 positively worded behavioural expectations that are taught, modelled, practiced, reinforced, and prompted consistently school wide with all students. At Tier 2, students at-risk or experiencing behavioural concerns are provided with supplemental interventions (e.g., psycho-educational group, mentoring) and their progress is monitored. Finally, at Tier 3, students who are exhibiting significant behavioural concerns, and those who have not sufficiently responded to Tier 1 and Tier 2 services, are provided with intensive supports, often including a functional behaviour assessment and individualized behaviour intervention plan.

Although these three tiers coalesce to form a cohesive and integrated continuum of supports in a school, this chapter will focus primarily on the foundational Tier 1.

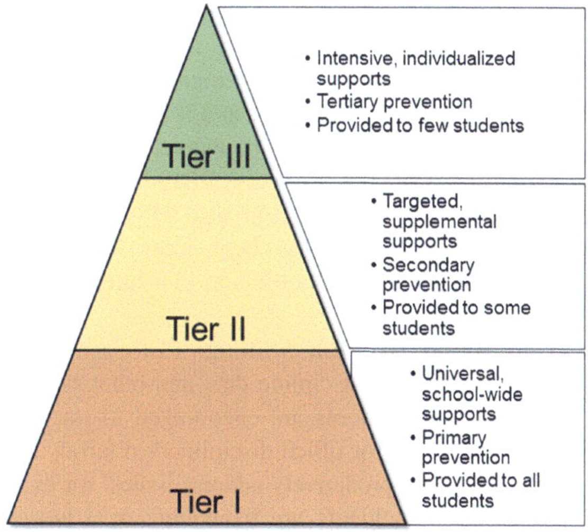

Fig. 5.1 Graphic representation of the Tiers of support in a PBIS framework

Applied at the school-level with all students, PBIS is undergirded by the premise that—much like academic content—behavioural expectations should be taught proactively and explicitly to all students. Additional critical components of PBIS include:

- **Building Leadership Team**: Although PBIS practices are implemented by all staff in a school, the planning and evaluation efforts should be guided by a building leadership team comprised of representative staff members. Because it is a systems change initiative rather than a specific curriculum, buy-in and input from stakeholders—staff, students, families—is important to the success of PBIS, and the inclusion of a parent or community representative on the leadership team is encouraged.
- **Behavioural Expectations**: A school identifies 3–5 positively worded, clearly stated, concise behavioural expectations that define what behaviours are expected in the school community. As one example, a school may select the three expectations: 'Be Safe, Be Responsible, and Be Respectful.'
- **Behaviour Matrix**: After agreeing upon the school's behavioural expectations, a behavioural matrix is developed. This matrix is a grid that operationally defines what the behavioural expectations look like in all school settings, such as bus, cafeteria, playground, classroom, and hallway. As one example, in the hallway 'Be Safe' might mean walking on one side of the hallway, keeping hands and feet to self, keeping your eyes forward, and listening to instructions from the teacher.
- **Teaching Behavioural Expectations and Routines**: Students are then taught what the expected behaviours look like and given opportunities to practice. Posters reminding students of the expectations may be displayed around the school as reminders. Refresher teaching sessions can be useful later in the school year.

- **Reinforcing Desired Behaviour**: All staff are involved in recognizing appropriate student behaviour that is consistent with school wide expectations. Although the type of reinforcement may vary by school, it often involves verbal praise or acknowledgement, and it may be paired with a tangible reinforcer (for example, a ticket that can be entered into a school raffle).
- **Discipline Policies**: Although PBIS is focused on fostering positive behaviour proactively, schools should also clearly and consistently define a range of consequences for problem behaviours, in a clearly articulated discipline policy. These consequences should aim to result in student learning and/or behavioural change.
- **Data-Based Decision Making**: PBIS schools should establish a systematic method of using discipline data and other behavioural data to make decisions. For example, schools are encouraged to track the time, location, reason, and type of offense for office disciplinary referrals and other disciplinary actions so they can more proactively address issues: for example, if data reveals that many behavioural incidents are happening in a loosely supervised area, additional supervision can be provided in that area. Schools are also encouraged to monitor the fidelity with which they implement PBIS practices, to inform further improvements in implementation.
- **Culturally Responsive Practice**: Although not mentioned in all PBIS research and guidance, we believe an essential core component of PBIS is ensuring that the features described above are all planned for and implemented with careful consideration of the cultural context of students, staff, and the school. We will explore this issue further later in the chapter.

Given the flexibility of the PBIS framework to adapt to locally established behavioural expectations and reinforcement procedures, PBIS is suitable for implementation across diverse geographic contexts. Over 23,000 schools in the U.S. are implementing PBIS (PBIS OSEP Technical Assistance Center 2017). Implementation has also been documented and discussed in several areas around the world including Canada (Kelm et al. 2014), Australia (De Jong 2005), the United Kingdom (Gore et al. 2013), and other European countries that are part of the European School Network (for example, in the Netherlands). Although there is evidence of PBIS-related trainings and discussions throughout other geographic locales, more research is needed to document implementation efforts in these areas.

Research on Effectiveness

Research suggests PBIS is associated with improvements in student prosocial behaviour (Bradshaw et al. 2012), perceptions of safety (Kelm et al. 2014), attendance (Freeman et al. 2015), and academic achievement (Horner et al. 2009). Furthermore, reductions in discipline referrals (Bradshaw et al. 2010), problem behaviours (Lassen et al. 2006), bullying (Kelm et al. 2014), and school suspensions

(Bradshaw et al. 2010) have also been associated with PBIS implementation. The impact of PBIS is not only on students, however. For example, increases in teacher self-efficacy (Kelm and McIntosh 2012), staff affiliation (Bradshaw et al. 2008), and staff perceptions of school safety (Horner et al. 2009), as well as decreases in administrator time spent on disciplinary issues (Scott and Barrett 2004), have also been related to PBIS implementation. Finally, some research on PBIS suggests it may reduce racial/ethnic disparities in school discipline, at least in the U.S. (Vincent et al. 2011a, b).

A recent synthesis of research on the effectiveness of school-wide PBIS—PBIS at Tier 1—revealed that, across 45 studies, most found either unanimously or predominantly positive outcomes of PBIS on office disciplinary referrals and student suspension (Noltemeyer et al. 2018). Despite the promise of PBIS on these behavioural outcomes, the findings related to academic outcomes were less consistent and warrant further investigation (Noltemeyer et al. 2018).

Culturally Responsive PBIS

Need for, and Description of, Culturally Responsive Practices in Schools

The effectiveness of programs implemented in schools is predicated on their ability to align with what is culturally relevant to the population of students being served. The importance of culturally relevant practices in schools has been theorized about and empirically tested for more than two decades (Brown-Jeffy and Cooper 2011; Dee and Penner 2017; Ladson-Billings 1995). A key impetus of such research is rooted in the search for clarity in contradictory results of ethnic minority youths' academic struggles juxtaposed against their social and cultural thriving. A primary assumption explaining that contradiction lies in the inter- and intra- group cultural differences that exist between teachers and their students, particularly beliefs about learning and how to teach. In the U.S., for example, those differences were, and continue to be, exacerbated by the fact that the vast majority of compulsory educators are white and female (U.S. Department of Education, Office of Planning, Evaluation and Policy Development, Policy and Program Studies Service 2016), with most students being identified as an ethnic/racial minority (Maxwell 2014). To be sure, we also see examples of the need for culturally relevant programming for youth in other parts of the world (Ajuwon 2008; Brake 2013; Woods 2009).

However, before considering the importance of curricular and pedagogical cultural relevancy in how and whether students learn, there are some foundational issues to consider in terms of what regulates basic human action. It has long been considered, at least in the Western world, that the regulation of human action is predicated on intrapersonal factors such as self-control (Mischel 2014). Specifically, one's self-control is what regulates how the person responds to their impulse to act. However, cutting edge research argues (and empirically supports) that human action is predicated not on internal factors alone, but rather, is the result of contextual factors (for example, the social milieu; see Lamm et al. 2017). Further, even some researchers that do emphasize internal factors (such as will-power) as the motivating force behind human action, also acknowledge the importance of context (for example, social support; see McGonigal 2011). Our goal in this chapter is not to settle this debate; rather, we simply want to highlight the importance of culture in human action.

Having said that, we argue that the effective implementation of a behavioural framework in school (e.g., PBIS) must also consider how relevant it is to the culture of students it serves. This is even more important knowing that PBIS does not focus solely on discipline, but also focuses on how to promote positive behaviour among students. Therefore, what constitutes positive behaviour and what is motivating (or reinforcing) for students will need to be relevant to their cultural values and how they think about and act in the social world.

Cultural Responsiveness and PBIS

Researchers have made recommendations and proposed frameworks for integrating culturally responsive educational practices and PBIS (Bal 2015; Bal et al. 2012, 2014; Banks and Obiakor 2015; Vincent et al. 2011a, b). It is important to note that some researchers and trainers deliberately avoid using the term *culturally responsive PBIS* (CRPBIS), arguing that to do so implies that CRPBIS is distinct from PBIS (Leverson et al. 2016). In this chapter, we use the term CRPBIS, while acknowledging that cultural responsiveness should be a core component of PBIS, and CRPBIS is not distinct from PBIS. This section reviews research and key themes related to CRPBIS.

CRPBIS emphasizes collaborative, culturally and contextually relevant data-based decision-making and practices to promote equitable systems and student outcomes. Collaboration in the CRPBIS context begins with the construction of PBIS teams that intentionally and actively involve a range of stakeholders, specifically members of historically marginalized groups that traditionally have little to no representation on school-based problem-solving teams (for example, low-income parents and students). CRPBIS teams determine culturally relevant positive behavioural standards and measures. These standards and measures then become the foundation of culturally relevant data-based decision-making.

Leverson et al. (2016) outlined five core components of CRPBIS: (1) identity (being aware of how identity influences classroom interactions); (2) voice (providing meaningful opportunities for parent and community engagement in PBIS); (3) a supportive environment (staff understand the school mission and work as a team to help each other accomplish it); (4) situational appropriateness (modifying one's behaviour when settings or contexts change); and (5) data for equity (trends in data regarding issues of equity or culture must be discussed).

Until recently, the CRPBIS literature has provided minimal guidance for "how to systematically incorporate cultural and contextual considerations and facilitate meaningful participation of families and community members" (Bal et al. 2014, 328). However, frameworks, technical guides, and empirical studies that intentionally address cultural responsiveness during the implementation of PBIS are emerging. The CRPBIS Project (see Bal et al. 2012) and the PBIS Cultural Responsiveness Field Guide (Leverson et al. 2016) are examples of projects and resources that have aimed to fill this gap.

Recommendations for Implementation

PBIS has been shown to positively impact student and staff outcomes. However, in order to maximize the potential of PBIS, it is essential to plan for and implement it in a culturally responsive manner. Although culturally responsive practices have certainly been included within the PBIS discourse, we argue that increased attention to this critical feature of PBIS is warranted. Cultural responsiveness should not be seen as an add-on or afterthought, but as something embedded within the planning and implementation process as a core component of PBIS. Key recommendations for schools seeking to implement CRPBIS in this way include:

- The PBIS leadership team that guides PBIS implementation and planning should be comprised of members from diverse backgrounds and roles. It is important for many voices to be heard.
- Behavioural expectations should be developed with strong community input (Greflund et al. 2014). The local context should always be kept in mind when identifying the expectations and determining how to teach and reinforce them.
- If any behavioural expectations differ between school and community contexts, staff should seek to navigate this in a respectful way. For example, staff can explicitly teach the differences in behavioural expectations, discuss the purpose of having that expectation in the school setting, and provide additional practice with that expectation (Leverson et al. 2016).
- Schools should strive for community engagement and participation in PBIS activities. As one example, McIntosh et al. (2014) describe how elders, chiefs, and other community members in an indigenous community were invited to participate in all PBIS assemblies and have representation on the school PBIS team.
- Schools should disaggregate their PBIS student data by student subgroups (for example, racial/ethnic, gender-based, income-based), and analyze and address the causes of any disparities in outcomes.
- Schools should engage in efforts to involve families in the PBIS process. This can be accomplished in many ways, such as including a family representative on the leadership team, including family perspectives when identifying behavioural

expectations for the school, and sharing information with families on how they can teach and reinforce the expected behaviours within the home setting.

- When teams assess their implementation of PBIS fidelity, and engage in action planning to improve implementation, cultural issues should be considered within this process. The Tiered Fidelity Inventory (TFI; Algozzine et al. 2014) is a frequently used fidelity assessment, and although it does not extensively assess cultural responsiveness, a TFI Cultural Responsiveness Companion tool (in Leverson et al. 2016) has been developed to supplement the tool and inform action planning.
- Staff should be encouraged to understand their own self-identity, the identities of the students and families they serve, and the community identity in their context (Leverson et al. 2016). It is also important for staff to understand implicit bias, and be aware of their own implicit biases.
- Professional development and coaching provided to staff should have cultural issues embedded within it as a core component, rather than added on as an afterthought.

Beyond incorporating these features into the PBIS framework, it is important for leadership teams to engage in a continuous process of data-based decision making and self-reflection to ensure that the practices are in fact producing the desired outcomes within all subgroups in the local population.

Acknowledgements We would like to acknowledge Catlyn Waltemire, graduate assistant at Miami University, for her assistance editing this chapter.

References

Ajuwon, P. M. (2008). Inclusive education for students with disabilities in Nigeria: Benefits, challenges and policy implications. *International Journal of Special Education, 23*(3), 11–16.

Algozzine, B., Barrett, S., Eber, L., George, H., Horner, R., Lewis, T., & Sugai, G. (2014). *School-wide PBIS tiered fidelity inventory*. OSEP Technical Assistance Center on Positive Behavioural Interventions and Supports.

Bal, A. (2015). *Culturally responsive positive behavioural interventions and supports*. Retrieved from http://www.wcer.wisc.edu/publications/workingPapers/papers.php.

Bal, A., Thorius, K. K., & Kozleski, E. (2012). *Culturally responsive positive behavioural support matters*. Tempe, AZ: The Equity Alliance.

Bal, A., Kozleski, E., Schrader, E., Rodriguez, E., & Pelton, S. (2014). Systemic transformation from the ground-up: Using learning lab to design culturally responsive schoolwide positive behavioural supports. *Remedial and Special Education, 35*(6), 327–339.

Banks, T., & Obiakor, F. E. (2015). Culturally responsive positive behaviour supports: Considerations for practice. *Journal of Education and Training Studies, 3*(2), 83–90.

Bradshaw, C. P., Koth, C. W., Bevans, K. B., Ialongo, N., & Leaf, P. J. (2008). The impact of school-wide positive behavioural interventions and supports (PBIS) on the organizational health of elementary schools. *School Psychology Quarterly, 23*(4), 462–473. https://doi.org/10.1037/a0012883.

Bradshaw, C. P., Mitchell, M. M., & Leaf, P. J. (2010). Examining the effects of schoolwide positive behavioural interventions and supports on student outcomes results from a randomized controlled effectiveness trial in elementary schools. *Journal of Positive Behaviour Interventions, 12*(3), 133–148. https://doi.org/10.1177/1098300709334798.

Bradshaw, C. P., Waasdorp, T. E., & Leaf, P. J. (2012). Effects of school-wide positive behavioural interventions and supports on child behaviour problems. *Pediatrics, 130*(5), 1136–1145. https://doi.org/10.1542/peds.2012-0243.

Brake, M. (2013). *Comparative youth culture: The sociology of youth cultures and youth subcultures in America*. Britain, Canada: Routledge.

Brown-Jeffy, S., & Cooper, J. E. (2011). Toward a conceptual framework of culturally relevant pedagogy: An overview of the conceptual and theoretical literature. *Teacher Education Quarterly, 38*(1), 65–84.

Dee, T. S., & Penner, E. K. (2017). The causal effects of cultural relevance: Evidence from an ethnic studies curriculum. *American Educational Research Journal, 54*(1), 127–166.

De Jong, T. (2005). A framework of principles and best practice for managing student behaviour in the Australian education context. *School Psychology International, 26*(3), 353–370.

Freeman, J., Simonsen, B., McCoach, D. B., Sugai, G., Lombardi, A., & Horner, R. (2015). An analysis of the relationship between implementation of school-wide positive behavior interventions and supports and high school dropout rates. *The High School Journal, 98*(4), 290–315. https://doi.org/10.1353/hsi.2015.0009

Gore, N. J., McGill, P., Toogood, S., Allen, D., Hughes, J. C., Baker, P., et al. (2013). Definition and scope for positive behavioural support. *International Journal of Positive Behavioural Support, 3*(2), 14–23.

Greflund, S., McIntosh, K., Mercer, S., & May, S. (2014). Examining disproportionality in school discipline for aboriginal students in schools implementing PBIS. *Canadian Journal of School Psychology, 29*(3), 213–235. https://doi.org/10.1177/0829573514542214.

Horner, R. H., Sugai, G., Smolkowski, K., Eber, L., Nakasato, J., Todd, A. W., & Esperanza, J. (2009). A randomized, wait-list controlled effectiveness trial assessing school-wide positive behaviour support in elementary schools. *Journal of Positive Behaviour Interventions*, 1–12. https://doi.org/10.1177/1098300709332067.

Kelm, J. L., & McIntosh, K. (2012). Effects of school-wide positive behaviour support on teacher self-efficacy. *Psychology in the Schools, 49*(2), 137–147. https://doi.org/10.1002/pits.20624.

Kelm, J. L., McIntosh, K., & Cooley, S. (2014). Effects of implementing school-wide positive behavioural interventions and supports on problem behaviour and academic achievement in a Canadian elementary school. *Canadian Journal of School Psychology, 29*(3), 195–212.

Ladson-Billings, G. (1995). Toward a theory of culturally relevant pedagogy. *American Educational Research Journal, 32*(3), 465–491.

Lamm, B., Keller, H., Teiser, J., Gudi, H., Yovsi, R. D., Freitag, C., et al. (2017). Waiting for the second treat: Developing culture-specific modes of self-regulation. *Child Development*. https://doi.org/10.1111/cdev.12847.

Lassen, S. R., Steele, M. M., & Sailor, W. (2006). The relationship of school-wide positive behavior support to academic achievement in an urban middle school. *Psychology in the Schools, 43*(6), 701–712.https://doi.org/10.1002/pits.20177

Leverson, M., Smith, K., McIntosh, K., Rose, J., & Pinkelman, S. (2016). *PBIS cultural responsiveness field guide: Resources for trainers and coaches*. OSEP Technical Assistance Center on Positive Behavioural Interventions and Supports. Retrieved from www.pbis.org.

McIntosh, K., Moniz, C. A., Craft, C. B., Golby, R., & Steinwand-Deschambeault, T. (2014). Implementing schoolwide positive behavioural interventions and supports to better meet the needs of Indigenous students. *Canadian Journal of School Psychology, 29*, 236–257.

Maxwell, L. A. (2014). *U.S. school enrollment hits majority-minority milestone*. Educational Week. Retrieved from http://www.edweek.org/ew/articles/2014/08/20/01demographics.h34.html.

McGonigal, K. (2011). *The willpower instinct: How self-control works, why it matters, and what you can do to get more of it*. New York: Penguin.

Mischel, W. (2014). *The marshmallow test: Understanding self-control and how to master it*. New York: Random House.

Noltemeyer, A., Palmer, K., James, A.G., & Wiechman, S. (2018). School-wide PBIS: A synthesis of existing research. *International Journal of School & Educational Psychology*. https://doi.org/10.1080/21683603.2018.1425169

Positive Behavioural Interventions, & Supports OSEP Technical Assistance Center. (2017). Retrieved fromhttps://www.pbis.org.

Scott, T. M., & Barrett, S. B. (2004). Using staff and student time engaged in disciplinary procedures to evaluate the impact of school-wide SWPBS. *Journal of Positive Behaviour Interventions, 6*(1), 21–27.

U.S. Department of Education, Office of Planning, Evaluation and Policy Development, Policy and Program Studies Service. (2016). *The state of racial diversity in the educator workforce*. Washington, D.C. Retrieved from https://www2.ed.gov/rschstat/eval/highered/racial-diversity/state-racial-diversity-workfoce.pdf.

Vincent, C., Swain-Bradley, J., Tobin, T. J., & May, S. (2011a). Disciplinary referrals for culturally and linguistically diverse students with and without disabilities: Patterns resulting from school-wide positive behaviour support. *Exceptionality: A Special Education Journal, 19*, 175–190.

Vincent, C., Tobin, T., Swain-Bradway, J., Randall, C., & Cartledge, G. (2011b). Toward a conceptual integration of cultural responsiveness and schoolwide positive behaviour support. *Journal of Positive Behaviour Interventions, 13*(4), 219–229. https://doi.org/10.1177/1098300711399765.

Woods, A. (2009). Learning to be literate: Issues of pedagogy for recently arrived refugee youth in Australia. *Critical Inquiry in Language Studies, 6*(1–2), 81–101.

Chapter 6
Toxic Teachers: A Bar on Positive Child Growth

Nilanjana Sanyal

Abstract Teachers are known to be the sculptors of children's personality by serving as effective 'role models.' This occurs by means of internalization of the values and teaching of teachers by students. This makes the personality of teachers serve as a radar for aligning children's growth and development along healthy lines. However, if teachers have 'toxic components' in their personality frames, owing to non-resolution of their own intra-personal conflicts, then the consequences on the fragile petals of children's mind frames are devastating, damaging the young 'seedlings' thoroughly. The fumes of toxicity of such teachers are likely to cause dents in the personality frames of children which might require therapeutic interventions to mend. The author attempts to identify the toxic components of unhealthy teachers in the educational set-up who deter children's development in the long run, with the help of supportive case studies so that rectifications may be put forward from the desk of the mental health practitioner. This would help children inhale fresh life-enriching air once again and instil positive growth.

Keywords Toxic teachers' personality · Role models · Growth Development · Children

Introduction

The blossoming bouquet of a child's development requires support, care, concern, exposure, and proper handling procedures, initially from informal family conditions and later, formally from school during the foundational years of life. Hence, the basic ambience of family and the quality experience in the classroom seem to be the two basic pillars of a future stable, well-adjusted personality of the child. In the educational context, the inter-connectedness of the teacher-personality and the learning ambience of the school classroom and hence the mode of grooming of the

---

N. Sanyal (✉)
Department of Psychology, University of Calcutta, 92 A.P.C. Road, Kolkata 700009, India
e-mail: sanyal_nilanjana2004@rediffmail.com

S. Deb (ed.), *Positive Schooling and Child Development*,
https://doi.org/10.1007/978-981-13-0077-6_6

children's personality is well-established. Good teaching requires a repertoire of appropriate interpersonal skills along with pedagogical ones (Fisher and Kent 1998). Educators seem to have an emerging recognition that the personality of a teacher and his attitude and an understanding of the layered child's mind are of paramount importance in ensuring proper social and emotional growth of students and in initiating adjustment in case of personality issues. Therefore, the desired personality of the teacher is a focal point of concern in the educational context and the direct influence of these adult personalities on the impressionable minds of children seems worthy of careful consideration.

Mental health practitioners believe that the personality of the teacher is an important determining factor of children's behavioural. Contextually, Ryan (1938) opines: "…In general, psychiatrists and mental hygienists agree that teachers play an important part in determining children's behaviour. Many of them put the school with its childhood associations next to the home as a significant factor in the development of personality, and consider the teacher second only to parent in influencing for good or evil the mental health of the child" (1938, 315). It is generally believed that there is no single teacher personality pattern that can be claimed as superior to all others, but rather there are several that are deemed desirable. Whatever the personality pattern might be, it is usually judged s desirable or undesirable in terms of the degree of effectiveness displayed by a teacher while working with children. Regarding the concept of an 'effective teacher,' it is agreed that such a teacher does not possess any one quality or trait that constitutes teaching effectiveness; but rather that he/she is expected to possess several desirable qualities to establish a harmonious teacher–student bond in the classroom, which is the outcome of the personality adjustment and orientation which the teacher has established in relation to him/herself and others (Del Popolo 1965). Hence, the teacher's personality, his/her perspective in life, adjustment pattern, and attitude towards children, are of supreme importance in the development of a healthy life platform and interactive personality mode in children. A teacher with negative personality qualities is predicted to incite misbehaviour on the children's part; integrative teacher-orientation is expected to usher in a cooperative, healthy behavioural mode in the child. The query is: when teachers with toxic personality are playing the part of negative role models, can we expect to have healthy child growth or are dents inadvertently caused in the pliable fresh minds of children, which will need therapeutic care to be altered? Isn't it an important issue to explore the consequences of toxic teachers and provide steps to assess them beforehand so that the initial years of life, when the child's personality is blossoming, can be full of fresh, life-enriching inspiration? Even if a toxic teacher exists in the child's environment, there must be ways and means of handling it. For children to emerge from this situation, courage is needed, with the help of teachers who are confidants, to overcome the powerful and destructive influence of toxicity in a teacher.

Teacher: A Radar or a Destroyer in the Railment of Child-Growth?

In a civilized society, exposure to formal education is expected to develop a repertoire of knowledge. This knowledge should not just be based on collecting information on selected areas of studies, but their absorption in the self-system, to know about life on earth, the world around us, and the inmates of the world as interactive agents. Understanding life as such, being realistic in orientation, and having a philosophy of one's own, ultimately seems to be the finished version of being educated. Hence, formal education is the first step to in grooming one's personality and here the teacher appears as the radar to follow. The teacher spreads the fabric of education before the students by presenting the contents of the subject as well as representing herself in the role model in a parental authoritarian frame to be followed in the context. The extent of subject-knowledge, the balance, and communication style, and personality of the teacher, thus, are important ingredients for the child's life to move in the right direction. The current educational scenario is studied to verify the impact of just the opposite of ideal conditions—specifically, teachers being immature and emotionally unstable, and inconsistent—on the developing mind of the school-goers. A teacher's toxic unstable personality must be unquestionably confronted to prevent pathological effects on students' behaviour.

It might be constructive to contextually examine a few sample student personalities, from the author's own practice as a psychodynamic psychotherapist.

Case I

A seven-year-old girl had been brought to the clinic with noticeable obsessive-compulsive features in her behaviour which could not be related to parental over-strictness or reprimands. Despite being a child in a nuclear family, and the parents being apparently free of any neurotic behaviours, she developed too much indecisiveness at any work and seemed to have a perfectionist streak. She seemed to lack self-confidence in anything she did and had a persistent approval-seeking attitude. A few months' therapeutic processing suddenly helped her to come out with an incident: of incontinence in urination in the class, followed by a severe rebuke by the teacher to leave the class and if possible, leave the school; a memory which made her shiver in the session. The incident had taken place at nursery level. She recalled the teacher as a 'terror' in her life.

Case 2

A pre-adolescent boy studying in a very renowned English-medium school in Calcutta was brought to the clinic with problems of inattention in studies, general depressive mood, not having interest in friends, and severe apathy towards school itself. He was the single child in an extended family set-up. His major interest area seemed to be eating. Being loved by everybody at home and receiving pampering on a regular basis, his over-eating tendency had resulted in his gaining weight; he was an over-weight boy. He was accustomed to friendly teasing and was not really interested in cutting down on his quota especially of junk food; but otherwise, he seemed to be a happy, mentally healthy child, having interest in studies, games, and other age-related activities. The sudden alteration in behaviour attracted everybody's notice. Family members tried their best to help him, but in vain. In therapy, he took time to open up, since he had an idea of the threat that the therapist was supposed to routinize his day and habit patterns and, in case he failed, he expected punishment. The therapist's assurance-filled communications ultimately helped him to locate his real problem-point. He spoke of a lady teacher, his class teacher at the moment, who never called him by name, but substituted it by uttering, "Oh you Fatso!" Day-in and day-out, he started feeling ridiculed by her, especially in front of his friends, some of whom started calling him the same. He said he could not talk about this to his parents, and kept his thoughts aside, but gradually he fell into a 'no-interest' mode regarding school and studies. His falling grades concerned everybody, but should we remain silent about the 'culprit' and her impact on him, which ushered in disturbances in character-frame? It is high time to speak of such issues in educational set-ups.

Case 3

A twelve-year-old girl was found to be extra restless in her general behaviour. She was refusing food and was reporting that none of her dresses seemed to suit her. She told her mother she found all her friends to be beautiful, and that she was the only ugly one. This was sudden and her mother could not relate it to any incident. Gradually, she noticed that her daughter was either in an absent-minded state or else in an irritated mood. Ultimately, clinical intervention helped her to open her injured mind. After school, a few girls used to stay back at the institute to take special class with a mathematics teacher. On certain days, her driver was late in picking her up and this was the time when the teacher would abuse her physically, with the threat that she would to face dire consequences, if she told anybody about it. The resultant pathology was shaking her. Do we feel her pain? Can we save such girls from having their mental petals be crushed by monsters in teacher roles?

Case 4

A boy of Grade V in a morning-section school was brought to the clinic with intense apathy towards school-going. He was a shy, introverted boy who abided by school rules and was basically an obedient child. He used to take regular piano lessons at home and was an avid music lover. The quality of sound from any object fascinated him. One day, during a lesson, he was called by the teacher a number of times. But he was thoroughly absorbed in watching something outside the window. Being non-responsive, he received physical beatings from the teacher as he could not explain what he was watching. His behavioural problem started from this point. In course of therapy, after months together, one day he was spontaneous in his transference reaction and uttered, "Had you been my teacher in school, I would have liked and enjoyed my school sessions." On being queried about his teacher, he could suddenly relate his school apathy to the incident, and described his emotions as follows:

> It was a rainy day. The weather was very pleasant and the surrounding greenery was looking very fresh. Suddenly I got stuck in a big leaf of a plant on the ground that held a few drops of rain. The droplets were moving a little on the leaf and somehow I felt a musical sound in it. It was a superb, fascinating feeling. I was watching it from my classroom window, sitting at the side of my desk. Suddenly, my Sir thrashed me hard. I was shocked. I could not answer him. Because of my fault, I was punished. I hate going to school and listen to him anymore.

Do teachers need to display understanding regarding the sensitive layers of young minds in class? Or else, because of our toxicity, do we crush the deep spontaneous beauty of a child's mind attuned with nature and life realizations of a different quality? These queries raise a demand to probe into the teachers' personality being an initiator or an impediment in children's growth.

Bullying Teachers: The First Sign of Toxicity in Personality

When one thinks about being bullied as a teenager, would one include teachers as the perpetrators? We grow up thinking that teachers are kind, trustworthy, and fair. Most are. But that's why the reports of educators singling out and berating students are troubling. This isn't people being sensitive or over-reacting to one-off comments. Bullying teachers are present in classrooms across the world with effects that are devastating to students' self-esteem.

A bullying teacher is typically defined as using a position of authority to either manipulate or belittle a student beyond what's accepted as normal discipline, according to Dr. Stuart Twemlow, who has researched this topic. It's important to remember that teachers are human, so they may lose their cool on a stressful day. But repeatedly lashing out is different. Name-calling, singling someone out, over-reacting to the point that a student is afraid, or physically intimidating or hitting a student, all count as bullying or abusive behaviours.

Primum non nocere. That phrase means 'First, do no harm,' and is often thought to be part of the Hippocratic Oath. It makes sense in the medical field where doctors must make decisions on how to treat patients. They want to do well: to cure their patients when possible, and make them as comfortable as possible, when a cure is not possible. But they also want to avoid harming their patients, making them worse off.

That phrase also makes sense in education. Ideally, teachers want to do well for their students; teach them, challenge them, inspire them. But if they can't do that, at the very least, they should not harm their students. A few teachers end up harming their students, but do so unintentionally. For instance, some teachers don't understand gifted children and so they don't understand the harm they can do by not providing the kind of academic environment these children need. But some teachers—thankfully a small number—seem to intentionally hurt their students. These are teachers one would call "toxic teachers".

What is a toxic teacher exactly? Briefly, a toxic teacher is one who poisons a child's mind. One would like to think that these toxic teachers don't actually mean to be harmful, but based on the behaviour, a psychologist would have to say that some of them intend to be hurtful. Does that indicate that they mean to cause harm? Toxic educators develop for a variety of reasons that usually stem from the current cloud of paranoia, fear, and frustration enveloping public education, but they need to fight the negativity! They're only hurting themselves and their students.

Teaching isn't combat. We're not in the classroom to humiliate and harden our students as if they're going into the cut-throat world of business, or getting ready for the next football game against a team with no losses. Our role should be to help them grow as genuine human beings by identifying what they do best and where they need to do more work. As reporter Charles Kuralt put it simply, "Good teachers know how to bring out the best in their students" (8). Who needs shame for that? Basically, teaching is essentially a signature tune of personality. The teacher adapts him/herself to teaching in a manner that is harmonious with his/her expressions toward life situations in general. Methods of teaching which are learned may influence teaching superficially but do link one's personality with that of children. It is the signature attitude, contents, and flair of one's personality that brings the teacher into the heart of children. The issue pinpoints the need to outline the desired-undesired personality aspects of teachers. Rizzo and Zabel (1988) felt that successful teachers appear to possess special personal and professional attributes. Chamberlain and Carnot (1974) opined that "good teachers are the first line of defence against delinquency" (8). Kauffman and Wong (1991) offered similar views stating that "generic teaching skills appear to be sufficient for dealing with typical behavioural problems. Nevertheless, different attitudes and additional skills may be required for effective teaching of students with behavioural disorders" (225). Hence, the desired and undesired traits of teachers' personality need to be demarcated.

Teacher Personality: Its Desirable Frame

Personality as a concept has a number of dimensions in its definition. In sum, it is thought to comprise all the varying past and present forces in one's life and in possessing certain traits which serve to condition the manner in which others react to the given one. Thus, it is something an individual diffuses in all of his contacts and appearances. It is the manner of one's walk and talk, one's means of give and take, the way one works or plays; that is, the tangible characteristics. Actually, personality seems to be a blend of developed traits—'surface traits'—and a personal philosophy of the person. This 'personal philosophy,'—'source traits'—(Barr 1952), is the individualistic perspective that, in the educational context, needs to be positive in teachers to usher in more positivity in the character development of students in general. Societal improvements begin there. This is growth in academics; this is growth in mental frames. Teachers, being the sculptor of the mental frames of children, at all levels, need to look into their own personality factors, locate any deviation there to correct them, or else try to improve on them to the best of their abilities. It is their integrated personality that cuts, shapes, and smoothens the fresh minds of children that ultimately takes the form of being the most 'effective one' in life. Hence, Gross (1954) attempted to derive a formula that can directly pinpoint a teacher's expected personality mould. Within the all-encompassing aura of teacher personality being an effective one, he came out with the question, "Did U?" to relate to keystones of great teaching.

To him, the teacher mentor should have the first D which stands for 'dynamic'. Dynamic teachers are found to stimulate mental activity in children by the movement of their minds as well as their bodies. The 'I' in the query is being 'ingenious'; where students look forward to attendance as each lesson seems to give a promise of being a new adventure, a fertile experience for any student. The ingenious teacher seems to have two qualities:

1. Having practice of pre-planning and;
2. Having insight.

Such a teacher is also marked by his control and a variety of methods. The second 'D' relates to being 'democratic'. Such a teacher knows how to be a leader, is able to retain the direction of the class, yet can delegate responsibilities and thereby help students to attain competency in problem-solving. The quality initiates the personal development of students. The 'U' in the process imparts the quality of being 'understanding'. The effective teacher must understand how his teachings will condition the students' growth and development and how his understanding must extend into the community: its history, customs, ideals, social arrangements, and avenues of communication. Not only the communication style, but such implications of dynamism, ingenuity, democracy, and understanding, lie in having an integrated personality set of students as outcomes of such exposures.

In the format of desirable traits of teacher's personality, Witty (1947) offered the following based on his study:

(i) *Cooperative, democratic attitude* that invited children's comments like, "The teacher believes everybody can do the work," or "Her room was filled with the golden sunshine of equality."
(ii) *Kindliness and consideration for the individual*: illustrated by a child saying, "She is kind and does not make a monkey out of you before everybody."
(iii) *Having wide interests* that called for such comments as, "He uses others' books, their textbooks and takes us on trips," or "She is that rare person, a well-rounded individual, with many facets to her personality.
(iv) *Teachers' general appearance and pleasing manner*: students are loud in saying, "She is kind, courteous and smiling," "She always dressed neatly and attractively and she sets an example for us."

(v) *Teachers' sense of humour*: drawing children's comment like, "We work hard, but have fun too," "She encouraged us to laugh with each other, never at each other."
(vi) The trait, *good disposition, and consistent behaviour* was indicated by saying, "She is always the same," "She has a smiling face, a kind manner and a pleasing voice."
(vii) *Interest in pupil's problems*: a stuttering child commented, "I shall never forget her because she has helped me over a period of self-consciousness, and my improvement is due to her making me feel at ease."
(viii) *Flexibility* had been considered by many saying, "She uses different ways to teach us to read."
(ix) *The use of recognition and praise* also seemed important in good teaching. "She praises when we do it right" children commented.
(x) *Unusual proficiency in teaching a particular subject.* A girl wrote, "Miss X did not teach me to read—it was like magic in reading."

The ample number of desirable teachers' personality traits has been in the opinion of a host of researchers in the line (McIntyre 1995; McIntyre and Battle 1998; Safran and Safran 1987; Storti 1994; Tannen 1990). Darling (1974) in a reverse direction reported that delinquent youths valued patient and accepting teachers who created opportunities for achievement, made the students adopt best efforts and held to clearly defined classroom rules. McIntyre in his different research findings (1991, 1996) found that urban socially maladjusted youths valued humorous, confident, 'street-smart' teachers who presented action-oriented lessons. Hence, the researchers emphasized the importance of maintaining a classroom-ambience characterized by understanding, security, warmth, and mutual respect. It is generally expected within the periphery of such a classroom, that children's needs, weaknesses, and desires would receive careful considerations that would ultimately result in a stable, non-toxic personality organization in blooming minds.

Toxicity in Teachers and Its Undesired Outcome

Sufficient researches on effective personality pattern of teachers have brought out significant point that there is one highly personal and special obstacle that confronts the teachers and prevent them from becoming well-integrated one is the core point of emotional immaturity in them. Among all adults, the pattern of personal adjustment depends in large measure upon the extent to which they can stay free from a number of persistent infantile reactions and emotional compulsions. Most of the time, adults are not aware of such shortcomings and may react as personality disordered individuals, who probably have no insight about mal-development in them. The nature of such imbalance may be in ego-syntonic or ego-dystonic frame, in both ways either affecting others or inculcating toxicity within one's personality frame. The expected infantile reactive mode or emotional compulsive tone in behavioural output generates toxicity which needs to be warded off to become an effective teacher and contribute to future nation-building. The balanced, effective teacher is a person whose companionship, counsel, and advice are highly sought by students. Toxic teachers have a sense of self-deprivation, denial, and abstinence as powerful elements in personality. which tend to alienate children and youth (Witty 1947). The following traits seem to have toxicity in their functional wing:

(i) Overt Narcissism: An entitled, agentic self-image of the teacher which seems to bear a high sense of superiority and hence a downward estimation of children's profile. The pattern is attention-demanding and commanding type. The reactive mode to any deviation from total surrender and submission may cause anxiety-provoking behaviour. The unpredictable teacher in such a personality-frame is a fearsome 'God' in the eyes of the child and is conceived as a constant terror in life.
(ii) Punitive Personality: Rigid, non-accommodative feature of a teachers' personality may seem to be toxic to children. Their sense of being powerful to lash out at students at any point appears dreadful to the young ones.
(iii) Angry Type: Overt aggressiveness of teachers in school situations of varied natures makes the teacher non-acceptable to children. In their common perception, he/she is the very strict type from whom reprimanding behaviour is easily apprehended. Teasing and bullying behaviour patterns get easily associated with such personalities.
(iv) Having Lack of Sense of Responsibility: Teachers who express less initiative in the task of teaching and accommodating children's limitations, are basically not comfort-generating persons in the school situation. There seems to be an instinctive sense in children to avoid such personalities.
(v) Anhedonic, Apathetic Teachers: Being partially withdrawn in life owing to any account of mental disorders, such teachers cannot adopt dynamism in their task. They behave like machines and cannot generate interest in studies or any other school work on the part of children.
(vi) Immaturity in Terms of Attention and Appreciation-Seeking: Being adults, one may have a sense of deprived self deep down and unknowingly behave in a regressive mode. Here attention and appreciation of personal contents are needed by them, rather than children in their most vulnerable emotional stage. If such teachers feel very much loved and demanded in school set-up, only then can they offer love and care to children. Since understanding such needs of an adult personality is beyond the means of children, they tend to be sufferers in unwanted teachers' hands.
(vii) Callous in Terms of Time Sense and Its Management: A disorganized teacher seems to have poor time-management. They tend to be more emotional and less rational in character-orientation. The ultimate hampered child-growth in such a hand is picking up a wrong role-model and losing control over self-demands easily.

(viii) Having Personality Disorder in Temperamental Frame: Being totally non-insightful regarding any specific disordered pattern, particularly of Cluster B and C variety, reflecting emotional immaturity, and over-anxiety may cause severe damage to children in any corrosive encounter with such teachers.

The Damage Due to Toxicity in Teachers

Therefore, the general effect on children of such toxic teachers can be multiple:

(a) Damaged self-esteem leading to self-destructive attitude-formation;
(b) Children may feel worthless, unlovable and inadequate in personal strength;
(c) They seem to develop burdens of guilt from over-criticism experience;
(d) Inherent sense of guilt with sense of worthlessness which may crush the possibility of having positive self-image;
(e) Strong anxiety-streaks, not having faith in anybody;
(f) May be withdrawn from their set of peers and the school environment;
(g) The lack of confidence and self-worth may colour the whole canvas of life with depressive tone;
(h) A child can also become reactive-type following toxic teachers' behaviour patterns.

The scenario is indeed very sad.

Maturity: The Only Alternative

It is necessary that teachers modify or correct these personality problems in the direction of emotional maturity, which is regarded as the most essential requirement for being a school teacher. Maturity is expected to be revealed in spontaneous and genuine responsiveness in interactive contexts. The private world of the adult teacher should have compatibility with the surrounding social life, and the personality system should be free of distorting emotional conflicts and complexes, while anxieties should be tempered with realistic outlooks. A mature teacher learns to live at peace with himself and others. He should have a spirit of friendliness, sympathetic concern, and genuine affection. Happiness and success in worthwhile endeavours in schools and challenging tasks are powerful contributors to wholesome personality development. A mature teacher is the building block of such a situation (Marsh and Houvar 1991; Murray et al. 1990). Renaud and Murray (1996) reported that highly extroverted teachers are viewed by students as friendly and easily approachable, which can possibly lead to stronger student-motivation and self-confidence and ultimately sketch the story of higher achievement.

Suggested Administrative Rectifications

A child is a precious asset not only of the family, but an important resource for the future of the whole nation. Inadvertent damage to his self-system is basically the loss of a national asset. In the present era of competition and excellence, attempts are ongoing to bring out the best in them and not to lose out on their potential due to negligence. It seems to be high time to take measures to save their bubbling energy, and to make them successful contributors in life. The scientific concerns regarding toxic personalities of certain teachers have come into the limelight. From the administrative point of view, certain steps need to receive consideration to rectify this situation. They are:

(i) During teacher selection procedure, the candidate's aptness to be a teacher should be assessed not only on the basis of academic skills but also on personality assessment in both projective and non-projective folds before being selected.
(ii) Personal unstructured interview sessions with a clinical psychologist are needed to feel the pulse of their personality and to tap their self-insight into their inner self.
(iii) In the interview process, certain created situations as examples should be included to map their reaction pattern.
(iv) Each applicant's frustration-toleration limit needs to be judged.
(v) Specific questions must include their personalized system of overcoming their burnout reactions, if there are any.
(vi) Teacher-training refresher courses must be arranged to improve teachers' hands-on-skills to tackle children at school.

Conclusion

To be a responsible and a mature teacher is a hard task to achieve. No self is totally devoid of its limitations. Understanding and acknowledging personal limitations is a positive personality frame product. Not everybody can be expected to have such balance; hence, behavioural disasters take place at times. Among all adults, personal adjustment depends in large measure upon a number of persistent infantile reactions and emotional compulsions. They need to free themselves from such immaturity which is the central source of their toxicity resulting in mis-matched behavioural style. This consideration is of utmost importance in the case of school teachers since they become the role models of students who accept them totally. The effective teacher is the one whose footprints children try to follow; they are the points of solace to pains of very young minds. Such a teacher's companionship is craved for, his advice most sought after; his care becomes the treasure in one's life. A real teacher is saluted, not rejected. His/her maturity commands the surrender of students; their toxicity is beyond conception.

References

Barr, A. S. (1952). The measurement of teacher characteristics and prediction of teaching efficiency. *Review of Educational Research, 22*(3), 169–176.

Chamberlain, L., & Carnot, J. (Eds.). (1974). *Improving school discipline*. Springfield, IL: Thomas.

Darling, G. (1974). The delinquent in the school. In C. Chamberlain & J. Carnot (Eds.), *Improving school discipline* (pp. 27–34). Springfield, IL: Thomas.

Del Popolo, J. A. (1965). Teacher personality: A concern of teacher education. *Peabody Journal of Education, 43*(1), 50–55.

Fisher, D. L., & Kent, H. B. (1998). Association between teacher personality and classroom environment. *Journal of Classroom Interaction, 33*(1), 5–13.

Gross, R. E. (1954). Did U? 4 traits of the great teacher. *The Clearing House, 28*(5), 287–289.

Kauffman, J., & Wong, K. (1991). Effective teachers of students with behavioural disorders: Are generic teaching skills enough? *Behavioral Disorders, 16,* 225–237.

Marsh, H. W., & Houvar, D. (1991). Students' evaluations of teaching effectiveness: The stability of mean ratings of the same teachers over a 13-year period. *Teaching and Teacher Education, 7,* 303–314.

McIntyre, T. (1991). Understanding and defusing the street-corner tactics of black socially maladjusted youth. *Severe Behavior Disorder of Children and Youth, 14,* 85–97.

McIntyre, T. (1995). Characteristics of a 'good teacher' as reported by emotionally and/or behaviorally disordered students. *Perception, 29,* 21–26.

McIntyre, T. (1996). Earning the respect of street-wise youngsters. *Reclaiming At-Risk Youth, 4,* 38–41.

McIntyre, T., & Battle, J. (1998). The traits of 'Good Teacher' as identified by African–American and White students with emotional and/or behavioural disorders. *Behavioral Disorder, 23*(2), 134–142.

Murray, H. G., Rushton, J. P., & Paunonen, S. V. (1990). Teacher personality traits and student instructional ratings in six types of university courses. *Journal of Educational Psychology, 82,* 250–261.

Renaud, R. D., & Murray, H. G. (1996). Ageing, personality and teaching effectiveness in academic psychologists. *Research in Higher Education, 37*(3), 23–340.

Rizzo, J., & Zabel, R. (1988). *Educating children and adolescents with behavioural disorders: An integrative approach*. Boston: Allyn and Bacon.

Ryan, W. C. (1938). *Mental health through education* (p. 315). New York: The Commonwealth Fund, Division of Publications.

Safran, S., & Safran, J. (1987). Teaches' judgments of problem behaviour. *Exceptional Children, 54,* 240–244.

Storti, C. (1994). *Cross-cultural dialogues*. Yarmouth, MG: Intercultural Press.

Tannen, D. (1990). *You just don't understand*. New York: Ballentine.

Witty, P. (1947). An analysis of the personality traits of the effective teacher. *The Journal of Educational Research, 40*(9), 662–671.

Chapter 7
Enhancing Education: Improving Learner Outcomes with Principles of Psychology

Anjali Gireesan

Abstract In our world, which is fraught with problems and fallacies, education is heralded as a beacon of hope and change. Some might say that this is vague and abstract, but this thought can be translated into reality by an effective symbiosis between the principles of education and psychology. Education can be seen as the administrator and psychology can be viewed as its efficient manager. Psychology, with its strong theoretical background and empirically verified principles, can play an important role in improving the process of education. This chapter is an endeavour to explore these concepts in the context of improving educational outcomes for all learners based on the ideology of various theories spelt out in Psychology. Education is a phenomenon whose success is dependent on many factors. Similarly, the antecedents and the consequences of the same are also manifested in many forms. In an endeavour to understand this properly, we rely on the characteristics of certain key players. These are children, parents, teachers, and the institutional and government policies, that integrate all these individuals into the framework of education. Teachers or educators play the role of enhancing the knowledge base, developing the current and future skills of children, and mediate the personality of children to adapt to different situations. From the pre-school period, children spend quality time with educators and peers who are very different from parents and family. Here, they get a more objective assessment of themselves and have clear parameters to understand their capabilities and efficiencies. Thus, school and the social agents associated with the institution become a very important part of a child's life.

Keywords School · Students · Education · Learner outcomes
Psychology

A. Gireesan (✉)
Defence Research and Development Organization (DRDO), New Delhi, India
e-mail: anjali.gireesan@gmail.com

S. Deb (ed.), *Positive Schooling and Child Development*,
https://doi.org/10.1007/978-981-13-0077-6_7

Positive Education: Introduction

The concept of positive education is a direct translation from Seligman's work, who is of the view that currently there is no overlap between the needs perceived of the children and the outcomes that a school provides for (Seligman et al. 2009). It has been defined as an educational approach directed towards acquiring traditional skills documented, as well as happiness. Positive education has progressive outcomes for both the teacher and the student communities. The implementation has been shown to reduce signs of stress and burnout among teachers, as well as to improve student achievement and motivation (Borkar 2016). The components of positive schooling include: care, trust, and respect by teachers and educators as a foundation; goals, and motivation of students as building blocks; and social contribution of the knowledge learnt, as the ultimate consequence of education (Snyder et al. 2010). Though there are multiple arguments in favour of, as well as against, this concept, it is increasingly gaining popularity. There is a need to determine what principles may be applied to facilitate the implementation of positive education and how the outcomes may be measured. One of the recent contributions in the field emphasizes on well-being literacy, taken as both a connecting and a measuring dimension of positive education (Oades 2017). This is heralded as an effective component because well-being, here, is considered as a long-term achievement of positive education rather than as a short-term effect of any school intervention targeted at well-being. Well-being will become a long-term achievement only if it becomes a part of school curriculum and not a subsidiary periodic event that takes place in educational institutions. In this chapter, we look at certain theories prevalent in Psychology that may help in manifesting positive education in different educational setups.

Piaget's Theory of Cognitive Development

Jean Piaget is considered to be a pioneer in eliciting the nuances of cognitive development, especially the progress that children make in this subtle but significant process. The framework given by Piaget is still followed in various disciplines of Psychology with its various modification. His theory rests on assumptions that children engage in the cycle of forming concepts, involving three important principles which are schemes, assimilation, and accommodation.

- **Schemes**: These are, essentially, the first steps directed towards forming a sense of the external world, initially, and the internal world, as the cognitive development progresses. Schemes are blueprints that are formed when a child encounters novel stimuli in the environment. For example, a child looking at a dog for the first time has a conceptualization that gradually takes in various aspects of the animal. In the beginning, it may just include the tail of a dog; anything with a tail is considered to be a dog.

- **Assimilation**: Assimilation is the process of collecting information about the new schemes that a child is encountering. For example, the scheme of 'ANIMAL' will involve information like four legs and one tail. This scheme is then applied in the environment and there are more numbers added in this category.
- **Accommodation**: Accommodation is the process of bringing change in the already assimilated scheme. This indicates that the cognitive development of a child is gradually becoming sophisticated. For example, all animals with four legs and a tail are considered to be 'dog'. As the child engages in accommodation, how two animals are different from each other is understood and there are, thus, modifications in the schemes.

Thus, Piaget gave an outline that may be used to understand the progress that the child makes in different tasks as the cognitive development moves in a positive direction. Another point that he emphasized was that the cognitive development of a child is not an independent process. It happens in direct correlation with the physical development of the child. The stage theory, thus, is an example that depicts thus notions. The four stages are as follows.

- **Sensorimotor Stage**: This stage is characterized by sophistication in cognitive skills through physical exploration of the world around the infant. It lasts from zero to two years of age. The child gains mastery over reflexes and learns to translate them into voluntary, goal-directed, and increasingly complex behaviours. By the end of the stage, the child learns object permanence, has inculcated the basics of experimental behaviour, and formal mental representation begins to emerge in the form of deferred imitation.
- **Pre-operational Stage**: This stage is characterized by Piaget as having more deficiencies than capabilities. According to him, the child here starts to operate on the world through faulty mental representations. The focus here is on initiation of gradually using mental representations to operate on the world, rather than using them correctly. Some of the deficiencies that require special mention are egocentric thought, centration, conservation, and transformation. But still, these deficiencies indicate increasing cognitive sophistication as the child now does not require physical exploration alone to assimilate and accommodate.
- **Concrete-Operational Stage**: This stage characterizes the early school years before the age of adolescence. Here, reasoning based on observation of facts starts to emerge. The child easily engages in inductive reasoning at this stage. This kind of reasoning helps in making generalizations. For example, in learning to solve arithmetic problems, the example of one addition problem may facilitate the solving of other addition problems as well which may involve different set of numbers.
- **Formal Operational Stage**: This stage is reached at adolescence and the cognitive sophistication that follows involves just qualitative changes. It is characterized by initiation formation of hypothesis and deductive reasoning which is a type of thinking that moves from universal to particular (Fig. 7.1)

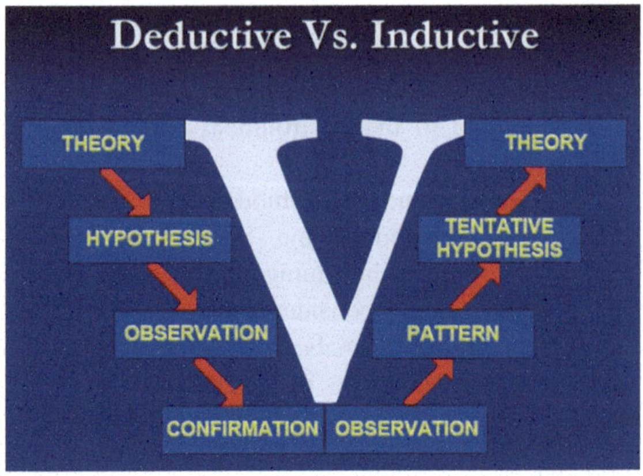

Fig. 7.1 Deductive versus inductive thinking

Educational Implications of Piaget's Theory

Piaget's theory of cognitive development has undergone many criticism and modifications but certain implications still remain true today as well. They are as follows:

- **Developmentally Appropriate Education**: A developmentally appropriate education caters to the physical, emotional, and cognitive development of the child in the context of maturation as supported by genetic endowment. For example, the current education system has the mathematics syllabus divided across different grades on the broad understanding of this framework. According to Piaget, each stage of cognitive development is characterized by a different mode of learning. In sensorimotor stage, physical exploration of objects needs to be facilitated whereas in formal operational stage, it is the hypothetical situations and experimentation of these that facilitates better education. This is often absent in the current educational system. Another problem that causes a hindrance to this kind of education is the teacher–student ratio in a classroom. For a developmentally appropriate education, an ideal ratio would be 1:10. But this seems to be impossible given the growing population and dearth of human resource to cater to this type of population. There is a need to revise the curriculum periodically on the principle of changing trends in the development of children rather than trends of society. For example, children are attaining puberty at a younger age now as compared to a decade ago. This will be accompanied by cognitive and emotional changes as well. Thus, the learning should take this trend into consideration. The Individualized Education Program (IEP) is a term that often appears in the context of children with special need. But every child needs to be considered special and has the right to IEP.
- **Speed of Cognitive Development**: The ignorance of understanding of the individual rate of maturation adds to the ineffective implementation of developmentally appropriate education. The emphasis on the child to solve complex

problems needs a proper understanding of the biological and environmental needs of the child. Each child will progress according to the interaction between these variables. So physical development of the child should be in tandem with the cognitive development. The unitary approach of the education system, concentrating on just one developmental aspect of the child, may not result in the outcome expected by the system.

- **Variation in Activities**: In our efforts to homogenize education and make it democratic, we have grossly ignored some fundamental principles of learning. Each child has a different way of adapting to the environment. While one child might do better at an audio-based activity, the other might be better at a pictorial activity. Thus, learning needs to be facilitated in such a way that appeals to different sensory systems and not just one. It might be difficult to introduce a topic using different modalities but the practice of it can involve activities of different kinds that are directed towards involving different sensory systems. For example, multiplication might be facilitated through pictorial representation of fruits, which are more familiar to the student, or it might be practiced by using varieties of dance steps. This way of learning also gives a choice to the child which often is perceived to be burdensome.
- **Importance of Self-initiation**: According to Piaget, education becomes a success only if it is self-initiated and children have a sense of ownership towards the knowledge acquired. In most of the classrooms today, the learning is passive which then goes unappreciated by students. For most of them, education is something that is compulsory and funded by their parents. In such a case, it becomes imperative that the learning is perceived to be earned and not just received. For example, the homework is aimed at learning at home as well. It will be more beneficial if homework becomes choice-based and each choice made needs to be earned through different protocols like answering a quiz. A pattern of such initiation in early foundation will result in more motivated and interested students in the advanced sector of education.

Vygotsky's Theory of Cognitive Development

Lev Vygotsky brought a very important part of the development to the forefront. He emphasized how the people surrounding children can facilitate a better cognitive development of the child. Though this also says that development is a function of the maturation of the child, the maximum potential of a child could be realized through active participation from the significant others with whom the child engages in an active social interaction. This zone of development is called the zone of proximal development (ZPD). Parents can take part actively in education by understanding different needs like autonomy, competence, and relatedness of their children. This may result in self-initiated regulatory behaviours at school (Grolnick 2009). Parental involvement and attainment are directly related to the education of young population (Huat See and Gorard 2015). Also, if parents are actively involved in the academics of their children, it may mitigate the adverse effects of irregular parenting styles practiced during early childhood (Monti et al. 2014). Similarly, teachers also play an important role in facilitating the education of children in a better way. The knowledge of teacher and motivation to teach is also related to student engagement (van Uden et al. 2014). Likewise, all people that a child interacts with in the surroundings becomes an important contributor of learning and hence education.

Educational Implications of Vygotsky's Theory

Like Piaget, there are certain things that we may include in the curriculum from Vygotsky's theory. They are as follows.

- **Encourage Pooling of Cognitive Resources**: There is a tendency in our academic curriculum to divide students into different groups based on their cognitive abilities. In certain schools, this also becomes the basis of dividing a particular grade into different sections. Though the intention behind such practice is to increase homogeneity in the classroom which may further facilitate better education, according to Vygotsky, such classification is of little use. The zone of proximal development that each child goes through is substantiated best by social interactions. In school, the probability of social interaction with peers is maximum. Heterogeneity in such interactions may thus facilitate a faster potential development in the ZPD rather than homogeneity. Also, during group activities in a classroom, such kind of cognitive pooling needs to be encouraged.
- **Scaffolding**: Scaffolding is any help provided by an expert in the ZPD. These are a series of instructions that the expert (parent, teachers) provides to the child in order to complete a task. The expert draws attention of the child to certain details that might facilitate this. For example, while making a puzzle, if the child is not able find a probable piece, the expert may draw attention to the shape of the piece or the detail of the picture. Scaffolding varies from culture to culture. The help that is needed by a child living in a tribal area may be very different from that of a child living in an urban area. This needs to be kept in mind when scaffolding is provided in the school setup where children from different backgrounds study together. It needs to be ensured that scaffolding is perceived to be helpful by the learner and there is a level of overlap between scaffolding provided in the school and what is being practiced at home.

Gagne's Nine Events of Instruction

Robert Gagne proposed nine pertinent events of instruction that are an important part of the teaching process. This is considered to be an excellent framework that systematically develops the topic to be covered and makes the teaching process comprehensive and complete (Khadooji et al. 2011). Though the professionals, practice these instructions in one or the other way, it is less conscious than effortful and goal directed. Spelling these events out adds to the enhancement of learning in a better way. The events have been found to be effective in teaching domain of various disciplines like nursing and clinical teaching (Miner et al. 2015) where student evaluation of teaching pedagogy showed significant improvement after the implementation of Gagne's framework. These instructions are constructed into a hierarchy aiding in completing the learning process.

1. **Gaining Attention**: The first event directly relates to employing techniques that help in gaining attention of the child. Gaining and sustaining attention in different environments is a function of learning performance for students (Kuo et al. 2017). This event is aimed at ensuring the initial reception of the child. There are different ways of doing it. For example, narrating the story of apple falling on the head of Newton, before directly starting with the definition of gravity. Stories encourage reflective practices in both children and teachers. Another way is to engage children in activities like throwing different things and observing where the object ultimately falls. This event needs to be made more theatrical and dramatic so that the learner's attention is fixed in the learning process. Following the same method for different activities makes the learner habituated to the process and the loss of novelty impacts gaining attention negatively. The novelty of the method may activate different reward centres in the brain which then acts as an intrinsic motivator for sustained attention (Foley et al. 2014).
2. **Informing Learners of the Objective**: This event is targeted at creating expectancies in the child for the proposed topic. The expectancy created is an important facilitator of learning motivation. It instils curiosity in the learning environment. In the absence of this stimulation, the student may become confused and engage in purposeless learning. The learning needs to be directed and focused so as to avail the potential benefits of education.
3. **Stimulating Recall of Prior Learning**: This step is not only important for attention but for facilitating memory as well. The two types of rehearsal that are crucial for the information to enter long-term learning are maintenance rehearsal and elaborative rehearsal. While maintenance rehearsal increases the capacity of short-term memory, elaborative rehearsal increases the probability of a piece of information to be remembered for a long time. This event of instruction is a manifestation of elaborative rehearsal where we connect the new information with already existing information. It forms an association in a way that increases neural connections in various regions of brain and thus decreases the vulnerability of forgetting.

4. **Presenting the Stimulus**: This event involves the introduction of the major topic and its different facets. Strategies that may improve selective perception, forms the content of this step. This phenomenon plays out in all of us automatically. We are able to focus our attention on certain things and not on others. The learning initiated in the classroom, thus, should avoid or reduce distractions to the maximum like unwanted noise and colour added to the environment. Also, the examples employed in the classroom should be pertinent to the topic and digression from the topic needs to be minimal.
5. **Providing Learning Guidance**: The focused perception of the topic is then followed by providing guidance as to how to enhance the learning. This is where the teaching modality takes centre stage. The instruction may take the manifestation of many forms involving both direct and indirect methods. This step is where the student semantically encodes information.
6. **Eliciting Performance and Providing Feedback**: These two events go hand in hand with each other. They involve a combination of different methods which give ways to observe the understanding of the learner and thus give feedback on the material learnt. The feedback operates on instruction methods like field visits, role plays, group discussion, critical analysis of the topic, and various other modalities. All these are considered to be active stimuli, aiding in eliciting response from the students. The student potential and motivation needs to be kept in mind when choosing between the options available for a particular topic.
7. **Assessing the Performance**: The practice done by the student is followed by an evaluation of the performance. Currently a common practice of this step is the tests and examinations prescribed in the curriculum of the academic set-up. Most of it capitalizes on the memory and writing capabilities of the student. This may need revision in time because assessment should be of more continuous nature, targeting various capabilities of the student.
8. **Enhancing Retention and Transfer**: This step is the most neglected one in our education system. Most of the learning is not followed up after the evaluation of it is over. For better and long-lasting learning, it is important that learning is observed in the surrounding and how it may be generalized in the surroundings around us. For example, the principles of mathematics taught remain in the textbooks for students unless they are followed up by being exposed to the utility of those principles in various professions.

Gagne also proposed the conditions of learning in which the learner progresses from a simple method of acquiring knowledge to more complex understandings of it. This involves skills of association, generalization, stimulus discrimination, and problem solving. This is also enhanced by the instructions provided by the teacher in the external environment in the student. Thus, Gagne emphasizes the importance of teachers, specifically in making the learning environment of the student more conducive and goal directed which is different from that of both Piaget and Vygotsky's approach.

Thorndike's Principles of Learning

Edward Thorndike is considered to be one of the pioneers in exploring and understanding the principles of learning. Though his principles are more freely associated with learning of human behaviour in different situations, they find applications in the field of educational psychology as well. The principles followed have been determined to contribute to the concept of positive schooling, specifically to that of contextualized teaching and learning (Saari 2016). These are basically a group of strategies targeted at specific interest of the student. His ideas and principles revolutionizes lexicography, curricular materials, and instruments used to look at individual differences in school settings (Mayer 2014). The principles are as follows:

1. **Law of Readiness**: Readiness refers to the action tendency of the student as well as that of the instructor. If either of them is not ready to learn then the learning is not considered to be fruitful. There are different resulting situations on the basis of this law:

    - *Student readiness negative (−) and teacher readiness positive (+)*: The learning environment that we generally see today across different classrooms falls in this category. The underlying causes may be many, ranging from attitude to motivation, but the result of this situation is that the learning process is hindered and will not progress in positive direction.
    - *Student readiness positive (+) and teacher readiness negative (−)*: This kind of classroom situation is harmful because a repeated pattern considerably decreases the motivation of the student to learn. Absence of teacher from the classroom or the teacher engaging the student in topics apart from the subject matter also depicts this situation. A repeated pattern impacts the learning process negatively.
    - *Student readiness positive (+) and teacher readiness positive (+)*: This is the ideal condition of learning wherein both the student and the teacher engage in goal directed process. The prevalence of such a situation depends on factors like motivation of the student and the teacher, and the experience of satisfaction by engaging in the learning process, which further increases the probability of incidence of this situation in the classroom environment.

2. **Law of Practice**: This law states that it is only with practice that the learning becomes more mature and internalized. Hence, practice should be an integral part of the learning process. This has been highlighted across different components of learning procedure. For example, attention is an important process of learning. Repeated exposure towards novel stimuli is essential for the learner to get habituated. Similarly, the memory process also capitalizes on this principle of use and disuse. A maintenance or elaborative rehearsal is needed for transferring the information from short-term memory to long-term memory, and neural connections are strengthened or weakened on the frequency of usage of certain learnt material. Hence, practice is an integral part of learning process.

3. **Law of Effect**: The law of effect is the most famous law propounded by Thorndike which relies on the perception of the consequences of learning. The learning becomes most effective when its result is considered to be pleasant and satisfying by the learner. In the absence of this condition, the learning will not be internalized and the connection between the learnt material and the learner will be weakened. Hence, it becomes the responsibility of the facilitator to promote events of satisfaction in the learning environment and reduce negative events that may create dissatisfaction in the learner. Events that promote the experience of satisfaction may include praise and appreciation by teachers and active class participation; and events that promote the experience of dissatisfaction may include shouting and chaos in the classroom and scolding of students.
   Apart from these three laws, there were further additions done later to the principles of learning. They are as follows.
4. **Law of Primacy**: This law states that what is learnt first needs to be correct and precise. The initial introduction of the topic needs to be in consonance with the facts about the topic because this information is difficult to correct later and may lead to incidences of confusion. Thus, the teacher needs to be careful in the initial days of learning.
5. **Law of Recency**: This law states that the topics learnt recently are more freely remembered than something which has been learnt in the past. This law emphasizes on eliciting connections between what is being currently learnt and what has already been learnt. Bringing this connection into light paves the way for better learning outcomes as compared to teaching new topics in isolation. This not only helps in managing retroactive interference, but also provides for more elaborative rehearsal which then ensures greater retention of the topics being learnt.
6. **Law of Intensity**: The intensity of the material used is another component that may facilitate better learning. This method indirectly points to the teaching pedagogy that may be used for eliciting the learning response desired by the teacher.

Educational Implications of Thorndike's Principles

Some of the educational implications of Thorndike's theory are as follows:

- Specific learning is more beneficial than general learning. The curriculum should be designed in such a way that interest of the student may be effectively invoked, maintained, and enhanced through suitable processes.
- Curriculum based on Thorndike's principles has often paved the way for metacognition in students. The learning strategies used by the students are examined in terms of the effectiveness in promoting learning. The process becomes more internalized and automatic with practice.

- Teachers may use these principles to enhance the learning process by keeping in context the attitude and motivation of students. It is also important to determine the readiness to learn in the student. Depending on the results, strategies may be adopted to bring all three to an optimal level, before initiating the learning process.

Conclusion

Positive education is a concept that may bridge the gap between actual needs of a child to be happy and outcomes provided by school curriculum. The principles and theories given by different theorists of Psychology may help in augmenting this process. While Piaget's theory emphasized developmentally appropriate education and self initiation, Vygotsky's theory may help in bringing together cognitive resources of peers, teachers, and parents to enhance the learning process of the child. Gagne's theory has implications for teachers and educators to make learning more effective. Thorndike's theory has educational implications for both teachers and students. All these principles together can contribute to different components of positive schooling and make education more purposeful

References

Borkar, V. N. (2016). Positive school climate and positive education: Impact on student's well-being. *Indian Journal of Health and Wellbeing, 7*(8), 861.

Foley, N. C., Jangraw, D. C., Peck, C., & Gottlieb, J. (2014). Novelty enhances visual salience independently of reward in the parietal lobe. *Journal of Neuroscience, 34*(23), 7947–7957.

Grolnick, W. S. (2009). The role of parents in facilitating autonomous self-regulation for education. *School Field, 7*(2), 164–173.

Huat See, B., & Gorard, S. (2015). The role of parents in young people's education—A critical review of the causal evidence. *Oxford Review of Education, 41*(3), 346–366.

Khadjooi, K., Rostami, K., & Ishaq, S. (2011). How to use Gagne's model of instructional design in teaching psychomotor skills. *Gastroenterology and Hepatology from Bed to Bench, 4*(3), 116.

Kuo, Y. C., Chu, H. C., & Tsai, M. C. (2017). Effects of an integrated physiological signal-based attention-promoting and English listening system on students' learning performance and behavioral patterns. *Computers in Human Behavior, 75,* 218–227.

Mayer, R. E. (2014). EL Thorndike's enduring. *Educational Psychology: A Century of Contributions: A Project of Division 15 (Educational Psychology) of the American Psychological Society*, 113.

Miner, M. A., Mallow, J., Theeke, L., & Barnes, E. (2015). Using Gagne's 9 events of instruction to enhance student performance and course evaluations in undergraduate nursing course. *Nurse Educator, 40*(3), 152.

Monti, J. D., Pomerantz, E. M., & Roisman, G. I. (2014). Can parents' involvement in children's education offset the effects of early insensitivity on academic functioning? *Journal of Educational Psychology, 106*(3), 859.

Oades, L. G. (2017). Wellbeing literacy: The missing link in positive education. In *Future directions in well-being* (pp. 169–173). Springer International Publishing.
Saari, A. (2016). Knowledge without contexts? A Foucauldian analysis of EL Thorndike's positivist educational research. *Studies in Philosophy and Education, 35*(6), 589–603.
Seligman, M. E., Ernst, R. M., Gillham, J., Reivich, K., & Linkins, M. (2009). Positive education: Positive psychology and classroom interventions. *Oxford review of education, 35*(3), 293–311.
Snyder, C. R., Lopez, S. J., & Pedrotti, J. T. (2010). *Positive psychology: The scientific and practical explorations of human strengths*. Sage Publications.
van Uden, J. M., Ritzen, H., & Pieters, J. M. (2014). Engaging students: The role of teacher beliefs and interpersonal teacher behaviour in fostering student engagement in vocational education. *Teaching and Teacher Education, 37,* 21–32.

Chapter 8
Strength-Based Approaches to Mental Health Promotion in Schools: An Overview

Shikha Soni and Noufal Hameed

Abstract Worldwide, approximately 10–20% of children and adolescents experience mental disorders, and half of all mental illness begin by age 14. About 75% mental illnesses start before the age of 24. Further, neuropsychiatric conditions are the leading cause of disabilities, across countries. Studies from around the world report that the majority of children and adolescents with mental health problems are affected in ways that their potential to live life to its fullest is not achieved. Also, they face several difficulties, compared to typically developing children, such as stigma, discrimination, poor academic achievement, etc. Recognizing this, many countries have taken up several initiatives for effectively dealing with the mental health issues of children at an early age. Such attempts, though in action for decades, were informed by what is known as 'deficit-based' mental illness prevention approaches. The past few years have seen a drastic shift in the focus of researchers and practitioners alike, who are working in the field of mental health, with the 'strength-based' mental health promotion approach gaining momentum. It is known that schools have the potential to be places where mental health issues can be addressed. The last couple of decades have seen a significant upsurge in attempts to utilize schools for promoting positive mental health. The present chapter will discuss in detail, the concept of mental health promotion and how schools can play a role in promoting positive mental health among children.

Keywords Mental health · Students · Schools · Strength-based approach

---

S. Soni (✉)
Department of Liberal Arts, Indian Institute of Technology Hyderabad, Hyderabad, India
e-mail: shikha1988@gmail.com

N. Hameed
Department of Clinical Psychology, National Institute of Mental Health and Neuro Sciences, Bangalore, India

S. Deb (ed.), *Positive Schooling and Child Development*,
https://doi.org/10.1007/978-981-13-0077-6_8

Introduction

It is easier to build strong children than to repair broken men

Frederick Douglas

Human development is a complex process and is defined as systematic continuities and changes in the individual that occur between conception and death (Shaffer and Kipp 2010). It is a co-construction of biological, cultural, and individual factors working together (Baltes et al. 2006). From a time when it was practice to divide the study of development into the study of physical growth and development, cognitive aspects of development, and psychosocial aspects of development, the current understanding has changed to see development as a holistic process with changes in any area influencing other areas (Sigelman and Rider 2009). Yet another important understanding about child development is the finding that all development occurs within a context, whether it be family, school, peer groups, or communities of various types. Further, these settings are influenced by several factors including historical, economic, social, and cultural factors. Another important change in our conceptualization of child development is the shift from the view of development as predominantly guided by innate mechanisms (Cosmides and Tooby 1997) to that of one involving a bi-directional influence between the genetic, neural, behavioural, and environmental factors (Shanahan et al. 1997). Hence, it is important to consider the concept of healthy child development in view of all these factors; for no development is possible without it.

The pertinent question then, is: What makes development healthy? Health is defined as "a state of complete physical, mental, and social well-being and not merely the absence of disease or infirmity" (WHO 2005). Further, health is not just about *not* having an illness, or about being able to cope adequately with all demands of daily life, but a state of balance to be achieved where there is an equilibrium within the individual, and between the individual and the social and physical environment (Sartorius 2006). Seen this way, providing a healthy development for children would mean that they are given opportunities for all-round development and not in merely in one area of life. As seen, development involves a mutual interaction between the physical, psychological, and social components. Further, the development of an individual is one where there is interaction among the contexts to which a child is exposed. Several studies show that school is a potential setting for promoting healthy child development. The present chapter is an attempt to provide the reader with a peek into the relationship between mental health, health, and the scope of using schools to achieve the objective of health. It also tries to provide a glimpse of how the concept of positive schooling can be related to mental health promotion.

For organizational purposes, we begin with an account of various mental health issues and the burden of mental health issues faced by children and adolescents of school-going age, followed by a section on various issues and challenges in dealing adequately with these issues. Following this, the concept of strength-based approaches to mental health promotion is given. This is followed by sections on the current evidence for mental health promotion in schools and a discussion on the scope of mental health promotion as a means for promoting positive schooling. Towards the end, the implications for the convergence of positive schooling and mental health promotion frameworks are given.

Promoting Mental Health in Schools

It was the Greek philosopher Plato who opined that "the purpose of education is to give the body and the soul all the beauty and all the perfection of which they are capable". The same was reflected in the words of Mahatma Gandhi when he said, "by education I mean an all-round drawing out of the best in child and man's body, mind, and spirit". Going through various perspectives about the purpose of education and schooling, there seems to have been an consensus on one aspect that the purpose of education and schooling is not just about the intellectual development of a child. Although there are varied opinions on how to achieve it, the common agreement is: education should provide a child with an opportunity to develop comprehensively as an adult. So, what is it that a school is supposed to strive for? In Bernard's opinion, the central theme of school and its surrounding community is the rights of the whole child, and all children, for survival, protection, and development (Bernard, as cited in Chabbott 2004). For him, it meant learning focused on strengthening the capacities of the children to act progressively on their own behalf through the acquisition of relevant knowledge, useful skills, and appropriate attitudes creating for themselves, and for others, places of safety, security, and healthy interaction. There is abundant literature on how a school can achieve this feat. One way is to provide the children with quality education which includes: (1) healthy and well-nourished learners who have family and community support; (2) safe, healthy, protective and gender-sensitive environments with adequate resources; (3) a curriculum reflecting the content and materials for the acquisition of basic skills; (4) child-centred teaching processes; and (5) outcomes that encompass knowledge, skills, and attitudes which are linked to larger, national level goals for education and positive participation in society (UNICEF 2002). It becomes obvious that the purpose of education and, in turn, the purpose of schools is to provide the students with opportunities so that healthy development becomes possible.

Before understanding the role of schools in promoting mental health, thus supporting healthy child development, we believe that several issues need to be taken into consideration. Of these factors, the most important is the burden of various mental health issues experienced by children and the related challenges in dealing with these issues effectively. Considering these, we would like to provide a short commentary on the burden of mental illness and related issues among children and adolescents, as well as related challenges. We believe that this would provide the reader with a perspective. Following this, the chapter gives a description of the concept of strength-based approaches to mental health promotion. Towards the end, the authors have tried to draw from the similarities between the concepts of positive schooling and mental health promotion.

Burden of Mental Health Issues During Childhood and Adolescence

Prior to the 1950s, congenital and acquired organ-system illnesses led the list of causes of morbidity and mortality among children and young people. These have become less important, largely owing to the advancements in the fields of medicine and biology (Palfrey et al. 2005). The decades 1960s–2000s saw the emergence of mental illness as the leading cause of morbidity and mortality, called the "new-morbidity", among children and young people (Palfrey et al. 2005). The first decade of the twenty-first century marked the emergence of the period called the "millennial-morbidity" (Palfrey et al. 2005), saw further rise in the importance of mental health within the child and adolescent mental health framework (Ravens-Sieberer et al. 2007).

In line with these findings, it is estimated that, worldwide, there has been an increase in the number of people experiencing some or other form of mental health issues. Studies from various countries show that, among those who are affected with different types of mental health issues, children and adolescents make a substantial number. Epidemiological data shows that, worldwide, 10–20% of children and adolescents experience mental disorders (WHO 2016). Further, one nationally representative study from the United States reveals that half of all time mental illnesses begin by the age of 14 years and 75% of people with adult-type psychiatric disorders would have the onset by 24 years of age (Kessler et al. 2005)

India shows similar trends in the number of children and adolescents experiencing mental health problems. For example, a large scale survey of 2064 children, aged 0–16 years, found a prevalence rate of 12.5% and 12.0% in 4–16-year-old children (Srinath et al. 2005). Another meta-analysis, including 16 community-based studies and seven school-based studies, reported a prevalence rate of psychiatric disorders of 6.46% in the community and 23.33% among school going children and adolescents (Malhotra and Patra 2014). Mental health issues such as substance abuse and dependence also seems to be very high among our adolescents. One study by National Sample Survey Organization of the Indian Government showed that about 20 million children of ages 10–14 years were estimated to be addicted to tobacco. And every year, about 5500 new users are added to this (Chadda and Sengupta 2002). Moreover, there is also a high rate of suicide among children and adolescents. In the United States, 52 per million adolescents within the age range of 12–17 years commit suicide, and about 33 children per million below 12 years kill themselves each year (Bridge et al. 2015). In India, youth in the age group 15–29 years accounted for the largest proportion (34.5%) of suicides (Crime in India, The National Crime Records Bureau Report 2009). Within the age range of 10–19 years, suicide accounted for about a quarter of all deaths in males and between 50% and 75% of all deaths in females, with an average of 148 girls per lakh and 58 per lakh boys committing suicide (Aaron et al. 2004).

The findings about current estimations of mental health problems among children and young people are under-recognized (Sourander et al. 2004) and may be higher than that reported in the current literature is also to be considered. Moreover, the number of students coming to college and school campuses is increasing (Hunt and Eisenberg 2010). This may either be a reflection of the increasing number of young population or, as reported by Hunt and Eisenberg (2010), a reflection of more students coming out with their problems than a real increase in the number.

Child and Adolescent Mental Health: Challenges

There can be no doubt as to the size of mental health issues among children and adolescents. Nevertheless, assuming that the issue lies only in numbers, the literature on child, adolescent, and youth mental health has a bigger story to tell, because, in matters of mental health, the challenges lie not just in tackling the numbers, but a variety of hindrances in reaching these affected children and adolescents. Any attempt at dealing with mental health issues among children and adolescents would not be complete, or even possible, without dealing with these hindrances. Understanding these challenges is crucial in our attempts at promoting healthy child development, irrespective of the setting. The following section is a glimpse of the complexity of the various challenges that lies in our way to provide opportunities for healthy development to our children.

As mentioned, the large number of young people experiencing some or other form of mental health issues, is a definite challenge to any community. Mental health begins in childhood and evolves over a period of time. However, unlike adult years, given the delicate nature of developments during childhood, it does not take a severe and long standing illness to bring about longer lasting and severely limiting impacts on the overall health of the individual (McGorry et al. 2007), leaving the affected individual socially isolated, stigmatized, and incapable of becoming a contributing member to the society (Waddell et al. 2007a, b). Further, unlike many of the severe and disabling physical illness which start late in life, the early beginning of mental health issues mean that the child suffers the maximum impact of disability when in the prime time of life, which is the time that they are usually most productive. Thus, a mental health issue which has an early onset can have a negative impact on a variety of life outcomes, including lower educational attainment, lower rates of employment, income, and standard of living (Kessler et al. 1995; Ettner et al. 1997; Bray et al. 2000; Fergusson et al. 2007; Avenevoli et al. 2008).

Closely related is the fact that, though mental health issues have an early onset, there is a significant delay between the time of onset and the first treatment contact. For example, in the United States, it was found that about 80% of those having a mental health problem eventually seek treatment, but it takes about a decade for the person to seek help from the time of onset of the illness (Olfson et al. 1998; Kessler et al. 1998). This delay in seeking help can lead to more severe clinical outcomes, increased severity of symptoms, and longer time of recovery and/or poor recovery. Furthermore, psychosocial problems and issues tend to accumulate over time (Deater-Deckard et al. 1998; Rönkä and Pulkkinen 1995). Besides the negative effects at the individual level, mental health problems take their toll on the family, and society at large, the costs of which lie largely outside the health care system.

These and a number of similar factors show the need for having an equal, if not enhanced, focus on providing platforms for promoting mental health of children in schools. Recent years have seen a drastic shift in the way education is viewed and the need for integrated care for children focusing on both intellectual development and overall development has gained the attention of governments and various other organizations around the globe. It also seems that promotion of mental health in schools can take our communities a long way in the attempts at converting schools to platforms for promoting healthy child development.

Strength-Based Approaches to Mental Health Promotion (MHP)

Before examining the role of mental health promotion in promoting positive schooling, it is useful to reflect upon the definition of the mental health promotion and the concept of strength-based approaches. Historically, the period of childhood and adolescence was seen as an age of vulnerability and problems. As epitomized in the "storm and stress" view of adolescence (Hall, as cited in Arnett 1999), this period came to be one with a focus on the various deficits that young people had. The most logical answer to deal with a period of problems was, then, to focus on the problems themselves. Thus, the traditional deficit orientation that came into existence largely organized itself around the identification, reduction, and prevention of factors that are understood as undermining healthy development, as well as the reduction and prevention of unhealthy behaviours (Benson et al. 2004). With the passing of years, this field of approaches, called the prevention approaches—with its implied interest in eliminating the onset of problems or minimizing their adverse consequences—grew and became institutionalized in terms of policy formulation and programmatic funding (Benson et al. 2004). Despite being a model with substantial influence across the globe (Olweus et al. 1999), the prevention approach was faced with a number of shortcomings.

One such shortcoming was evident from the fact that, by focusing on what was wrong with people, the policies and programmes failed to understand and utilize strengths and protective factors (Alvord and Grados 2005), which in turn created a 'deficit cycle' creating a dependency on the experts and professionals. Further, focusing only on the problems could lead to potential stigmatization (Small and Memmo 2004). Also, a narrowed focus on the problems led to a proliferation of programmes that are specific to separate problems, leading to lesser appreciation of the shared risk, protective, and promotive factors (Guerra and Bradshaw 2008). Most importantly, the prevention approach failed to pay attention to normal, healthy development (Cowen 1994). Yet another criticism made against the problem focused approaches was the argument that just eliminating the problems does not guarantee that the child will go on in a healthy developmental trajectory (Roth and Brooks-Gunn 2003).

Strength-based approaches, as opposed to the deficit-approach, begins asking 'what is right with people?', and adds external sources of support when needed. This, in turn, leads to a more holistic focus and allows the individual to explore further and create positive expectations leading towards individual empowerment and decreased dependence on the 'experts'. For example, positive youth development approach, a prominent strength-based paradigm, views the individual as naturally competent and as having an inclination towards prosocial engagements (Damon 2004) which is seen even in childhood. It further focuses on the positive aspects of health, such as assets and strengths, than on deficits and needs (Jané-Llopis et al. 2005), and also on individual and community-level capacity building by enhancing the innate ability of the people to achieve and maintain good mental health (Pollet 2007). It is also believed that the best way to prevent youth from experiencing problems is by helping them to achieve their full potential (Small and Memmo 2004) where they achieve their potential when there is an alignment between their personal strengths and the community that they belong to (Seibereisen and Lerner 2007). Moreover, the belief in the inherent trust in each young person, and his/her capacities, and an understanding that each person is doing his/her best in light of their experiences to date, the strength-based approach is able to bifurcate the problem from the person (Rapp et al. 2006; Alvord and Grados 2005) leading to a change in the concept of 'person as the problem'. When an individual is led to believe in his own strength and ability, and their efforts are acknowledged, and their experiences are validated, there is a possibility that labels will be avoided, and the person will feel motivated and interested to be more engaged. Another point in favour of a strength-based approach is that activities and programmes that foster positive mental health also help to prevent mental illness (Jané-Llopis et al. 2005) indicating the preventive role of the same.

There are a number of strength-based approaches across countries. These programmes include approaches such as Appreciative Inquiry, Asset-based Community Development, Community Development, Developmental Assets, Positive Youth Development, Resilience, Social Development, Sustainable Livelihoods, and Youth Engagement and so on. These programmes focus on various positive attributes such as capacity and intentionality, meaningful participation, solutions and potentials, opportunities for skill building, personal relationships (Cooperrider et al. 2003; Chaskin et al. 2001; Scales et al. 2006; Hamilton et al. 2004; Masten et al. 1990; Chambers and Conway 1992).

Similarly, the strength-based approaches to MHP aim at promoting mental health by focusing on the strengths of the individuals. For example, MHP is defined as the creation of individual, social, and environmental conditions that are empowering, and enable optimal health and development and involve individuals in the process of achieving positive mental health and enhancing quality of life (Jané-Llopis 2007). Further, MHP aims to achieve wellness for the entire population by addressing the determinants of mental health and relies on the collaboration of all sectors of community: individuals, families, and communities (Jané-Llopis et al. 2005). Mental health promotion, thus, focuses on creating environments for individuals that are conducive for mental health and well-being (GermAnn and Ardiles 2009). Creating such environments, that are supportive for promotion of mental health, requires action on the many social and economic determinants of mental health, including healthy child development, employment and working conditions, social support networks, income and social status, and education (GermAnn and Ardiles 2009). Despite some disagreements on a number of issues—what actually constitutes mental health promotion, its role in overall health promotion, and where it stands in relation to mental illness prevention—there is agreement that positive mental health is the desired outcome of the mental health promotion interventions (WHO 2002). In short, mental health promotion focuses not on incapacity, but on the strengths of the individuals, and on nurturing what is best within each individual (Pape and Galipeault 2002).

Considering the fact that the various personal, social, and environmental factors influence the mental health and illness of individuals in any given community, the World Health Organization (2005) has outlined three main objectives for mental health promotion which includes: (1) the development and maintenance of healthy communities; (2) fostering of each individual's ability to deal with the social world; and (3) promoting the individual's ability to deal with thoughts and feelings, and the management of life and emotional resilience. Mental health promotion aims to achieve these objectives through a number of strategies. A few such strategies are outlined by WHO (2016), two of which have direct implications for child and adolescent mental health and well-being: providing support to children, which may include skill building programmes and child and youth development programmes; and mental health promotional activities in schools which are aimed at implementing programmes that promote ecological changes in schools and creating child-friendly schools.

These suggest that there is a definite need for addressing mental health needs of the young people in every community. It is also clear that providing adequate care for individuals cannot be complete by focusing only on mental health issues. It is also evident from the above sections that mental health promotion can be a useful tool in overcoming a number of shortcomings inherent in the mental illness prevention approaches. Despite all these advantages of mental health promotion approach, one should also ensure that it works and that there is enough evidence to say that mental health promotion actually delivers what it proposes to deliver, for any approach is as good as the evidence that it has. Considering this, the following section provides a glimpse into the existing literature on the evidence base for the success of mental health promotion approaches in schools.

The Scope of Mental Health Promotion in Schools: What Does the Evidence Say?

There are clear evidences for the advantages of mental health promotion in different settings, including schools. It is to be noted that there are thousands of school mental health programmes and they go by various names: mental health, 'social and emotional learning', 'emotional literacy', 'emotional intelligence', 'resilience', 'life skills' and 'character education' (Weare 2010). Further, these initiatives may be universal in nature (targeting all the children) or focus on a particular group of children (high risk children, for example). The universal programmes are based on whole school approach and are aimed at building a positive, safe environment with the objective of building coping and social skills which, in turn, enhance competence, self-esteem, self-control, leading to improvements in school achievement and in mental health (Jané-Llopis et al. 2005). Such programmes are effective in promoting mental health by influencing curriculum and school policy, ensuring inclusion of teachers, students, and parents in mental health promotion activities (Keleher and Armstrong 2005). They also require significant changes in the existing systems and support from school authorities (Severson and Walker 2002). On the other hand, targeted programmes are those intended at children who have high risk of experiencing some form of mental health issues. Such programmes target children who are experiencing high levels of distress, children and adolescents from immigrant families (Barrett et al. 2001), refugee children (Barrett et al. 2000) and children suffering the effects of parental divorce (Wolchik 1993) or death of a parent (Sandler et al. 1992), and so on.

A number of effectiveness studies, reviews, and meta-analyses have shown the efficacy of both universal and targeted mental health promotion initiatives. For example, the Fast Track PATHS, a universal social-emotional learning programme resulted in reduced aggression, hyperactive-disruptive behaviours, and improvement in social competence, prosocial behaviour, and improved academic engagement (Conduct Problems Prevention Research Group 2010). Yet another study evaluated another universal school-based programme, designed to prevent depression in adolescents, and found significantly lower levels of depressive symptomatology and hopelessness, at post-intervention and 10-month follow-up in the programme participants, compared to the control group (Shochet et al. 2001). Another study which examined the effects of a teacher consultation and coaching programme, delivered by school and community mental health professionals, found that the intervention was effective across multiple domains including teacher–student relationship closeness, academic self-concept, and peer victimization (Cappella et al. 2012). One of the most influential and most widely discussed studies in the field of youth mental health is the 4-H programme. Findings from this decade long study involving more than three thousand students show that the participants in the programme are more likely to contribute to society and engage in civic activities, show increased academic achievement, and to show healthy life choices compared to non-participants (Lerner et al. 2008).

In India, two models proposed by NIMHANS (National Institute of Mental Health and Neurosciences) Bangalore are-based on the life skills approaches. Cascade Model of Life Skills Education by Department of Psychiatry, aims to train teachers as life skills facilitators, highlighting peer learning and group involvement (Bharath and Kumar 2008). The themes outlined were nutrition, hygiene, academics, interpersonal, relationships, substance use, gender issues, career, and social responsibilities, which were found to enhance the student–teacher interaction and self-esteem (Bharath and Kumar 2010). Another Model of promotion of mental health and psychological well-being of adolescents also includes resiliency with other themes like suicide prevention, awareness about mental illness, exam pressure and school related issues, self-image, parents related issues, sexual abuse and harassment, peer pressure, adolescent issues and sexuality, sexual abuse, substance abuse and alcohol, HIV and AIDS sexuality Values and Life skills, making a career plan and gender-related issues, to promote positive mental health (Vranda 2015).

A review of 31 school-based universal mental health promotion studies (Adi et al. 2007) found that the programmes show evidence for short-term effectiveness in reducing stress, and improved coping, conflict-resolution, and social problem solving, social awareness and emotional literacy in the long term. The review also provides good evidence to support multi-component programmes, covering classroom curricula and the school environment, which include significant teacher training and development and support and training for parenting. Another review of 84 research reports with 127 treatment-control comparisons on social skills training to prevent anti-social behaviour and promote social competence, showed a small but significant overall effect of the interventions in areas which included aggressions, delinquency, disruptions, social interaction skills, pro-social behaviour, self-control or social problem solving (Beelmann and Lösel 2006). Another review of 19 studies aimed at emotional and social learning with a universal approach, showed the strong and significant impact of many programmes on social and emotional skills and attitudes to self and others, along with strong support for universal programmes (Diekstra and Gravesteijn 2008). A review of 526 universal positive youth development programmes looking into the effect of the interventions on schools, families, and communities, found that changing social systems affecting children and adolescents can be successful (Durlak and Weissberg 2007).

One review of 44 studies on school-based violence prevention programmes for children at risk for aggressive behaviour, showed that school-based violence prevention programmes are useful in reducing aggressive and violent behaviours in children who already exhibit such behaviour, irrespective of whether the programmes focused on skills training of non-response, or social skills training or changes in the social contexts (Mytton et al. 2006). Another review of 80 studies on social and emotional learning programmes for students who are already showing early signs of emotional and behavioural problems, found the programmes to be effective in improving attitude towards, self, school, and others, and improved social and emotional skills compared to the non-participants (Payton et al. 2008). The authors also reported that the programmes showed effects whether delivered by school personnel or non-school personnel. They further recommended such programmes as options for promoting youth well-being and adjustment. In a systematic review of 52 systematic reviews and meta-analyses of mental health promotion programmes in schools reports a wide range of beneficial effects on children, families, communities, and on mental health, social, emotional, and educational outcomes (Weare and Nind 2011). The review also identified a number of characteristics associated with effective interventions including, teaching skills, focusing on positive mental health, balancing universal and targeted approaches, starting early with the youngest children and continuing with older ones, operating for a lengthy period of time and work from a multimodal/whole-school approach.

The literature is filled with evidences for the usefulness of mental health promotion in school settings, for a wide variety of age groups (Browne et al. 2004; Pollett 2007), and for both high risk and no risk participants. However, as mentioned before, the process of adopting such initiatives is time consuming as well as requiring adequate resources. A number of studies, however, show that even in limited settings, such as schools, implementing mental health promotion programmes are feasible. Further, it is also found that providing quality school mental health promotion programmes, building capacity in the education sector, as well as developing assessment strategies for complex, school level changes can be achieved (Rowling 2007).

As seen above, there indeed are a wide variety of benefits to mental health promotion efforts in school settings. Barring a number of potential difficulties, it also seems that mental health promotion in schools can be achieved. When looked at from a positive schooling perspective, there seems to be tremendous potential for a convergence of mental health promotion programmes and initiatives with that of providing positive schooling thus promoting healthy child development. This is not to suggest that the potential benefits of mental health promotion are the only reasons for suggesting school-based mental health promotion. There are a number of other factors that make it crucial to promote mental health in schools. The following section discusses a number of other reasons why mental health promotion needs to be included in the school setting, along with how mental health promotion and positive schooling can go hand in hand.

Mental Health Promotion and Positive Schooling: Scope for Convergence

For the majority of individuals who have gone through schooling, the experience was of getting degrees and preparing for a career and making the future 'safe'. Unfortunately, a number of teachers and school authorities hold the same viewpoint, where the focus remained on 'teaching' students. However, recent times have seen a revival in the true objective of education, and the idea of holistic development of the children was gaining momentum. There was increasing understanding that promoting healthy development requires providing adequate care to the mental health needs of the children. Thus, the importance of school for mental health was realised, and also the possibilities that schools hold for promoting mental health has been evident for some time, with a surge of research in the area in the last two decades (Weare and Nind 2011).

Why is it that school is so important in promoting mental health for children? One reason is that, as mentioned earlier, there are a large number school-going children and adolescents who are experiencing some form of mental health issues. Worldwide, 91% of primary-school-age children were enrolled in school in 2013 (UNICEF 2016) and even in West and Central Africa, where enrolment is the lowest, 74% of them enrolled in school. Considering the fact that a majority of children who do seek help for mental health issues receive their care through the education sector and also that schools are the most common point of entry for them (Farmer et al. 2003), this provides the school an unparalleled potential for reaching them at a very early age. It is also suggested as a strategy, to provide mental health services in schools to have a larger impact on public health and to reach to maximum children (Huang et al. 2013). Furthermore, for children belonging to less optimal psychosocial backgrounds, where the available support for healthy growth and development is either non-existent or minimal, schools can be a big support. Also, many schools already provide some form of social and emotional support services. In the United States, for example, 63% of schools provide prevention services, 59% provide programmes intended at behavioural issues, and about three-fourth of the schools have programmes aimed at promoting safety and prevent drug-use (Foster et al. 2005). In addition, schools are considered accessible and relatively stable sites where interventions to promote mental health can be located (Bond et al. 2007). A school is a place where students come from a number of different places and hence is a common platform (Short and Talley 1997). Such common platforms make the implementation of various programmes feasible.

Along with wide-spread depression and also minimal increase in happiness, Seligman et al. (2009) provided one more reason for using positive principles in schools. They reported that, based on their observations, there is a synergy between well-being and better learning. This way, even if one assumed that the sole purpose of schools was to promote learning—which is the traditionally expected outcome of schooling—the positive interventions are relevant and important. For example, positive mood, which is an objective and outcome of positive interventions, improves attention (Fredrickson and Branigan 2005), stimulates creativity (Estrada et al. 1994), and holistic thinking (Kuhl 2000).

It is important that children are provided with all possible avenues for healthy development. During early childhood, a number of factors contribute to the healthy development of the child. A few such factors include: ability and confidence to explore new things, ability to cope with changes, emotional regulation skills, freedom to explore the world around, choice making, and problem solving skills, and a sense of uniqueness (Kiefer et al. 2004). For a child—beginning from birth, and spanning through early and middle childhood—social support, a key contributor to resilience and thus to mental health, comes from primary caregivers or parents (Pilowsky et al. 2004). As children become older, the sources of support extend to include more and more people from outside family and, once they start schooling, the school becomes the main setting for promoting mental health. During these years, the whole world of the child undergoes a dynamic shift, including expanded opportunities for extra and co-curricular activities, friendships that become prominent, and an increasingly complex social and academic environment (Lavoie et al. 2016).

Research evidence shows that a curriculum and school policy that engages the children, parents, and the teachers, are more effective than programmes focusing on specific topics in promoting healthy child development (Keleher and Armstrong 2005). Also, as we have seen, since the majority of children worldwide attend schools during childhood and adolescence, they spend a considerable amount of time in academic institutions. For example, it is reported that children in East Asian countries spend about 208 days in schools on average in an academic year, whereas in United States it is 180 days (Lee and Barro 2001). It is 240 days on average in Indonesia, 220 days in Korea, about 200 days in South Africa, 190 days in Britain, and 187 days in Singapore (Parinduri 2014). Thus, students' day-to-day interactions with peers and others become an increasingly important factor of student well-being. Similarly, in a study conducted among parents and educators, promotion of well-being and character was reported to be an important aspect of schooling (Cohen 2006). It seems that school, indeed, is a potential setting where there is huge scope of contributing to our efforts for promoting healthy child development (Weist 2005).

Positive Schooling

Human societies, past and present, had invested a great deal in educating their children. Despite the fact that the efforts and resources put into promoting education vary among societies, there was never a question about the importance of education. By extension, schools became an integral part of most societies. Even from ancient times, education was always thought as something that has to reach the whole individual, and not just information. Sri Aurobindo, the great Indian philosopher, believed that 'true and living' education helps an individual to realize and bring out the full potential that he is endowed with, helps a man to enter into his right relation with life, mind and soul of the people to which he belongs and with that of great total life, mind, and soul of humanity of which he himself is a unit and his people or nation a living, separate and yet inseparable member (Aurobindo, as cited in Sahu 2002).

Going by this concept where education is meant to help an individual recognize and achieve his full potential and to come into a harmonious relation with humanity as a whole, one might feel that, at present, the whole education system is on a different track. However, with recent developments in the field of child and adolescent development, and increasing understanding of the need for a holistic care for the children, the concept of positive schooling is gaining increased attention from different sectors.

Snyder et al. (2010) provide a visual representation of their concept of positive schooling. They define positive schooling as "an approach to education that consists of a foundation of care, trust, and respect for diversity, where teachers develop tailored goals for each student to engender learning and then work with him or her to develop the plans and motivations to reach their goals" (Snyder et al. 2010). They talk about the components of positive schooling using the image of a school building. As shown in the definition, the foundations of positive schooling are formed out of care, trust, and respect for diversity. They propose that it is crucial to have a caring and trusting atmosphere which is supportive as only in such an environment can children flourish. Highlighting the need for having a sense of caring, they add that students need teachers who are responsive and available. Only when such a secure base is available, is exploration possible and children are able to find ways to their own goals of life (Shorey et al. 2003).

At the ground level, there is a plan and motivation and these are driven by goals (first floor). They suggest that there is a need for careful planning process on the part of instructors while teaching. Also, motivation is the companion to planning. Teachers can be the models for the students by being motivated themselves and making the lesson plans and goals interesting. They recommend using materials that are relevant for the students, taking 'risks' and trying new approaches, and use of praise as potential strategies by which student motivation can be improved. Goals, or the content, are represented by the first floor. By providing means of targeting students' learning efforts, goals are especially helpful if decided on in mutual agreement between the teachers and students (Snyder et al. 2010). Further, setting up of goals becomes more effective when they are set as reasonably challenging and tailored for students' needs and the attaining of the new goals stretch their efforts. They also strongly recommend students be given a say in regard to their teachers' conduct of classes (Snyder et al. 2010). Above the first floor is 'hope'. When careful planning is done, students and teachers are motivated, and goals are set, a spirit of inquiry becomes evident and the learning expands, leading to a sense of empowerment, and students become lifelong problem solvers. This learning of how to learn, according to Snyder et al. (2010), creates a sense of hope in the students, and a hopeful child continues learning long after he finishes schooling, and never stops learning. Finally, a child who is motivated and empowered with hope, goes on to the recognition of the world beyond self and the school, and become part of the larger society where he or she will share his or learning (Snyder et al. 2010). Thus, positive schooling leads to the process where the child goes back to the community to which he or she belongs and contributes to its various causes, whether it be teaching other children or sharing one's insights (Snyder et al. 2010).

Promoting a positive school climate is considered integral to the provision of positive schooling to the students. For example, positive school climates are considered powerful as they meet the student needs of belonging, commitment, and autonomy (Narvaez 2010). It is further observed that, in a research on student motivation and learning, a school climate characterized by higher levels of support and expectations for both achievement and behaviour produces the best results.

Mental Health Promotion and Positive Schooling: Scope for Convergence

One cannot fail to notice the similarity between the way purpose of education is conceptualized and what positive schooling envisages to achieve. This section tries to look at the scope of strength-based approaches to mental health promotion in promoting positive schooling, thus helping reach the true goal of education: ensuring healthy child and adolescent development. Mental health promotion and positive schooling have many parallels. For instance, the essential features of Positive Youth Development paradigm (PYD), which is a strength-based programme, are: (1) positive and sustained adult-youth relations; (2) life-skill building activities; and (3) opportunities for youth participation in and leadership of valued family, school, and community activities (Lerner 2004). In the same way, positive schooling requires that teachers become trusted and available adults for students, promoting a sense of security, and a key component of school climate is the relationship between students and adults, and also the relationships between schools, families and their communities. Moreover, one of the fundamental principles of positive youth development is promoting synergy between the resources within each individual, along with those developmental assets available in the community. Like the strength-based approaches, positive schooling also focuses a lot on the individual strengths and abilities (Snyder et al. 2010).

A positive school climate promotes academic achievement, school safety, reduces drop outs, and improves healthy interactions and well-being (Cohen and Geier 2010); various strength-based approaches also show similar findings. Quality education also demands safe and healthy environments, so do strength-based approaches. The 2004 Hay Group study of 134 schools in England showed that the successful schools were those who had a more demanding culture; they showed a hunger for improvement, promoting excellence, and help for every child (Fullan 2001). Mental health promotion, or strength-based approaches in general, starts from the premise that each child has an inherent capacity to learn and also emphasizes individual capacity and intentionality (Cooperrider et al. 2003). Positive schooling also involves providing quality education where the teachers adopt a student-centred approach for teaching and one where the students have adequate opportunities to voice their opinions about a number of relevant issues (Snyder et al. 2010).

Similarly, strength-based approaches seek active involvement of the students in the learning process and provide opportunities for child participation (Lerner 2004). Further, the concept of empowerment, described in the positive schooling literature, is also seen prominently in strength-based approaches. For instance, one of the key principles of effective mental health promotion programme is identified to be its focus empowerment (Barry 2007). Such a philosophy dictates that programmes be delivered in a manner where there is active participation of the users in gaining understanding. Like positive schooling, mental health promotion approaches also have a collaborative nature.

Ultimately, it is also seen that the purpose of education, the objective of positive schooling, and strength-based approaches, are one and the same: to create healthy individuals who not only excel in their own way, but also go on to become active and contributing members to the society to which they belong; at the foundation of positive schooling and mental health promotion is the same goal of optimal development.

Positive Schooling and Mental Health Promotion: A Note of Caution

Despite the fact that there are a number of benefits for adopting mental health promotion strategies in schools in an attempt to promote overall well-being of children, a few things need to be take into consideration. For one, despite the evidences that are outlined, we still need to have more evidences to say that mental health promotion programmes are truly beneficial (Spence and Shortt 2007). There also is a question about the quality of the programmes and programme implementation where there are reports that a number of programmes are not showing impact due to lack of consistent, rigorous, and faithful implementation (Weare and Nind 2011). Also, even in the event that an evidence-based programme is developed, it does not guarantee success unless executed well (Durlak et al. 2011). Another concern over the implementation of mental health promotion programmes is seen in the concern by many parents that these programmes will teach values that are not concomitant with the values that the parents wish to instil in their children (Arthur 2005).

There also is the worry of wasting precious resources of time and money or that such programmes may even worsen the students' achievement by distracting their attention from academic subjects (Benninga et al. 2006). Further, in situations where many basic needs of the children are not met—for example basic infrastructure such as clean water, toilet facilities, and basic materials for study—there is the question of whether time and resources should be invested on this. Adding to this, in the event that the programme does not produce desired results, funding bodies, organizations, staff, community stakeholders, and students, lose what they have invested, financially, and emotionally (Pluye et al. 2004).

Further, for a mental health promotion programme to be effective, it seems that working on skills alone is not enough; for optimal outcomes, the skills work needs to be embedded in a whole-school multi modal approach which, in turn, requires significant changes in the overall system of a particular school (Weare and Nind 2011). Furthermore, for schools to become actively involved in mental health promotion and to achieve positive schooling practices, it requires allocations of substantial resources in terms of professional development, developing curriculum, and also working with students in new ways (Slee et al. 2012). Another key issue is that it often becomes difficult to manage the transition between the development of a programme with a positive outcome evaluation and sustaining the programme in other settings, especially for longer periods of time (Slee et al. 2012). In addition, even within settings that are similar, structural affordances and constraints of educational organizations may influence the outcome of a programme (Resnick 2010).

Conclusion

Promoting healthy child and adolescent development is a priority for any community. Considering the fact that children, in most communities, spent a considerable amount of time in schools and educational institutions, it is crucial that attempts are made to utilize the time spent there in creating an environment of support and care where our children can thrive and achieve their best. The high rate of prevalence of mental health issues, as well as the limitations of a purely prevention-oriented approach in dealing with mental health issues, calls for changes in the school ethos to focusing on the strengths of students, and creating a positive school climate. Strength-based approaches, and mental health promotion, seem to be potential candidates to create a positive school culture, thus providing the children an opportunity for holistic development. We all have the responsibility to shape our nation. Schools, to achieve their true purpose, have to change and adapt to the newer approaches. Each one of us has the duty to do what is within our capacity to mobilize the potential lying dormant in schools; for our hope for the future lies in the children of today.

References

Aaron, R., Joseph, A., Abraham, S., Muliyil, J., George, K., Prasad, J., Bose, A., et al. (2004). Suicides in young people in rural southern India. *The Lancet, 363*(9415), 1117–1118.

Adi, Y., Killoran, A., Janmohamed, K., & Stewart-Brown, S. (2007). *Systematic review of the effectiveness of interventions to promote mental well-being in primary schools: Universal approaches which do not focus on violence or bullying*. London: National Institute for Clinical Excellence.

Alvord, M. K., & Grados, J. J. (2005). Enhancing resilience in children: A proactive approach. *Professional Psychology: Research and Practice, 36*(3), 238.

Arnett, J. J. (1999). Adolescent storm and stress, reconsidered. *American Psychologist, 54*(5), 317–326.

Arthur, J. (2005). The re-emergence of character education in British education policy. *British Journal of Educational Studies, 53*(3), 239–254.

Avenevoli, S., Knight, E., Kessler, R. C., & Merikangas, K. R. (2008). Epidemiology of depression in children and adolescents. *Handbook of Depression in Children and Adolescents*, 6–32.

Baltes, P. B., Reuter-Lorenz, P. A., & Rösler, F. (Eds.). (2006). *Lifespan development and the brain: The perspective of biocultural co-constructivism*. Cambridge University Press.

Barrett, P. M., Moore, A. F., & Sonderegger, R. (2000). The FRIENDS programme for young former-Yugoslavian refugees in Australia: A pilot study. *Behaviour Change, 17*(3), 124–133.

Barrett, P. M., Sonderegger, R., & Sonderegger, N. L. (2001). Evaluation of an anxiety-prevention and positive-coping programme (FRIENDS) for children and adolescents of non-English-speaking background. *Behaviour Change, 18*(2), 78–91.

Barry, M. M. (2007). Generic principles of effective mental health promotion. *International Journal of Mental Health Promotion, 9*(2), 4–16.

Beelmann, A., & Lösel, F. (2006). Child social skills training in developmental crime prevention: Effects on antisocial behaviour and social competence. *Psicothema, 18*(3).

Benninga, J. S., Berkowitz, M. W., Kuehn, P., & Smith, K. (2006). Character and academics: What good schools do. *Phi Delta Kappan, 87*(6), 448–452.

Benson, P. L., Mannes, M., Pittman, K., & Ferber, T. (2004). Youth development and public policy. In R. M. Lerner & L. Steinberg (Eds.), *Handbook of adolescent psychology* (pp. 781–814). Hoboken, NJ: Wiley.

Bharath, S., & Kumar, K. V. (2008). Health promotion using life skills education approach for adolescents in schools-development of a model. *Journal of Indian Association for Child and Adolescent Mental Health, 4*(1), 5–11.

Bharath, S., & Kumar, K. V. (2010). Empowering adolescents with life skills education in schools—School mental health program: Does it work? *Indian Journal of Psychiatry, 52*(4), 344.

Bond, L., Butler, H., Thomas, L., Carlin, J., Glover, S., Bowes, G., & Patton, G. (2007). Social and school connectedness in early secondary school as predictors of late teenage substance use, mental health, and academic outcomes. *Journal of Adolescent Health, 40*(4), 357–e9.

Bray, J. W., Zarkin, G. A., Dennis, M. L., & French, M. T. (2000). Symptoms of dependence, multiple substance use, and labor market outcomes. *The American Journal of Drug and Alcohol Abuse, 26*(1), 77–95.

Bridge, J. A., Asti, L., Horowitz, L. M., Greenhouse, J. B., Fontanella, C. A., Sheftall, A. H., et al. (2015). Suicide trends among elementary school—Aged children in the United States from 1993 to 2012. *JAMA Pediatrics, 169*(7), 673–677.

Browne, G., Gafni, A., Roberts, J., Byrne, C., & Majumdar, B. (2004). Effective/efficient mental health programmes for school-age children: A synthesis of reviews. *Social Science and Medicine, 58*(7), 1367–1384.

Cappella, E., Hamre, B. K., Kim, H. Y., Henry, D. B., Frazier, S. L., Atkins, M. S., et al. (2012). Teacher consultation and coaching within mental health practice: Classroom and child effects in urban elementary schools. *Journal of Consulting and Clinical Psychology, 80*(4), 597–610. https://doi.org/10.1037/a0027725.

Chabbott, C. (2004). *UNICEF's child-friendly schools framework: A desk review, report to UNICEF.*

Chadda, R. K., & Sengupta, S. N. (2002). Tobacco use by Indian adolescents. *Tobacco Induced Diseases, 1*(2), 111.

Chambers, R., & Conway, G. (1992). *Sustainable rural livelihoods: Practical concepts for the 21st century*. UK: Institute of Development Studies.

Chaskin, R., Brown, P., Venkatesh, S., Vidal, A., & Chaskin, R. (2001). Community capacity and capacity building: A definitional framework. *Building Community Capacity*, 7–26.

Cohen, J. (2006). Social, emotional, ethical, and academic education: Creating a climate for learning, participation in democracy, and well-being. *Harvard Educational Review, 76*(2), 201–237.

Cohen, J., & Geier, V. K. (2010). School climate research summary: January 2010. *School Climate Brief, 1*(1), 1–6.

Conduct Problems Prevention Research Group. (2010). The effects of a multiyear universal social-emotional learning program: The role of student and school characteristics. *Journal of Consulting and Clinical Psychology, 78*(2), 156–168. https://doi.org/10.1037/a0018607.

Cooperrider, D. L., Whitney, D. K., & Stavros, J. M. (2003). *Appreciative inquiry handbook* (Vol. 1). Berrett-Koehler Publishers.

Cosmides, L., & Tooby, J. (1997). *Evolutionary psychology: A primer.*

Cowen, E. L. (1994). The enhancement of psychological wellness: Challenges and opportunities. *American Journal of Community Psychology, 22*, 149–179.

Crime in India, The National Crime Records Bureau Report. (2009). Ministry of Home Affairs, Government of India.

Damon, W. (2004). What is positive youth development? *The Annals of the American Academy of Political and Social Science, 591,* 13–24.

Deater–Deckard, K., Dodge, K. A., Bates, J. E., & Pettit, G. S. (1998). Multiple risk factors in the development of externalizing behaviour problems: Group and individual differences. *Development and Psychopathology, 10*(3), 469–493.

Diekstra, R. F., & Gravesteijn, C. (2008). Effectiveness of school-based social and emotional education programmes worldwide. *Social and Emotional Education: An International Analysis*, 255–312.

Durlak, J. A., & Weissberg, R. P. (2007). The impact of after-school programmes that promote personal and social skills. *Collaborative for Academic, Social, and Emotional Learning (NJ1).*

Durlak, J. A., Weissberg, R. P., Dymnicki, A. B., Taylor, R. D., & Schellinger, K. B. (2011). The impact of enhancing students' social and emotional learning: A meta-analysis of school-based universal interventions. *Child Development, 82*(1), 405–432.

Estrada, C. A., Isen, A. M., & Young, M. J. (1994). Positive affect improves creative problem solving and influences reported source of practice satisfaction in physicians. *Motivation and Emotion, 18,* 285–299.

Ettner, S. L., Frank, R. G., & Kessler, R. C. (1997). The impact of psychiatric disorders on labor market outcomes. *ILR Review, 51*(1), 64–81.

Farmer, E. M., Burns, B. J., Phillips, S. D., Angold, A., & Costello, E. J. (2003). Pathways into and through mental health services for children and adolescents. *Psychiatric Services, 54*(1), 60–66.

Fergusson, D. M., Boden, J. M., & Horwood, L. J. (2007). Recurrence of major depression in adolescence and early adulthood, and later mental health, educational and economic outcomes. *The British Journal of Psychiatry, 191*(4), 335–342.

Foster, S., Rollefson, M., Doksum, T., Noonan, D., Robinson, G., & Teich, J. (2005). School mental health services in the United States, 2002-2003. *Substance Abuse and Mental Health Services Administration.*

Fredrickson, B. L., & Branigan, C. (2005). Positive emotions broaden the scope of attention and thought-action repertoires. *Cognition and Emotion, 19*(3), 313–332.

Fullan, M. (2001). The change. *Educational Leadership, 59*(8), 16–20.

GermAnn, K., & Ardiles, P. (2009). *Toward flourishing for all: Mental health promotion and mental illness prevention policy background paper.* Vancouver, BC: Pan-Canadian Steering Committee for Mental Health Promotion and Mental Illness Prevention. Retrieved from BC Mental Health & Addiction Services. http://www.bcmhas.ca/NR/rdonlyres/90672D9C-AFC9-4134-B52D-B956C12A4E56/35226/TowardFlourishingBackgroundPaperFinalApr09.pdf.

Guerra, N. G., & Bradshaw, C. P. (2008). Linking the prevention of problem behaviours and positive youth development: Core competencies for positive youth development and risk prevention. *New Directions for Child and Adolescent Development, 2008*(122), 1–17.

Hamilton, S. F., Hamilton, M. A., & Pittman, K. (2004). Principles for youth development. *The Youth Development Handbook: Coming of age in American Communities, 2,* 3–22.

Huang, K. Y., Cheng, S., & Theise, R. (2013). School contexts as social determinants of child health: Current practices and implications for future public health practice. *Public Health Reports, 128*(6_suppl3), 21–28.

Hunt, J., & Eisenberg, D. (2010). Mental health problems and help-seeking behaviour among college students. *Journal of Adolescent Health, 46,* 3–10.

Jané-Llopis, E. (2007). Mental health promotion: Concepts and strategies for reaching the population. *Health Promotion Journal of Australia, 18*(3), 191–197.

Jané-Llopis, E., Barry, M., Hosman, C., & Patel, V. (2005). Mental health promotion works: A review. *Promotion & Education, 12*(2_suppl), 9–25.

Keleher, H., & Armstrong, R. (2005). *Evidence-based mental health promotion resource.* Melbourne: Report for the Department of Human Services and VicHealth.

Kessler, R. C., Berglund, P. A., Demler, O., Jin, R., Merikangas, K. R., & Walters, E. E. (2005). Lifetime prevalence and age-of-onset distributions of DSM-IV disorders in the national comorbidity Survey Replication. *Archives of General Psychiatry, 62*, 593–602.

Kessler, R. C., Foster, C. L., Saunders, W. B., & Stang, P. E. (1995). Social consequences of psychiatric disorders, I: Educational attainment. *The American Journal of Psychiatry, 152*(7), 1026.

Kessler, R. C., Olfson, M., & Berglund, P. A. (1998). Patterns and predictors of treatment contact after first onset of psychiatric disorders. *American Journal of Psychiatry, 155*(1), 62–69.

Kiefer, H., Cohen, N., & Pape, B. (2004). Handle with care: Strategies for promoting the mental health of young children in community-based child care. Canadian Mental Health Association.

Kuhl, J. (2000). A functional-design approach to motivation and self-regulation. In T. M. Boekaerts, P. P. Pintrich, & M. Zeidner (toim.) *Handbook of self-regulation*.

Lavoie, J., Pereira, L. C., & Talwar, V. (2016). Children's physical resilience outcomes: Meta-analysis of vulnerability and protective factors. *Journal of Pediatric Nursing, 31*(6), 701–711.

Lee, J. W., & Barro, R. J. (2001). Schooling quality in a cross-section of countries. *Economica, 68* (272), 465–488.

Lerner, R. M. (2004). *Liberty: Thriving and civic engagement among America's youth*. Thousand Oaks, CA: Sage Publications.

Lerner, R. M., Lerner, J. V., & Phelps, E. (2008). *The positive development of youth: Report of the findings from the first four years of the 4-H study of positive youth development*. Medford, MA: Institute for Applied Research in Youth Development, Tufts University.

Malhotra, S., & Patra, B. N. (2014). Prevalence of child and adolescent psychiatric disorders in India: A systematic review and meta-analysis. *Child Adolescent Psychiatry Mental Health., 8* (22), 8.

Masten, A. S., Best, K. M., & Garmezy, N. (1990). Resilience and development: Contributions from the study of children who overcome adversity. *Development and Psychopathology, 2*(4), 425–444.

McGorry, P. D., Purcell, R., Hickie, I. B., & Jorm, A. F. (2007). Investing in youth mental health is a best buy. *Medical Journal of Australia, 187*(7), S5.

Mytton, J. A., DiGuiseppi, C., Gough, D., Taylor, R. S., & Logan, S. (2006). School-based secondary prevention programmes for preventing violence. *The Cochrane Library*.

Narvaez, D. (2010). Building a sustaining classroom climate for purposeful ethical citizenship. In: *International research handbook on values education and student well-being* (pp. 659–673). Netherlands: Springer.

Olfson, M., Kessler, R. C., Berglund, P. A., & Lin, E. (1998). Psychiatric disorder onset and first treatment contact in the United States and Ontario. *American Journal of Psychiatry, 155*(10), 1415–1422.

Olweus, D., Limber, S., & Mihalic, S. F. (1999). *Blueprints for violence prevention, book nine: Bullying prevention programme*. Boulder, CO: Center for the Study and Prevention of Violence.

Palfrey, J. S., Tonniges, T. F., Green, M., & Richmond, J. (2005). Introduction: Addressing the millennial morbidity—The context of community pediatrics. *Pediatrics, 115*(Supplement 3), 1121–1123.

Pape, B., & Galipeault, J. P. (2002). Mental health promotion for people with mental illness: A discussion paper. *Mental Health Promotion Unit of Health Canada*.

Parinduri, R. A. (2014). Do children spend too much time in schools? Evidence from a longer school year in Indonesia. *Economics of Education Review, 41*, 89–104.

Payton, J., Weissberg, R. P., Durlak, J. A., Dymnicki, A. B., Taylor, R. D., Schellinger, K. B., et al. (2008). The positive impact of social and emotional learning for kindergarten to eighth-grade students: Findings from three scientific reviews. Technical Report. *Collaborative for Academic, Social, and Emotional Learning (NJ1)*.

Pilowsky, D. J., Zybert, P. A., & Vlahov, D. (2004). Resilient children of injection drug users. *Journal of the American Academy of Child and Adolescent Psychiatry, 43*(11), 1372–1379.

Pluye, P., Potvin, L., Denis, J. L., & Pelletier, J. (2004). Programme sustainability: Focus on organizational routines. *Health Promotion International, 19*(4), 489–500.

Pollett, H. (2007). Mental health promotion: A literature review. *Ottawa, Ontario: Canadian Mental Health Association.* Retrieved February, 29, 2009.

Rapp, C. A., Pettus, C. A., & Goscha, R. J. (2006). Principles of strengths-based policy. *Journal of Policy Practice, 5*(4), 3–18.

Ravens-Sieberer, U., Auquier, P., Erhart, M., Gosch, A., Rajmil, L., Bruil, J., et al. (2007). The KIDSCREEN-27 quality of life measure for children and adolescents: psychometric results from a cross-cultural survey in 13 European countries. *Quality of Life Research, 16*(8), 1347–1356.

Resnick, L. B. (2010). Nested learning systems for the thinking curriculum. *Educational Researcher, 39*(3), 183–197.

Rönkä, A., & Pulkkinen, L. (1995). Accumulation of problems in social functioning in young adulthood: A developmental approach. *Journal of Personality and Social Psychology, 69*(2), 381.

Roth, J. L., & Brooks-Gunn, J. (2003). What exactly is a youth development program? Answers from research and practice. *Applied Developmental Science, 7*(2), 94–111.

Rowling, L. (2007). School mental health promotion: Mind matters as an example of mental health reform. *Health Promotion Journal of Australia, 18*(3), 229–235.

Sahu, B. (2002). *The new educational philosophy*. New Delhi: Sarup & Sons.

Sandler, I. N., West, S. G., Baca, L., Pillow, D. R., Gersten, J. C., Rogosch, F., et al. (1992). Linking empirically-based theory and evaluation: The Family Bereavement Programme. *American Journal of Community Psychology, 20*(4), 491–521.

Sartorius, N. (2006). Lessons from a 10-year global programme against stigma and discrimination because of an illness. *Psychology, Health & Medicine, 11*(3), 383–388.

Scales, P. C., Benson, P. L., Roehlkepartain, E. C., Sesma, A., & van Dulmen, M. (2006). The role of developmental assets in predicting academic achievement: A longitudinal study. *Journal of Adolescence, 29*(5), 691–708.

Seligman, M. E., Ernst, R. M., Gillham, J., Reivich, K., & Linkins, M. (2009). Positive education: Positive psychology and classroom interventions. *Oxford Review of Education, 35*(3), 293–311.

Severson, H. H., & Walker, H. M. (2002). Proactive approaches for identifying children at risk for socio-behavioural problems. *Interventions for Children With or At Risk for Emotional and Behavioural Disorders*, 33–53.

Shaffer, D. R., & Kipp, K. (2010). Introduction to developmental psychology and its research strategies. In D. R. Shaffer & K. Kipp (8 Eds.) *Developmental psychology: Childhood and adolescence* (pp. 1–39).

Shanahan, M. J., Valsiner, J., & Gottlieb, G. (1997). *Developmental concepts across disciplines* (pp. 13–71). Comparisons in Human Development: Understanding Time and Context.

Shochet, I. M., Dadds, M. R., Holland, D., Whitefield, K., Harnett, P. H., & Osgarby, S. M. (2001). The efficacy of a universal school-based programme to prevent adolescent depression. *Journal of Clinical Child Psychology, 30*(3), 303–315.

Shorey, H. S., Snyder, C. R., Yang, X., & Lewin, M. R. (2003). The role of hope as a mediator in recollected parenting, adult attachment, and mental health. *Journal of Social and Clinical Psychology, 22*(6), 685–715.

Short, R. J., & Talley, R. C. (1997). Rethinking psychology and the schools. *American Psychologist, 52*(3), 234–240.

Sigelman, C. K., & Rider, E. A. (2009). Developmental psychopathology. In Life-span human development (6th ed., pp. 468–495). Belmont, CA: Wadsworth Cengage Learning.

Silbereisen, R. K., & Lerner, R. M. (2007). Approaches to positive youth development: A view of the issues. *Approaches to Positive Youth Development*, 3–30.

Slee, P. T., Dix, K. L., & Askell-Williams, H. (2012). Whole-school mental health promotion in Australia. *The International Journal and Education, 3*(2), 37–49.

Small, S., & Memmo, M. (2004). Contemporary models of youth development and problem prevention: Toward an integration of terms, concepts, and models. *Family Relations, 53*(1), 3–11.

Snyder, C. R., Lopez, S. J., & Pedrotti, J. T. (2010). *Positive psychology: The scientific and practical explorations of human strengths*. Sage Publications.

Sourander, A., Multimäki, P., Santalahti, P., Parkkola, K., Haavisto, A., Helenius, H., et al. (2004). Mental health service use among 18-year-old adolescent boys: A prospective 10-year follow-up study. *Journal of the American Academy of Child & Adolescent Psychiatry, 43*(10), 1250–1258.

Spence, S. H., & Shortt, A. L. (2007). Research review: Can we justify the widespread dissemination of universal, school-based interventions for the prevention of depression among children and adolescents? *Journal of Child Psychology and Psychiatry, 48*(6), 526–542.

Srinath, S., Girimaji, S. C., Gururaj, G., & Seshadri, S. (2005). Epidemiological study of child & adolescent psychiatric disorders in urban & rural areas of Bangalore, India. *Indian Journal of Medical Research, 122*(1), 67.

UNICEF. (2002). *Adolescence: A time that matters*. UNICEF.

UNICEF. (2016). *The formative years: UNICEF's work on measuring early childhood development*.

Vranda, M. N. (2015). Promotion of mental health and well-being of adolescents in schools—A NIMHANS model. *Journal of Psychiatry, 18,* 303. https://doi.org/10.4172/2378-5756.1000303.

Waddell, C., Hua, J. M., Garland, O. M., DeV Peters, R., & McEwan, K. (2007a). Preventing mental disorders in children: A systematic review to inform policy-making. *Canadian Journal of Public Health/Revue Canadienne de Sante'e Publique*, 166–173.

Waddell, C., Peters, R. V., Hua, R. M., & McEwan, K. (2007b). Preventing mental disorders in children: A systematic review to inform policy-making. *Canadian Review of Public Health, 98,* 166–173.

Weare, K. (2010). Mental Health and social and emotional learning: Evidence, principles, tensions, balances. *Advances in School Mental Health Promotion, 3,* 5–17.

Weare, K., & Nind, M. (2011). Mental health promotion and problem prevention in schools: What does the evidence say? *Health Promotion International, 26*(suppl_1), i29-i69.

Weist, M. D. (2005). Fulfilling the promise of school-based mental health: Moving toward a public mental health promotion approach. *Journal of Abnormal Child Psychology, 33*(6), 735–741.

Wolchik, S. A., et al. (1993). The children of divorce parenting intervention: Outcome evaluation of an empirically-based programme. *American Journal of Community Psychology, 21*(3), 231–293.

World Health Organization. (2002). *The world health report 2002: Reducing risks, promoting healthy life*. World Health Organization.

World Health Organization. (2005). *WHO global atlas of traditional, complementary and alternative medicine* (Vol. 2). World Health Organization.

World Health Organization. (2016). *World Health Statistics 2016: Monitoring health for the SDGs sustainable development goals*. World Health Organization.

Chapter 9
The Critical Role of Schools in Adolescent Mental Health Care: Organizing Systems and Developing Pathways

Chetna Duggal and Lamia Bagasrawala

Abstract Adolescence is a period of rapid psycho-social development offering great opportunities for identity exploration, critical thinking, and skill-building. As adolescents strive to fulfil the tasks of this exciting yet challenging period, the strain on existing internal and external resources, and the demand for supportive systems, increases. The absence or inaccessibility of such supportive and care mechanisms can have a significant impact on the emotional and social well-being of adolescents. In India, this is visible in the increasing prevalence of suicides, and the prevalence of mental health concerns, among adolescents. This, coupled with the shortage of mental health professionals and insufficient mental health care services in India, calls for integration of mental health with other primary systems of care and support. Schools are one such system catering to a large group of children and adolescents. This chapter, therefore, aims to highlight the significant mental health concerns experienced by adolescents, and to discuss the potential of a school as a site for mental health advocacy and care. It is argued that, as a microcosm of society, schools can create a mentally healthy climate for students by changing the discourse from an illness-based approach to a well-being model. This chapter further proposes the idea of schools adopting a multi-level approach and mobilizing resources for mental health promotion, prevention, and intervention. For this, the roles and responsibilities of different stakeholders—school leaders, parents, teachers, peers, and mental health professionals—in the Indian context, are discussed and the importance of collective efforts is emphasized.

Keywords Mental health · Schools · Adolescents · School climate
Intervention · Promotion · Prevention · Advocacy

C. Duggal (✉)
School of Human Ecology, Tata Institute of Social Sciences, Mumbai, India
e-mail: chetnaduggal@gmail.com

L. Bagasrawala
Mumbai, India

S. Deb (ed.), *Positive Schooling and Child Development*,
https://doi.org/10.1007/978-981-13-0077-6_9

Introduction

Adolescence is a period of transition from childhood to adulthood. As adolescents transition into adulthood, they experience a wide range of physical, emotional, and social changes. Physiologically, with the initiation of puberty, adolescent boys and girls experience bodily changes, coupled with reproductive and sexual development. Erikson's theory of psychosocial development also emphasizes adolescence as a crucial period of identity development. At this time, individuals explore their social roles, discover their sexual identity, and develop life goals. If they experience role confusion, or are unable to develop an integrated sense of self, they may experiment with different lifestyle choices, be unable to pursue their goals, and may experience psychosocial distress. It is important, therefore, for adolescents to receive adequate and appropriate support to navigate this stage successfully.

In addition to psycho-social development, studies from neuroscience show that, during adolescence, the brain goes through rapid changes, both in structure and function. During this period, higher level cognitive abilities—such as planning, decision making, and reasoning—begin to develop. This is because the prefrontal cortex, associated with the development of these abilities, goes through the process of pruning. The unused neural connections are eliminated and the white matter in this region increases (Steinberg 2012). This period is also characterized by increased activity of dopamine, which plays a critical role in how individuals experience pleasure and reward. This is important in understanding the increase in sensation-seeking and risky behaviours—such as rash driving, substance abuse or adventure sports—among adolescents.

Neurologically, the connections between the prefrontal cortex (the cognitive parts of the brain) and the limbic system (the structures dealing with emotions) are also strengthening during adolescence. This has great implications on how adolescents process emotions, make meaning of emotional experiences, and regulate emotions. It is also important to note that these neurological changes do not happen at the same time. While cognitive processes may develop by mid-adolescence, brain regions involved in emotion regulation may continue to develop until late adolescence. This implies that young adolescents may have strong intellectual understanding but may take longer to develop socio-emotional skills. This may explain why adolescents are often easily influenced by peer pressure and engage in risky activities like drug use or unsafe sexual experimentation (Steinberg 2010).

While adolescents experience, and sometimes struggle to deal with, these changes, they are also continuously influenced by socio-cultural expectations and experiences. This is particularly evident in the process of gender intensification during adolescence. The gender intensification hypothesis states that young boys and girls begin to demonstrate sex-typed behaviours and traits peculiar to masculinity and femininity during adolescence (Galambos et al. 1990). This may be attributed to the process of gender socialization within families and society. While factors like family context and individual characteristics play a role in this process, there is considerable research and evidence which shows that boys and girls face pressure to conform to gender roles and adopt stereotypical gender-role attitudes and behaviours during early adolescence (Priess et al. 2009). Such pressures can be extremely challenging for young individuals, as they try to fit into culturally sanctioned roles and identities.

The psychological experiences of adolescents are influenced by their biological and genetic factors and the larger socio-cultural system. There are a range of factors that may either facilitate the process of healthy development or hinder this process. While some adolescents may adapt to these bio-psycho-social changes with or without social support, some others may experience distress and difficulties in coping with the demands of this life stage. It becomes critical therefore to understand the psychological concerns that adolescents are likely to experience and strengthen the ecosystem to help them transition through this period smoothly.

Adolescent Mental Health

In India, approximately 20% of the population is between the ages of 10 and 19 years (Census 2011). By 2020, it is predicted that India will have the highest percentage of young people in the world, with 34.33% of its total population between the ages of 15 and 24 years (Government of India 2017). India is likely to be one of the youngest nations in the world by 2020. It is important to invest in the health of these young individuals who will take up the role of a productive taskforce in the economy.

The World Health Organization aptly states that adolescence is a period of "tremendous growth and potential" but also that of "considerable risk" (WHO 2016). These risks, if left unaddressed, can have a lasting impact on the individual's life. As identified by UNICEF (2011), mental health problems, specifically depression, are one of the largest contributors to the global burden of disease on young people in the age group 15–19 years. Suicide, another relevant mental health problem, is the second leading cause of death among adolescents between 15 and 19 years of age, globally (WHO 2014). The developmental trajectory of psychological disorders further shows that most adult mental health concerns often have their onset during adolescence (Jones 2013). This data highlights the immediate need to address adolescent mental health concerns worldwide. This urgency has been identified by organizations like the United Nations and World Health Organization on multiple occasions. Recently, to mark the World Health Day 2017, the WHO declared 'Depression' as the theme and identified adolescents and young adults as an important target group.

Prevalence of Adolescent Mental Health Concerns in India

The prevalence of psychological disorders among adolescents in India over the last fifteen years presents a diverse picture. The Census (2011) reports that 1,10,189 adolescents between the ages of 10 and 19 years in the country have a mental illness. The data from epidemiological studies—conducted in community settings and schools using self-report inventories and clinical screening instruments—show a varied prevalence rate of mental illness among adolescents ranging from 0.20% (National Sample Survey Organisation 2003) to 45.8% (Arun and Chavan 2009). This variation may be attributed to the wide range of psychological disorders assessed across various studies, the difference in sampling and data collection processes, settings of the study, as well as variation in defining psychological disorders and mental health concerns.

In the recent National Mental Health Survey (NIMHANS 2016), it was found that 7.3% of adolescents in the age group 13–17 years, across four States of India, were experiencing some psychological disorder with depression, agoraphobia, intellectual disability, autism spectrum disorder, anxiety and psychotic disorders being the most common in this age group. This data is congruent with prevalence rates obtained from other epidemiological studies. Depression is very common among adolescents with prevalence rates as high as 37% (Chandrashekarappa et al. 2016) and 10.3% (Mishra and Sharma 2001). Anxiety related disorders such as generalized anxiety (6.7%), Obsessive Compulsive Disorder (OCD) (7.8%), and panic attacks (15.7%) have also been found to be highly prevalent among adolescents (Chandrashekarappa et al. 2016). Apart from emotional concerns, adolescents also experience behavioural problems like Conduct disorder (16.7%) (Reddy et al. 2011), Attention deficit Hyperactivity Disorder (ADHD) (4.3%) (Patil et al. 2013) and Oppositional Defiant Disorder (ODD) (0.9%) (Srinath et al. 2005). Psychotic symptoms and disorders are also prevalent (1.87%) (Gaur et al. 2003) in this age group.

Substance abuse is another commonly reported mental health problem among Indian adolescents. Alcohol use (15%) (Jaisoorya et al. 2016) and addiction to drugs like *ganja* and marijuana (8.18%) (Sharma and Chaudhary 2016) is common among teenagers in schools, in urban and rural India. In addition to these common mental disorders, with the rise in technological advancements and the arrival of the digital age, adolescents are increasingly using the internet; thus, addiction to internet is also on the rise (Goel et al. 2013; Jhala and Sharma 2017).

Other common psycho-social concerns experienced by adolescents include peer-related problems contributing significantly to difficulties in everyday life: friendships and classroom interactions (Bhola et al. 2016; Reddy et al. 2011) as well as feelings of loneliness and worry (Samanta et al. 2012).

The trends from epidemiological studies therefore show that clinically diagnosable common mental disorders such as depression, anxiety, behavioural concerns, substance abuse and psychosis and psycho-social concerns seem to be common among adolescents in India. These psychological disorders and concerns are found to be prevalent among both boys and girls, and there is an absence of any conclusive data on the gender differences, if any, at the national level.

The Lancet Commission report (2016) states that suicide is the leading cause of death among adolescent boys and girls in India. The National Crime Records Bureau reports that suicide rates among adolescents and youth in the age group 15–29 years has been increasing every year. The rates increased from 3.73 to 3.96 per 1,00,000 population between 2002 and 2011 (as cited in Singh and Gururaj 2014). India has been reported as having the highest suicide rate (35.5%) for individuals between the ages 15 and 24 years, according to the WHO report on preventing suicide (WHO 2014). In India, academic stress has been identified as a key factor, placing many students at risk for suicide. In Kota, where the maximum number of students in the country flock to receive coaching for medical and engineering exams, the suicide rates are recorded to be as high as 17 suicides in 2016 (Hindustan Times 2017).

The prevalence data presents the crucial need to address these adolescent mental health problems. In doing so, it is important to recognize that some factors within the larger ecosystem can alleviate mental distress while some can increase the risk of developing a mental disorder. For example, factors such as family and social support (Mehta et al. 2015), secure parenting, and positive learning environments within school (WHO 2012), are protective factors in preventing adolescents from experiencing psychological disorders. However, factors like death of parents, poor financial circumstances at home (Bhola et al. 2016), as well as adverse learning environments, peer pressure, and difficulties at school (WHO 2012), can place adolescents at a higher risk for developing mental disorders.

Conceptualizing Adolescent Mental Health Concerns Along a Continuum

As seen above, the concerns that students experience are complex, and across multiple domains including emotional, interpersonal, behavioural, and social. The signs, symptoms, and manifestations of each of these concerns vary greatly and so does the impact on the individual's functioning and well-being. It is important therefore to conceptualize mental health along a spectrum ranging from well-being, at one end, to mental illness on the other. This understanding of mental health, as seen in Fig. 9.1, helps to identify the services and systems required to address adolescent needs at different points along the continuum. This model has been developed by combining the mental health wellness continuum of the Rural Adversity Mental Health Program (2015), Australia, with the adaptation of the Institute of Medicine mental health intervention spectrum (Mrazek and Haggerty 1994).

Adolescents, who may be emotionally healthy and adapting well to their social context, may not be in need of mental healthcare services. However, these young

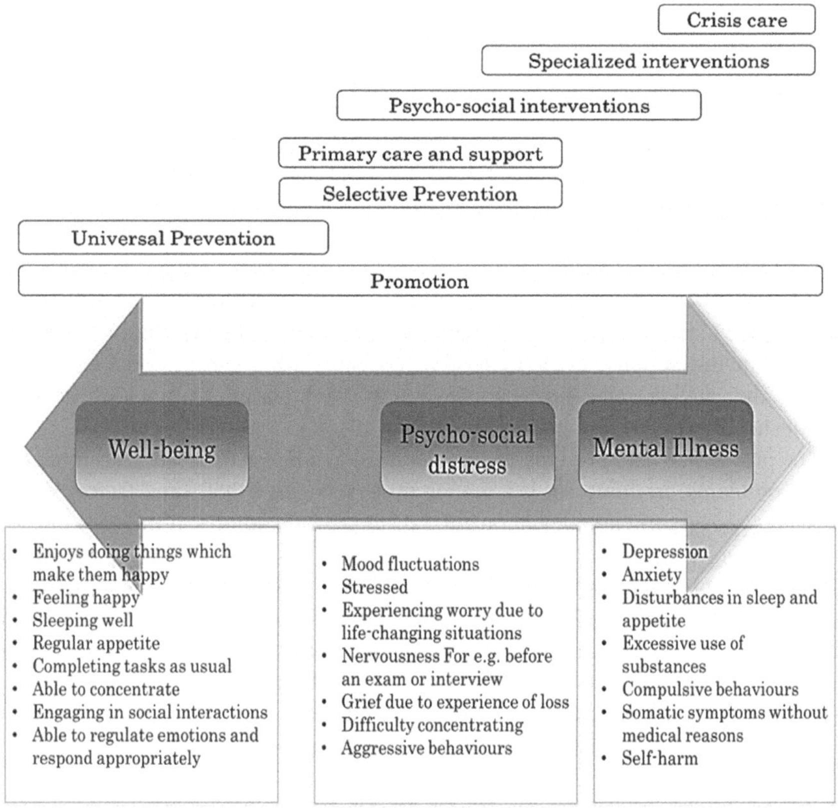

Fig. 9.1 Mental healthcare continuum and services along the continuum

individuals require continuous support and a safe environment to maintain their emotional state of well-being and prevent them from sliding to the other end of the spectrum. Adolescents who may experience some psycho-social concerns—such as exam anxiety or difficulty in a romantic relationship—are likely to feel distressed and in need of special support to feel better. This support, provided by structures within the microsystem, will help the adolescents to cope with the difficult circumstances and prevent them from experiencing mental illness. The other end of the spectrum includes common and severe mental disorders such as depression, psychosis, substance abuse, and self-harm. Adolescents experiencing such concerns are in need of specialized mental health services including psychotherapy, crisis care, or in some cases, psychiatric medication. In such situations, it is important to ensure that once the problem is addressed, efforts are also made to prevent the young individual from experiencing similar concerns in the future and to enhance his/her well-being. In this chapter, the role of a school in addressing mental health needs along the continuum, and the possibilities of strengthening systems within the school to provide healthcare services ranging from promotion to specialized care, will be discussed.

Schools as Mental Healthcare Sites

Schools are one of the most integral structures of a child's ecological system. In addition to the primary contribution of schools in providing literacy, numeracy, and scientific knowledge, schools play an important role in children's emotional and social development (Greenberg et al. 2003; Sylva 1994) and psychological health. The experience children have at school not only influences their development trajectory but also plays a role in later life outcomes. For instance, the long-term negative impact of bullying in schools on emotional well-being as adults (Wolke and Lereya 2015), as well as the long-term positive influence of school-based early childhood emotional and social programmes on social adjustment (Barnett 1995), has been well documented. This shows that the school plays a significant role in the development of individuals, as well as the larger society and community.

The role of a school in a child's life is comprehensively explained by the ecological systems theory. As stated in the ecological systems theory of human development (Bronfenbrenner 1979), school is one of the most significant structures in the child's microsystem, along with the family and neighbourhood. These structures in the child's immediate environment interact with one another to influence the child's development. Bronfenbrenner (1979) identifies the relationship between the school and the home as a significant factor influencing the child's ability to learn. The school system is further influenced by social norms and cultural values which are part of the exo-system and macro-system. While the school can play a major role in nurturing children and integrating them into the society, schools also have the potential to emulate and echo social discrimination and exclusion (Morrison 2002). It is, therefore, important to review and strengthen the role of schools as a primary microsystem in promoting child development and creating a safe environment that creates emotionally resilient and mentally healthy individuals.

Over the last decade, globally, there has been considerable focus on the role of education and schooling in furthering development. The United Nations' Sustainable Development Goals (SDGs) identifies the need to "ensure inclusive and equitable quality education for all" as one of the key goals and an important instrument in attaining the other SDGs (UNESCO 2017). The goal clearly states that a safe, non-violent, inclusive, and effective learning environment, along with opportunities for skill-development, is required for sustainable development. This essentially means that the focus is not merely on academic outcomes but also on engaging the learner and empowering them in skills and competencies required in the twenty-first century (UNESCO 2017). Schools are, therefore, not merely academic institutions but spaces contributing to the holistic development of the individual.

The idea of utilizing schools to facilitate adolescent well-being has gained much popularity over the years. There is consistent evidence over the years on the impact of psychological distress and mental health on academic outcomes among school students (Sylva 1994), especially adolescents (McLeod et al. 2012; Rothon et al. 2009). Studies have found that immediate and long-term life satisfaction have been negatively associated with adolescent mental health concerns (Guneya et al. 2010; Nishida et al. 2016) and positively associated with self-esteem and healthy peer relationships during adolescence (Huang et al. 2014). This has made it imperative for schools worldwide to give prime importance to the mental health and well-being of their students.

Mental health programmes at various levels within the school have been implemented globally for years. Schools are home to a large number of adolescents and, as discussed earlier, have a profound impact on the individual's life (Hendren et al. 1994). From school-based health centres to multi-tiered systems of support, schools around the globe are adopting different practices to provide social, emotional, and behavioural assistance to students. Mental health care services globally, have been found to be more effective when provided in students' natural environment, such as schools (Atkins et al. 2000), and when integrated with their learning environment. In addition to affordable and easily accessible services, school-based mental health care is also found to be effective in educating teachers about their own mental health and its impact on students (Chamberlin 2009). School-based services are effective in early identification, diagnosis, and treatment of children and adolescents (Committee on School Health 2004). In a meta-analysis of school-based mental health programmes, it was found that students in schools with a social and emotional learning programme showed an increase in performance on standardized scores as compared to students in non-intervention schools (as cited in Fazel et al. 2014). The need and benefits of school-based programmes have been acknowledged and documented globally.

The key question, however, is that, in an education system which is strongly driven by academic performance, where does the mental health of adolescent students fit in? As discussed above, the mental and emotional well-being of students is extremely important, not only from a public health perspective, but also from the academic viewpoint. It is important, therefore, to identify ways of converging mental health and education in India to promote adolescent mental health support in schools. This will also help address the huge treatment gap that the Indian mental health system is grappling with. In India, the National Mental Health Survey (NMHS) (NIMHANS 2016) reports that 9.8 million adolescents between 13 and 17 years of age are in need of mental health interventions. However, there is a dearth of mental health professionals, with numbers as low as 3800 psychiatrists and 898 clinical psychologists (Government of India 2014). Therefore, it is inevitable and critical to involve the Indian Education system, which caters to a large section of the Indian adolescent population, to help bridge this treatment gap. Schools are, therefore, an essential site, not only for mental health intervention, but also to support adolescent mental health needs along the mental health spectrum.

Mental Health Care in the Indian School Education System

According to the UNICEF data on attendance rates, between the years 2009 and 2015, 85% of primary school-age children and 61% of secondary school-age children are attending schools worldwide (UNICEF 2016). In India, there are approximately 13,06,992 schools providing primary, secondary, and high school education to students and approximately 212,748,064 students are enrolled across these sections in urban and rural areas (Government of India 2009a, b). With education policies like the Sarva Shiksha Abhiyan (2001) and the Right of Children to Free and Compulsory Education Act (RTE) (2009), education in schools has received great priority in the last decade and half in India. The RTE makes schooling and education free and mandatory for those between 6 and 14 years of age. The number of students enrolling in schools is also on the rise, with a 12.53% increase in the school enrolment rate from 2002 to 2009, as reported by the All India School Education Survey (The British Council 2014). As of 2014–15, 78.5% students are enrolled in secondary schools in India (Government of India 2016), making it inevitable to explore the critical role of schools in student well-being.

In order to understand the role of schools in the Indian context, it is important to acquaint oneself with the vast schooling system, the existing frameworks for student mental health, and the contextual factors influencing the system. The school education system in India is one of the largest and complex systems in the world (The British Council 2014). Such a composite system can be better understood along two major dimensions: affiliation to educational boards and school ownership.

Classification of Schools Based on Educational Board Affiliation

Most schools in India are governed by different curriculum bodies and boards, including the State Government boards, Central Board of Secondary Education (CBSE), Council for the Indian School Certificate Examination (CISCE), National Institute of Open Schooling Board (NIOS), International Baccalaureate (IB), International General Certificate of Secondary Education (IGCSE), and Cambridge International Examinations. The needs and concerns of students across these boards are quite different, as each board caters to distinct socio-economic strata. Having said that, the resources and systems in each board to address these needs are also very different, making the system elaborate and multifaceted. The Council of

Boards of School Education in India (COBSE) is a voluntary association of all school boards in India including the State boards, CISCE, CBSE, and NIOS. Established in 1979, the COBSE works in collaboration with the Ministry of Human Resource Development (MHRD), Government of India, and other national level educational agencies like the National Council of Educational Research and Training (NCERT), National University of Educational Planning and Administration (NUEPA), and National Council of Teacher Education (NCTE). COBSE is involved in curriculum planning, exam framework development, setting educational standards, evaluating schools and coordinating between different boards. While COBSE acts as an apex body, each of these boards attempts to address the education and development needs of the students in different ways. The teaching and learning processes, school environments, and learning outcomes, are defined differently across these boards. In addition to the vast diversity in the academic curriculum, there are significant differences between boards in the curriculum for socio-emotional development.

The importance of socio-emotional development in education has been acknowledged at the policy and framework level in India. This is reflected in the series of different programmatic initiatives within the country over the last three decades. In 1978, the Ministry of Education had introduced 'Socially Useful Productive Work (SUPW)' as part of its endeavour to promote Gandhian values among school students. While most schools stopped including it in the curriculum, the CISCE council has made SUPW and community service mandatory for high school students. At the national level, the Adolescence Education Programme (AEP) was launched in 2005 as a partnership between the NCERT, MHRD, and United Nations Population Fund (UNFPA). The AEP was developed in response to the recommendations enlisted in the National Curriculum Framework (NCF) (2005). The NCF highlights the need for holistic development, and building life skills, and identifies mental health as one of the many areas of focus within school. However, the NCF does not identify mental health as a separate component, and does not provide any guidelines to promote or address mental health concerns in schools. The framework describes the need for school counselling but only in the context of career guidance and reducing academic stress related to Grade 10 and 12 Board examinations. At the programmatic level, the AEP aims specifically at empowering adolescents by imparting knowledge about adolescence and adolescent-related concerns—like substance abuse and developing life skills—to protect them from risky situations. The AEP has been conceptualized as a programme to be implemented by agencies such as the Kendriya Vidyalaya Sangathan, Navodaya Vidyalaya Samiti, NCERT, CBSE, and others. In 2005, the CBSE board designed a life-skills curriculum for Grades 6–10, along with reference manuals for teachers to execute the curriculum in school. This curriculum focuses on the core life skills provided by the WHO.

While socio-emotional learning has been identified as a significant aspect of schooling across educational boards and by the Government, the programmes and frameworks do not have a strong mental health mandate and coverage. These programmes have been developed for adolescents in secondary or high school, and include components on interpersonal relationships, physical growth, safety, emotion regulation, and prevention of HIV/AIDS. As might be evident, the focus of the programmes is mainly limited to growing-up issues, safety, peer-related issues, and academic stress. However, apart from prevention of substance abuse, these programmes do not include a strong mental health component. Other common mental health concerns, or topics related to counselling and help-seeking, are not included in these programmes. In the current system, therefore, the educational boards are offering multiple opportunities for schools to promote and strengthen students' social and emotional skills. However, they do not provide learning standards, quality guidelines, and review mechanisms to assess the impact of the programmes (Singh and Menon 2015). Therefore, while programmatic initiatives have been planned, these have not been designed as sustainable models that can be implemented, and lack a mental health approach and mandate. This is a major gap and challenge in the current school education system in India that must be overcome to address adolescent mental health concerns discussed in the previous section.

Classification of Schools Based on Ownership

The complexity of challenges in integrating mental healthcare with the education system increases when the segregation of schools according to their ownership is taken into consideration. The ownership of the school determines the availability and accessibility of resources and provisions within the school and its impact on student well-being. In India, some schools are run by the government while others are managed by the private sector. Among the government schools, some are managed by the central or state governments—such as the Kendriya Vidyalaya, Military schools, and so on—and others are funded by the local governing bodies such as the Zilla Parishads, Panchayats, and so on. Among private schools, some are completely funded by private sector organizations or Trusts, while others are managed privately but receive financial aid from the government. Although the total number of public sector schools is much higher, constituting about 78% of all schools in India, the enrolment rates in higher grades is greater for private sector schools (The British Council 2014).

In addition to these categories, over the last decade, the public-private partnerships (PPP) in school education have also strengthened. The PPP model can help address many existing challenges in the Indian schooling such as quality, affordability, and access (Chaudhry and Uboweja 2014). For instance, the central government's Model school scheme and collaborations with non-profit organizations, like the Akanksha Foundation, are efforts in this direction to provide innovative, effective, and affordable education for all.

The government, private, and PPP schools differ greatly from each other. The fee structure, infrastructure, teaching and learning processes, and curriculum, across these schools varies greatly, and so do the needs of the students they cater to (The British Council 2014). The picture gets more complex when the system is reviewed along the axes of geographical location, urban versus rural setting, strength of the institution, availability of skilled teaching faculty, characteristics of school leadership, and involvement of community in school decision making. This variation is reflected in the diverse challenges, discussed below, that schools experience, depending on their ownership, cultural setting, and the socio-economic background of students.

Private schools in India are more likely to have better amenities and infrastructure as compared to public schools. Private schools have better access to toilets, drinking water, libraries, and electricity connections, and more teachers, as compared to government schools (Singh 2013). However, they are also likely to have more students in the classroom. Enrolment in government schools is reducing and, while the pupil-teacher ratio is acceptable as per the RTE (2009) norms (30:1), multi-grade classrooms are also very common. Teachers in government schools are teaching two or more grades in a single classroom in both urban (Singh and Sarkar 2012) and rural (Bhattacharjea et al. 2011) areas. This makes the teacher's task more complex, as they have to consider variability in age, diversity in ability, and curriculum appropriateness. It is important to note that the RTE (2009) does not provide any provisions for multi-grade classrooms.

Corporal punishment is another major concern among government and private schools. According to the Young Lives school survey (2010–11), in Andhra Pradesh, students in private schools, and those residing in urban areas, reported higher levels of corporal punishment than their counterparts in government schools, and those residing in rural areas (Morrow and Singh 2014). Similar differences in the prevalence of corporal punishment between public and private schools have also been found in another study of adolescents in Pondicherry (Deb et al. 2017).

Teaching and the attitudes of teachers is also found to be different across schools. The Young Lives School Survey (2010–11) found that 23% of students in government schools perceive their teachers to be biased, compared to 14% in recognized private unaided schools. This is likely to impact the classroom environment and the student–teacher relationship, which is integral to the learning process. Students are likely to learn better if teachers are motivated and happy in their workspaces. Teachers' motivation is highly linked to their beliefs about the school. However, it was found that only 50% of teachers in government schools thought highly of their schools, compared to 80% of teachers in recognized private unaided schools. The survey also found that teacher absenteeism was higher in public schools. However, dismissal of teachers by higher authority was high in private schools, but nil in public schools. The authors deliberate that the permanent nature of employment and poor supervision in public schools, could result in less accountability among teachers (Singh and Sarkar 2012).

Current Status of Mental Healthcare in Indian Schools: Needs and Challenges

In India, the concept of school-based mental health services is not new. The review conducted by Bharath et al. (2008) highlights various school mental health programmes initiated over the years. According to the review, one of the first such programmes was initiated by the Child Psychiatry Unit, NIMHANS in 1976. The programme involved training school teachers in child and adolescent mental health across thirteen sessions. Over the years, NIMHANS has conducted many skill development trainings for teachers and developed and executed life skills education curriculum. In Mumbai, a school mental health clinic was established in early 1980s, to address the psychological needs of school-going students. The clinic offered a student-enrichment programme to students performing poorly in the academic sphere. Similarly, many other projects and programmes have been implemented in various regions including Mangalore, Chennai, Delhi, and Kerala. However, most of these programmes have either worked with specific target groups or were short-term projects, not integrated with the school curriculum. This review also put forth the need for a comprehensive and holistic school mental health programme for all students of the school (Bharath et al. 2008). In light of this need, and the existing school enrolment data reviewed earlier, it is important to maximize the potential of schools in enhancing student mental health.

As discussed in the previous section, Indian schools have a huge untapped potential to promote and enhance mental health of large numbers of adolescents. Schools provide easy access to infrastructure and skilled human resources, making them a potential site for implementing mental health programmes and interventions. However, this is only one aspect of the larger picture and the current status of Indian schools is not all promising. The Indian school education scenario is multi-layered and multi-dimensional. At the national level, the Indian school education system is a myriad of complex structures with varying needs and demands. The availability and accessibility of resources across all these schools is inequitable, and so are their capacities to address student needs. The variability is also reflected in the wide range of decision-making agencies and boards and the diversity of stakeholders across these schools. This, coupled with the lack of implementing provisions and a monitoring agency, makes the picture seem rather alarming.

Despite these complexities, schools have made an attempt to introduce mental health as a key component in education through programmes like the AEP and CBSE life-skills education. However, there is absence of national-level data on the progress and impact of both these programmes. In such a situation where review mechanisms are not systematically included in the programme framework, there is no substantial way of identifying strengths of these programmes, the challenges encountered in implementing them and the outcomes for students and schools. This makes the scenario more challenging in the absence of any documented evidence on school-based mental health programmes for adolescents in India.

When all these challenges are viewed in the context of the wide spectrum of mental health concerns that adolescents are experiencing, the task at hand seems insurmountable. In order to address the heterogeneous needs of this group discussed earlier, it is essential for schools to provide mental health services across all levels of care, including mental health promotion, prevention, and intervention. This will ensure that all students in the school receive adequate and appropriate support required to transition smoothly into adulthood. In view of the treatment gap, it is essential to include all stakeholders of the school community including teachers, leaders, and staff, in providing school-based mental healthcare services to students. Therefore, on a closer look, school-based mental healthcare in India would need to be an intricate web of complex structures with a large human capital and a strong vision for adolescent well-being. The unique challenges that the Indian school education system faces can be addressed by a model that is as inclusive and flexible to accommodate the diverse conditions of the schooling system and needs of the students.

Globally, school-based mental healthcare services are categorized into three models (Committee on School Health 2004). The first model is a school-supported mental health model which includes services provided by the school counsellor, social worker, and an in-school mental health clinic. The second model is the community connections model, whereby the school seeks mental health services from an offsite counsellor, professional, or agency, who delivers the services to the school contractually. And the third model is the comprehensive integrated model, which addresses mental health needs of the entire school by including prevention programmes, referrals, direct mental health services, as well as involvement of families and caregivers. In the Indian context, in view of the challenges and concerns discussed above, the third model seems like the best fit. It is, therefore, critical for school-based mental health care services in India to include four key characteristics, derived after reviewing the existing system and needs. These are: a guiding framework, an integrated model, a multi-level approach, and optimal utilization of existing resources.

Since the diversity across schools in India is so wide, one programme cannot meet the needs of all students. It is essential for the model to serve as a guiding blueprint that schools can adopt and implement creatively to meet their requirements. The mental health programmes must not run parallel with the academic curriculum but must be integrated into the learning environments for highest impact. These services are designed for the entire adolescent school-going population and therefore demands a multi-level approach, which not only focuses on providing interventions to those in need but also on enhancing the well-being of all students. And lastly, the model must ensure that the entire school community is involved in this process to reduce dependency on specialized care. Such a model will guide the designing and development of effective school-based programmes. The next section of the chapter will describe one such model, the World Health Organization (WHO) integrated model for school mental health. The model reflects all the four characteristics discussed above and can serve as a suitable framework in the Indian context.

An Integrated Approach to School Mental Health: The WHO Model

As learning institutions, schools must provide a safe and enriching environment to students to facilitate academic achievement and social, psychological, and emotional development. Schools are not public health centres and will therefore not focus merely on interventions such as counselling and psychotherapy. In order to address the heterogeneous needs of young students, the school has to adopt a multi-level approach along the continuum of care.

The World Health Organization's (WHO) whole-school approach to mental health is an integrated, multi-level model. In this chapter, the model will be specifically used as a framework to address needs of the adolescent school-going population in India. The model (Fig. 9.2) consists of four levels of intervention corresponding to different levels of care beginning with health promotion and primary prevention (Levels 1 and 2), secondary prevention (Level 3) and tertiary prevention (Level 4).

In the model, Levels 1 and 2 involve and impact the entire school community. Efforts at Levels 3 and 4 are more specialized, and often require participation of relatively few stakeholder groups. A school has multiple stakeholders influencing the students' development in different ways, including school leaders, members of the management, teaching and non-teaching staff, parents, families, caregivers, older and junior students, peers, consultants, vendors such as bus staff and canteen

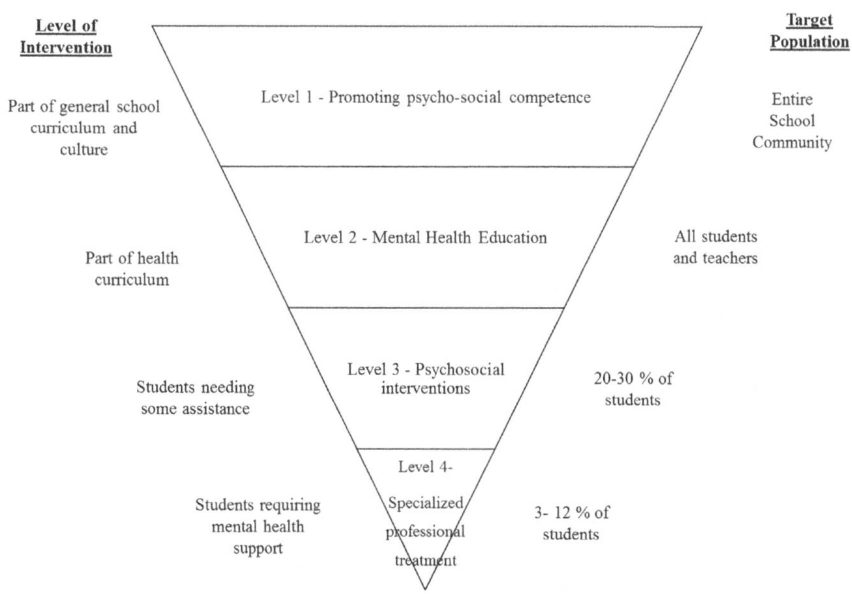

Fig. 9.2 WHO whole-school approach to mental health (Adapted from Hendren et al. 1994)

staff, and other members of the local community. For this chapter we will focus on three prominent stakeholder groups in the school: school leadership, educators, and mental health professionals. In most schools, the leadership consists of members of the Board and the school principal, vice-principal and/or coordinators and head of departments. Educators include all the teaching faculty in the school, subject teachers, and non-academic subject teachers like music and art faculty. Mental health professionals in schools are often limited to school counsellors or psychologists. While this section will elaborate on the role of counsellors, we do recognize that counsellors must work in collaboration with remedial educators and special educators.

The components under each level and role of different stakeholders, beginning from the top of the model, will be discussed followed by a few examples of effective and creative initiatives and programmes undertaken at that level globally and in India. The discussion on each level is concluded by few remarks about the scope of implementing similar initiatives in India.

Level 1: Promoting Psychosocial Competence

The first level of the model focuses on mental health promotion and development of psycho-social competencies. This implies creating a safe and secure school environment that fosters socio-emotional growth, positive relationships, and a general sense of well-being. This level includes two components: creating a safe climate and developing socio-emotional skills. Each of these components has been implemented across various schools internationally, and there is substantial evidence to support the impact of these practices on student well-being.

Components Under Level 1

The first and most prominent component of the entire model is the process of establishing a positive school climate. School climate refers to the "quality and character of the school" (National School Climate Council 2007). The climate reflects the experiences of various stakeholders in the school including teachers, students, and other staff, as well as the values, norms, relationships, learning practices, and structures of the school. A positive school climate facilitates holistic development of students through respectful relationships, desirable modelling from educators and leaders, and involvement and engagement of all stakeholders in achieving the school's vision. Such an environment encourages young students to initiate leadership and contribute productively to society. It is within such an atmosphere that students can begin to see the school as a microcosm of their society. Reviews of programmes and practices around the world show that a positive school climate and culture, have lasting impact on student development, and are integral to the process of mental health prevention (Weare and Nind 2011).

Another important element of promoting mental health is socio-emotional skill development. These skills are often called life skills. The WHO identified some core life skills which include decision making, problem-solving, critical and creative thinking, communication and interpersonal relationships, self-awareness, empathy and skills required to cope with emotions and stressors (Hendren et al. 1994). While some of these skills are geared towards prevention of undesirable behaviours or outcomes—such as unwanted pregnancy, substance abuse, HIV/AIDS, bullying, and so on—some skills strengthen certain personality aspects, like confidence and self-esteem (Hendren et al. 1994). An effective practice at Level 1 may include communication skills training or conflict resolution programmes to prevent bullying (Morrison 2002). The impact of life skill development includes better adjustment and relationships with school teachers, peers, and prosocial behaviour (Srikala and Kumar 2010) as well as better academic outcomes (Hendren et al. 1994).

Role of Stakeholders at Level 1

At this level, the role of school leadership is extremely crucial. School leaders who believe in the organizational values and ethos are more likely to be motivated and driven to collaborate with students and teachers to promote a safe school climate. The school principal and the leaders can become champions for mental health by creating whole-school systems and policies that align with the school values. Creating a safe climate requires the entire school community to participate and this is possible only under the guidance of a strong, considerate, and enthusiastic leadership which believes and uphold the school's vision. Along with the responsibility of mentoring and steering the activities at this level, leaders may also have to make systemic arrangements like creating a time-table for life skills education (Meenakshi and Narayana 2013), inviting experts to develop the curriculum and train the school staff, as well as creating systems to review the impact of these sessions. In Indian schools, since teachers often experience work stress, the school leaders will have to identify ways of inviting the teachers on board and distributing the work load equitably among all staff members. The school leaders may also develop pathways to reach out to parents and involve them in the process of curriculum development and execution.

While the leaders play a crucial role in strategizing, designing and creating structures to implement activities and programmes at this level, school educators will be involved in executing these plans. They will work collaboratively to develop whole-school activities and practices that promote a safe and positive school climate. They will develop lesson plans and classroom activities to strengthen the school climate and create a positive learning environment. They will encourage students to follow the school values through effective modelling. They will also initiate contact with families through regular parent-teacher meetings, interactions, or parent visits during school annual days, to involve them in promoting school culture. Educators will also provide inputs in developing the life skills curriculum and integrating it with the subject curriculum. For example, a social sciences teacher may discuss the skill of responsibility in the context of citizenship and civic duties.

School counsellors at Level 1 will assist the school leadership in planning and designing a whole-school approach to enhance the school climate. School counsellors will also assist educators in developing lesson-plans that are inclusive, ensuring that all student voices are heard and respected. If the school has a full-time counsellor, he/she may design the life-skills education curriculum for each grade, and help the educators in facilitating these plans. However, in the absence of a school counsellor, this task can be outsourced to off-site mental health professionals.

Examples of Existing Initiatives

The most recognized and evidence-based model that promotes psycho-social competencies within schools is the 'Collaborative for Academic, Social, and Emotional Learning (CASEL)'. The CASEL framework promotes the need for holistic development with an approach to create positive and safe learning environments. CASEL identifies the importance of a safe school climate and suggests that a school climate which communicates values like honesty, respect, and responsibility, along with certain themes that present the purposefulness of schooling, is one of the five key characteristics of a school that demonstrates social, emotional, and academic excellence (Elias et al. 2008). CASEL was founded in 1994 and, in 1996, it moved to the University of Illinois, Chicago, under the leadership of Dr. Roger Weissberg. CASEL works across three domain areas: research, practice, and policy. It works with classrooms and schools to develop evidence based SEL practices. Currently, CASEL also offers online resources and guidelines as well as standards for developing SEL practices with a focus on collaboration. In 2017, team members from CASEL, along with other authors, conducted a meta-analysis of 82 different SEL interventions. The study found significant positive impact of the SEL intervention on students' academic performance, socio-emotional skills, attitudes, and well-being indicators. The authors also found that students who had received the SEL interventions reported significantly lower levels of emotional distress, drug use, and conduct problems (Taylor et al. 2017).

There are many other programmes which have been initiated at the school-level to promote positive learning environments. One such programme was the campaign titled 'All kinds of kinds' initiated in 2013 in North Park Jr High School, New York, as an endeavour to respect the diversity in school. The school students and teachers created a video highlighting their differences to the soundtrack of Miranda Lambert's 'All kinds of kinds'. This video was followed by creating a picture path along the school hallways with pictures of all students holding up their 'all kinds of kinds' sign. The programme also included a 27-min-long video about bullying, showing how bullying can be physically and emotionally hurtful. The video, which uses the song 'Bruises' by Train, was inspired by Dr. Brene Brown's Daring Greatly, and imparts a powerful message on vulnerability. The programme had a positive effects on the students' behaviour as well as the school climate. Suspension rates in and out of school decreased by 28 and 78% respectively, and school discipline referrals reduced by 60% after the implementation of the program. Absenteeism rates of staff also reduced. Students demonstrated better scores in reading and math. The programme content was also made available as a curriculum that schools can refer to and teach, to address issues of bullying in the school. The programme received much acclaim and is now practiced across many schools in USA.

Current Status and Future Possibilities in India

The significance of a positive school climate has been highlighted in the NCERT framework for Education in Values in School. The framework suggests creating a school climate that promotes values, positive communication, and freedom of expression, and is free of stereotypes and gender-bias, for holistic development of students. At the same time, there are many life-skills education (LSE) programmes which are implemented across schools in India. LSE has also been recommended by the National Mental Health Policy 2014, and is included as an important component of the national adolescent health strategy, or the Rashtriya Kishore Swasthya Karyakram (RKSK). The District Mental Health Programme (DMHP) also includes LSE for adolescents in Grades 8, 9, and 10, which covers topics similar to the CBSE life-skills curriculum such as sexual health, interpersonal relationships, and career guidance.

The school mental health model implemented by 'Expressions India' a Delhi-based organization (Bharath et al. 2008) is one of the initiatives towards enhancing school climate. The model provides scope for assessing students' emotional, social, and behavioural needs, as well as builds capacities of school teachers, counsellors, and parents, through workshops and training programmes. The model also incorporates the component of student leadership, by identifying peer mentors who can be trained to impart life skills education. A study found that adolescents participating in this life-skills programme scored significantly higher on self-esteem, emotional adjustment, as well as levels of empathy (Yadav and Iqbal 2009). While this programme has been reviewed, there is absence of documentation of short and long-term impact of other adolescent centric life-skills education programmes in India.

There is consensus among policy-makers, school boards, and the government in promoting positive learning environments and adolescent skill-building programmes. However, the challenge in the Indian context is to design a programme that is contextually relevant. In order to establish a positive learning environment, schools in India will have to replace certain redundant and harmful teaching practices with positive instructional strategies. For instance, to address corporal punishment and punitive practices, teachers have to be encouraged to explore alternative methods of disciplining, such as positive reinforcement and behavioural management strategies. Teacher trainings and school mandates on the use of restorative practices will be the first step in this direction. Schools can create platforms for student–teacher interactions to strengthen their relationship. Addressing issues of labelling, prejudices, and biases among the teaching community (Tammana 2016) is also an important component of creating a safe school climate in Indian schools. Simple practices like displaying posters of respectful language, and identifying discriminatory and hurtful words and phrases, can reduce hate language in the school premises, and promote a culture of mutual respect. This will require dedicated efforts by the school leaders to steer such practices and motivate their staff and students to sustain it.

The increase in number of LSE programmes shows that the need for socio-emotional skill development has received great prominence. However, the challenges are in executing the programmes effectively and assessing them. It is important to identify how these different bodies and boards can work collaboratively. How does the DMHP LSE programme compare to the CBSE life-skills curriculum and the AEP? What are the provisions to ensure that DMHP LSE will be implemented across schools affiliated to all boards? How will teachers be trained in implementing these sessions? These are key questions that need to be answered to address the existing challenges. The DMHP currently measures the impact of LSE by reviewing the number of teachers trained and the number of schools covered by the outreach program. However, specific impact indicators to assess shift in students' knowledge, attitudes, and behaviours have to be developed.

At Level 1, therefore, the needs and challenges in Indian schools are very unique to the context, and require collaborative efforts from schools, educational boards, as well as the government, in eliminating unsafe teaching practices, promoting a positive learning culture, developing a common framework for life-skills education across all school boards, and developing systems to implement these programmes and monitor them regularly.

Level 2: Mental Health Education

The second level in the WHO model is aimed at creating awareness, and reducing the stigma associated with mental health and mental illness in schools, by providing accurate and appropriate information to students and teachers. At this level, school interventions focus on two broad objectives: Generating awareness and reducing stigma, and mental health education.

Components Under Level 2

Stigma around mental health, and discrimination against those with mental illness, are huge challenges in the Indian and global public health sector. This often becomes a huge barrier in seeking help for mental health concerns (Lyon et al. 2016). Since schools are a reflection of the larger socio-cultural system, it is unfortunate that the stigma and discrimination around mental health is also very common in schools. One way of addressing this is to create awareness about mental health and mental illness through classroom discussions, documentary viewing, or displaying posters about content related to mental health such as stress, psychological and emotional concerns during adolescence, puberty and its effects, role of the brain, seeking assistance, and other similar topics (Hendren et al. 1994). Charts and factsheets, about mental health problems and mental illnesses among adolescents in India, can help students understand the intensity of the problem. Awareness campaigns will address any biases or misconceived notions within the community. Schools can also create awareness about mental healthcare services and professionals. Providing information about counselling, medication, and other forms of mental health services, will reduce the stigma associated with help-seeking. Schools may also provide students and families with a list of service providers in and around the school. This will encourage students to develop a non-judgmental attitude towards mental health services, and motivate them to seek help for their concerns.

Another important component at Level 2 involves educating the students, teachers, and school community on mental health and mental illness. These sessions can be conducted by the school counsellor, or a trained mental health professional, with the aim to empower the school to make informed decisions about students' mental health. Mental health education will focus not only on mental illnesses but also provide strategies to help students enhance their psychological well-being. This ensures that students can relate to the content and translate the learnings in their daily life. It is important for these sessions to be integrated with the whole-school curriculum or included as part of the general health curriculum.

Role of Stakeholders at Level 2

The programmatic interventions at this level require equal involvement of school leaders, educators, and counsellors. School leaders will identify platforms and forums in the school for mental health awareness. Along with the educators, they will identify activities that can be conducted across the whole school to reduce stigma around mental health. School leaders will also play a critical role in introducing mental health as part of the curriculum in the school. Such a move may face resistance from teachers, parents, or the community, because of the stigma associated with it. It will be important for school leaders to gather sufficient data and evidence to support their decision, and discuss the same with parents and teachers during formal meetings and interactions. School leaders will oversee the process of curriculum designing and development to ensure that it is contextually relevant and age-appropriate. They will create training schedules and trainers to equip teachers with the knowledge and skills. School leaders will also play a role in reviewing the programme regularly and monitoring its progress.

School educators will play an important role in designing and implementing activities to generate awareness about mental health. However, before they can contribute to this process, they must receive adequate information and training. The current teacher-training courses in India do not have a component on adolescent mental health. It is important, therefore, to build the capacities of the educators before they can become the agents for accurate knowledge. They can mobilize students and champions from all grades to organize events and activities to create mental health awareness. For instance, educators can help students design a small booth in the school where they ask students to complete a short quiz on myths and facts about mental health. This will help reach out to large numbers of students, and demystify the idea of mental health. Since educators interact regularly with students, they can help make the curriculum specific to students' needs. At the classroom level, educators can initiate simple strategies like the check-in ritual (University of Michigan 2015) to encourage students to recognize their feelings, and create a safe space for them to talk about emotional experiences. At this level, educators will be involved in executing the plans and engaging in knowledge building with students in the classroom.

The school counsellor's role at this level is extremely important in designing and developing the content for all activities. The counsellor, or a trained mental health professional, will provide expert inputs and knowledge in developing resource materials for whole-school awareness activities. The counsellor will also lead the process of developing a school-based mental health curriculum that is appropriate and relevant to the students. For example, in a community where substance abuse among high school students is high, the mental health curriculum for middle school students can aim to provide information about substance abuse and its effects. It is extremely important for counsellors to work collaboratively with educators and leaders. If the school has a full-time counsellor, he/she may also utilize classroom spaces for small group discussions, role-plays, and other methods of providing information about specific mental health concerns, mental healthcare services, and ethics involved in mental healthcare, such as confidentiality. Counsellors can also develop a directory of service providers around the school as a resource for students and families. If a school does not have a counsellor, the school can connect with off-site or consulting professionals for the same.

Examples of Existing Initiatives

There are very few programmes which focus on providing mental health education and addressing stigma around mental illness within schools. One such programme is the Breaking the Silence (BTS), initiated in 1991 in USA. BTS teaches students about mental health, encourages them to seek help, and breaks the stigma associated with it. BTS was initiated as part of a campaign to end discrimination, launched by the non-profit organization National Alliance on Mental Illness (NAMI). It was only in 1999 that the paper 'Breaking the Silence: Teaching the Next Generation about Mental Illness' was published and the programme was implemented across various States. So far, BTS has made its presence felt across various countries—including Japan, Armenia, Ireland, Canada, Australia, and others—through its lesson plans and posters. It also provides resources, presentations, and teaching videos online. Let's Talk Mental Illness (LTMI) is a part of the BTS programme, and involves a presentation featuring a first-person narrative by someone living with a mental illness. The objective of LTMI is to destigmatize and change students' perceptions about mental illness. While the programme has expanded and reached out to many students, there is absence of data on the impact of the program.

Current Status and Future Possibilities in India

Mental health education has not received much prominence in Indian schools. Most organizations that provide mental health education sessions often offer it as workshops, seminars, or conferences. However, long-term continuous programmes on mental health education and awareness building are not available. 'Reach Out' was a student-led effort in this direction in a school in Mumbai. Reach Out created awareness about mental health concerns and mental well-being among adolescent students in the school. As part of the programmes, students conducted classroom interactions, created awareness on social media through a Facebook page, and also developed manuals to share information about common adolescent mental health concerns. While the impact of this programme is not documented yet, it serves as a great example of mental health education within a school.

In the absence of such programmes and initiatives, and the increasing number of adolescents experiencing mental health concerns, the need for immediate action at this level is strong. So far, most programmes and interventions, recommended in policies and implemented across schools, have focused on socio-emotional skill development. However, this leaves out the large number of adolescents experiencing common mental illnesses, and those at risk for suicide, and other severe mental illnesses. Programmatic initiatives at this level are therefore significant to change the discourse around mental health in schools. This will be possible only if mental health finds a mention in the policies and educational frameworks. It is important for the NCF and educational boards to include mental health education as part of the curriculum of the school.

In India, the stigma around mental health is a huge problem, contributing negatively to help-seeking behaviours as well as treatment prognosis (Shidhaye and Kermode 2013). It is important, therefore, to create programmes that will break these barriers to help-seeking. In addition to mental health education, schools also need to generate awareness about mental healthcare. Misconceptions about counselling and the role of a school counsellor abound in Indian schools and these need to be addressed. The nature of schools and contexts also varies widely in India and it is important for programmes to be aligned with the students' socio-cultural environment. For example, sessions on substance abuse may focus more on alcohol and smoking for students in the urban private schools, and more on use of *ganja* and tobacco, in rural government schools.

Another major challenge in the Indian context is the dearth of mental health professionals. It is important therefore for schools to establish networks of mental health professionals and organizations, NGOs, and academic agencies which can provide services to the school at this level. Schools can then outsource the process of content design, development, and execution. Adopting a cascade model, whereby schools can invite mental health professionals to train the school teachers, can also be effective in the Indian schools.

Therefore, at present, Indian schools need to establish systems and mandates to initiate and effectively implement activities at this level. This will lay the foundation and encourage schools to participate at this level.

Level 3: Psychosocial Interventions

The first two levels of the WHO model promote mental well-being in the entire school community. However, there is a significant section of students in the school who may be experiencing psycho-social distress associated with exams, academic pressure, friendships, romantic relationships, bullying, or conflicts at home. Level 3 aims to develop interventions to address the needs of these students. While these students need support and assistance, they may not require long-term specialized care such as psychotherapy or psychiatric intervention. The two key components under this level are: early identification and preventive systems.

Components Under Level 3

At this level, interventions are designed to identify and address the needs of students who are experiencing distress or at the risk of a psychological concern. The school community can be educated in identifying signs and symptoms of common adolescent psycho-social concerns. For example, teachers may be asked to observe students who are neglected or isolated by their peers, or any sudden behavioural changes in the student. A student who is experiencing problems in a romantic relationship, may suddenly become withdrawn and not participate in class. If such behaviour persists for some time, it can be a red flag. Similarly, a sudden drop in academic performance may also be an indicator of psychological distress. Early identification ensures that the student's distress can be managed before it becomes a clinical concern. Once identified, the student can be referred to the appropriate professional for help. The school leaders, teachers, and counsellors, must design a protocol to be followed once these students are identified.

Apart from early identification, this level also includes interventions at the preventive level for students who are at high risk for developing a mental health concern. The school must develop systems to ensure that these students receive adequate support and assistance to alleviate the distress. Students must be helped to develop self-regulation skills which will help them address similar concerns in the future. For instance, students who engage in aggressive behaviours, or find it difficult to resolve conflicts, may be provided with support in communication skills and anger management strategies. Teachers can be educated in identifying students who are more vulnerable, or are at higher risk of experiencing psychological distress, such as students coming from poor economic conditions, families witnessing domestic violence or those who have a physical disability. Creating safe spaces for discussions or facilitating small group sessions are effective interventions to target common adolescent concerns in the school at this level without relying on specialized services.

Role of Stakeholders at Level 3

At this level, although the entire school community is not influenced or involved, all stakeholders play very crucial roles. School leaders become more supervisory as compared to the previous levels. They will collaborate with the teachers and school counsellor to develop a systematic protocol to address students' concerns. Questions like 'What are the steps involved in the referral process? How can students refer themselves? Which concerns are likely to be resolved by the teachers?' will be pertinent to this process. Once the systems have been established, school leaders will supervise these processes regularly, through update meetings with school educators and counsellors. School leaders will also create specific schedules and make arrangements to train the teaching and non-teaching staff in early identification and prevention.

School educators will be involved in identifying students who require support and will follow set procedures to ensure that the assistance is provided. In the absence of a school counsellor, teachers may even provide some support to students. It is essential, therefore, for teachers to be trained in basic skills required as first respondents.

The school counsellor, at this level, will work collaboratively with teachers to develop a robust system for identification and referral, while ensuring that professional ethics such as confidentiality are maintained. The counsellor will be involved in designing and facilitating preventive and supportive programmes for students who are experiencing distress.

Examples of Existing Initiatives

Many schools internationally provide specific in-school and after school programmes and services to assist students experiencing psycho-social distress. 'Turning the Tides for children and families (TTT)' is a similar programme initiated by the New Jersey Department of Children and Families. TTT is a school- and community-based psycho-social intervention offering after school programmes to students. One of the programmes it offers is called the Skills for Psychological Recovery (SPR) and involves skill-building for teens and their families. Another programme called 'Sources of Strength' is a peer-leader programme which encourages middle and high school students to seek help from adults during crisis. These programmes are offered for free to the schools. While this intervention was developed in response to specific needs of students and families post a disaster in New Jersey, it is an example of how schools can outsource psycho-social interventions in the absence of in-school mental health professionals.

Current Status and Future Possibilities in India

Among school-going adolescents in India, psycho-social concerns related to relationships, academic stress, peer pressure, and bullying are highly prevalent. While these issues may present themselves differently across these schools, it is important to acknowledge that these concerns can cause significant psychological and emotional distress. While some of these problems, such as bullying, can also be addressed by initiating structural changes in the school under Level 1, it is equally important to provide support and help to students who are experiencing such distress.

In India, at present, school-based counselling is the only system in place to address the needs at this level. However, this is insufficient as most schools still do not have a school counsellor. Despite measures to increase mental health services in schools—such as the CBSE mandate to appoint a school counsellor in every school—the picture doesn't look too promising. According to reports, a survey conducted by the Associated Chambers of Commerce and Industry of India in the Delhi-NCR region found that only three percent of the private schools had a school counsellor (The Hindu 2016). This makes it advisable to devise alternate strategies to address the psycho-social needs of students in schools.

One way of addressing the existing gap, is by building capacities of teachers as first-level respondents. Teachers in schools can be trained to identify students in need of help and provide psychological first aid (PFA) whenever required. PFA is common in regions affected by conflict. For instance, a PFA workshop was conducted for teachers, journalists, and other common people in Kashmir, by Help Foundation and Directorate of Health Services Kashmir (Mushtaq 2016).

A manual for training schools in Psychological First Aid has been developed by the Ministry of Education, Government of Liberia, in collaboration with UNICEF and USAID, and includes components of early identification, assessment, and providing immediate support and care to students in need. Similar manuals and training resources can be developed by the government to ensure uniform training practices across India. Schools can also create documents which identify risk factors relevant to their context, and warning signs of various mental health concerns, to help teachers identify students who are in need of help. Schools require continuous support at this level to train staff and build knowledge on mental health and psycho-social interventions. Collaborations with mental health professionals and NGOs are crucial at this level.

Another significant step that Indian schools can take is to develop mentoring systems in the school to create support networks for students in distress. For instance, schools can develop a teacher-mentoring programme which trains teachers in basic skills required to address adolescent needs. Students can be informed about the role of the teacher-mentor who will listen and provide a comforting space to the student. They will carry out a risk assessment, also identify the level of distress experienced by the student, and may choose to provide some strategies to alleviate this distress. Teacher-mentors will not substitute as counsellors, but will serve as mediating agents who can also refer students to in-school or off-site counselling if required. Similarly, schools can also create spaces for peer mentoring. For example, the RKSK has a component on peer education, whereby adolescent girls and boys are trained as mentors for other adolescents. Schools in India can create a system along similar lines and equip young students with mental health knowledge and skills to support their peers.

The needs at the third level, although specific to a few students in the entire school, can be difficult to meet, and require systemic changes and involvement of various stakeholders. In Indian schools, it is therefore important to strengthen the capacities of teachers and students and establish partnerships with external agencies to meet these needs.

Level 4: Specialized Professional Treatment

The fourth level of the WHO model involves targeted action to support students who are experiencing significant psychological distress, mental health concern/s, or clinically diagnosable psychological disorders. Although a relatively small section of the adolescent school-going population experiences these concerns, the impact of such experiences on the student's life can be long-term and debilitating to say the least. It is important therefore to ensure adequate and appropriate services at this level.

Components Under Level 4

This level aims to provide specialized care to students who may experience significant distress which impacts their daily functioning and performance. Addressing the needs of these students in the school can be done in three ways: appointing a full-time counsellor to provide in-house counselling to the students; partnering with an agency or NGO that can provide similar services in the school; or referring identified students to off-site mental health professionals. The services offered at this level include counselling, psychotherapy, any traditional forms of therapy that are practiced in the culture, and psychiatric medication. It is also important for the school to develop a system to provide crisis intervention for students reporting abuse or those engaging in self-harm. Following a set protocol at such times reduces panic and helps address the students' concerns effectively.

Role of Stakeholders at Level 4

Although the focus of this level is on specialized care, the role of all the stakeholders remains equally important in developing the systems conducive for such care. The school leaders will identify the resources available in the school to provide specialized services. For instance, the school leaders can ensure that the school has a counselling room, assessment tools, referral sources, and so on. School leaders will also supervise and receive regular updates of the progress in therapy and ensure that students are receiving appropriate care as deemed necessary by the counsellor. They may also ask the educators to make specific provisions in the classrooms to meet the students' needs. However, if the school does not have a counsellor, the school leaders will initiate and establish referral networks. School leaders can also lead a team of teachers who can supervise and monitor the process of referrals and follow-ups.

The educators can assist the counsellors by referring students who they identify as being at risk for a mental health concern. They may provide written observations of the student to facilitate the intervention. Educators may also incorporate suggestions provided by the counsellors in the classroom arrangements or teaching methods to help the student.

Since these students require professional support through counselling or psychotherapy, the role of the counsellor is crucial at this stage. The counsellor will be involved in conducting an informal and formal assessment of the student, as well as designing an intervention plan. If the student requires psychiatric help or long-term psychotherapeutic assistance, the school may refer the child to agencies or off-site mental health practitioners. If the student's concerns are not too severe, yet demand urgent attention, the school counsellor can provide evidence-based interventions to the student. The counsellor may also decide to involve the student's parents and/or caregivers at some point during this intervention. The counsellor will also keep a set of self-help resources and helpline numbers that can be provided to students as additional support. The counsellor may also provide group-based interventions if required.

Examples of Existing Initiatives

While services at this level are often school specific, the Los Angeles Unified School District, (LAUSD), covering over 900 schools, has designed a system to provide mental health services, as well as crisis counselling, to students in need. Through School Mental Health (SMH), a collaboration of mental health professionals under the LAUSD, school students are provided with clinical services and medical support services through clinics and wellness centres. SMH works in collaboration with the school principal, teachers, staff, parents, and other stakeholders and provides services ranging from Tier 1 universal services to Tier 3 intensive care. SMH also clearly outlines the procedures for referral, including intake and assessment processes. Such a system seems extremely useful when specialized care has to be provided in the absence of resources within the school.

Current Status and Future Possibilities in India

Adolescent mental health concerns do not find a mention in the Indian education frameworks and agendas. Except for the CBSE mandate for school counsellors, there are no other provisions by the school boards or the government to address the needs of students experiencing psychological distress. As discussed earlier in the chapter, the number of students experiencing common mental disorders such as Depression and anxiety, and the number of students attempting suicide, is extremely high in India. Therefore, schools need to ensure adequate services to students for such concerns.

To be able to execute effective interventions at this level, schools must focus on providing evidence-based interventions and assessing the impact of the same. Such services can be provided by professionals trained in mental health or psychology. However, often there aren't any mental health professionals in schools. This is one of the largest challenges that the Indian schools face at this level. This makes it difficult for schools to provide mental health interventions at Level 4 within the school. It is important, therefore, for schools to partner with offsite mental health professionals and agencies. At the same time, it is also the responsibility of mental health professionals to reach out to local schools, offer their services to school boards, and promote school-based mental health services (Srikala and Kumar 2010).

Another challenge in the Indian context is the lack of specialized professional training in adolescent and school mental health. Degree programmes and professional courses in psychology at the undergraduate and graduate level in India, include a very small component of adolescent mental health. Topics related to school mental health are often not included in the course curriculum. Therefore, counsellors often find it difficult to design and develop school-based programmes and provide student-centric services.

In addition to these challenges, the ambiguity about the role of school counsellor in Indian schools makes the picture more complex. School counselling is still in its nascent stages and as a result, the role of a counsellor is still evolving in many schools. In most schools, the counsellor is often involved in teaching and student management activities and is also given other school duties. This leaves very little room in the counsellor's time-table to facilitate individual and group therapy or counselling interventions. It is important, therefore, for the educational boards, as well as policy-makers, to establish guidelines to assist schools and mental health professionals in identifying the role of a school counsellor.

Thus, at Level 4, the task for Indian schools is complex. While schools require to develop their own pathways to provide effective mental healthcare services to students who are experiencing psychological distress, the larger systems and frameworks also need to develop specific guidelines to assist schools in addressing the needs at this level.

The four levels of intervention discussed above are designed to serve as one integrated model for school mental health. While each level focuses on specific areas of mental health promotion, prevention, and intervention, it is recommended that schools focus on all the levels. It may be likely, however, that a school may decide to begin by implementing interventions at one particular level which the school identifies as an urgent need. Schools must begin by mapping their existing systems and processes to identify areas of strength and those which require attention. For example, in schools where corporal punishment is still common, efforts at Level 1, to promote a restorative system and safe climate, may be most useful for the school. Similarly, a school which has a robust life-skills education curriculum in place, may want to focus on incorporating a mental health curriculum too. It is, therefore, important to refer to this model as a framework which guides the designing and planning of a school mental health program.

Conclusion

Adolescents in India are the potential future leaders of the country. However, the current status of adolescent mental health in India is very disquieting. There is an urgent need for concerted efforts towards developing mechanisms and utilizing existing systems to strengthen the protective factors and reduce the risks that adolescents are experiencing. Schools are an effective and efficient platform to initiate this overwhelming task of enhancing adolescent mental health. By adopting a multi-level, collaborative approach, schools can become active spaces for mental health promotion, prevention, and intervention.

This is only the first step towards developing safer and positive schools which promote adolescent well-being, and provide maximum opportunities for them to grow and excel. While there is sufficient evidence for the effectiveness of school-based mental health programmes globally, it is important to generate similar evidence in India. As schools implement this model, it is important for school leaders to adopt a systemic perspective and ensure that the practices are ecologically relevant. Schools must also attempt to set up mechanisms to assess their efforts by developing impact indicators and documenting the reviews. Such a method will help establish an evidence-based and sustainable model with a promise of scalability.

The need and significance of school-based mental health services and socio-emotional learning is well reflected in the policy documents and national level frameworks in India. However, collaborative efforts have to be made to translate these guidelines into effective programmatic interventions. This demands convergence between various ministries at the Central and State government level, as well as partnerships between academic institutions, NGOs, private sector, and the community. The roles of various stakeholders, including mental health service providers, the local, State, and Central government bodies, as well as resource-rich schools, will have to be identified and enlisted. This will help generate pathways and opportunities for liaising to mobilize resources adequately and equitably across schools.

In addition to programmatic development at the school level, in India, there is also a significant need for a monitoring and guiding body at the district, State, and national levels that can help schools in effective implementation. For instance, in Ontario, the School Mental Health-ASSIST (SMH-ASSIST) is an implementation initiated in 2011, to assist schools to promote mental health, and provide support to students experiencing mental health concerns. The ASSIST framework is oriented towards promotion, prevention, tiered intervention, and scaling up of programmes in schools, by providing continuous support to school leadership, building capacities, providing resources, and assisting in designing evidence-based programmes for schools. While the COBSE serves as an apex body in the Indian Education system, a separate body that oversees school-based mental health services, and works collaboratively with all boards, can be designed and created.

When questions of impact, assessment, equity, and collaborative leadership are introduced, the discourse on school mental health becomes more complex and challenging. But these are pertinent questions that need to be addressed within schools, at community gatherings and at national-level debates. The answers will present themselves as we initiate this movement, one school, district, and State at a time.

References

Arpan. (n.d.). *Annual Report 2015-2016*. Arpan.

Arun, P., & Chavan, B. (2009). Stress and suicidal ideas in adolescent students in Chandigarh. *Indian Journal of Medical Sciences, 63*(7), 281–287.

Atkins, M. S., Adil, J. A., Jackson, M., McKay, M. M., & Bell, C. C. (2000). An ecological model for school-based mental health services. In *3th Annual Conference Proceedings a System of Care for Children's Mental Health: Expanding the Research Base* (pp. 119–122).

Barnett, W. S. (1995). Long-term effects of early childhood programmes on cognitive and school outcomes. *The Future of Children, 5*(3), 25–50. Retrieved from http://www.jstor.org/stable/1602366.

Bharath, S., Kumar, K. K., & Mukesh, Y. P. (2008). Clinical practice guidelines for school mental health program. *Indian Journal of Psychiatry*.

Bhattacharjea, S., Wadhwa, W., & Banerji, R. (2011). *Inside primary schools a study of teaching and learning in rural India*. ASER.

Bhola, P., Sathyanarayanan, V., Rekha, D. P., Daniel, S., & Thomas, T. (2016). Assessment of self-reported emotional and behavioral difficulties among pre-university college students in Bangalore, India. *Indian Journal of Community Medicine, 41*(2), 146–150.

Bronfenbrenner, U. (1979). An ecological orientation: Purpose and perspective. In U. Bronfenbrenner (Ed.), *The ecology of human development experiments by nature and design* (pp. 3–15). Harvard University Press.

Center for Mental Health in Schools. (n.d.). *Mental health in schools: An overview*. Retrieved from School Mental Health Project, UCLA. http://smhp.psych.ucla.edu/aboutmh/mhinschools.html.

Chamberlin, J. (2009, January). Schools expand mental health care. *Monitor on Psychology, 40*(1). Retrieved from American Psychological Association. http://www.apa.org/monitor/2009/01/school-clinics.aspx.

Chandrashekarappa, S. M., Ramakrishnaiah, N. M., Ram, D., & Manjunath, R. (2016). Mental Health among adolescent girls—An effort to know the association of mental disorders with socio-demographic variables. *International Journal of Medical Science and Public Health, 5*(11).

Chaudhry, S., & Uboweja, A. (2014, March). Public-private partnerships in school education—Learning and insights from India. Central Square Foundation.

Committee on School Health. (2004). School-based mental health services. *Pediatrics, 113*(6), 1839–1845.

Deb, S., Kumar, A., Holden, G., & Rowe, L. S. (2017). School corporal punishment, family tension, and students' internalizing problems: Evidence from India. *School Psychology Internationa, 38*(1), 60–77.

Elias, M., Parker, S. K., Weissberg, R., & O'Brien, M. (2008). Social and emotional learning, moral education, and character education: A comparative analysis and a view toward convergence. In L. Nucci & D. Narvaez (Eds.), *Handbook of moral and character education* (pp. 248–266). New York: Routledge.

Fazel, M., Hoagwood, K., Stephan, S., & Ford, T. (2014). Mental health interventions in schools—Mental health interventions in schools in high income countries. *Lancet Psychiatry*, 377–387. https://doi.org/10.1016/s2215-0366(14)70312-8.

Galambos, N. L., Almeida, D. M., & Petersen, A. C. (1990). Masculinity, femininity, and sex role attitudes in early adolescence: Exploring gender intensification. *Child Development, 61*(6), 1905–1914. https://doi.org/10.2307/1130846.

Gaur, A. D., Vohra, A., Subash, S., & Khurana, H. (2003). Prevalence of psychiatric morbidity among 6 to 14 years old children. *Indian Journal of Community Medicine, 28*(3), 133–137.

Goel, D., Subramanyam, A., & Kamath, R. (2013). A study on the prevalence of internet addiction and its association with psychopathology in Indian adolescents. *Indian Journal of Psychiatry, 55*(2), 140–143. https://doi.org/10.4103/0019-5545.111451.

Government of India. (2009a). *Classwise enrolment in different categories of schools (Provisional data)—Eighth All India School Education Survey*. Retrieved from Open Government Data Platform India. https://data.gov.in/dataset-group-name/eighth-all-india-school-education-survey.

Government of India. (2009b, September). *Pre-primary education and alternative schooling—8th All India School Education Survey (8th AISES)*. Retrieved 2017 June, from Open Government Data Platform India: https://data.gov.in/catalog/pre-primary-education-and-alternative-schooling-8th-all-india-school-education-survey-8th.

Government of India. (2014, December). *Mental health institutions in the Country*. Retrieved from Press Information Bureau, Ministry of Health and Family Welfare, Government of India: http://pib.nic.in/newsite/PrintRelease.aspx?relid=112890.

Government of India. (2016). *Educational statistics at a glance*. New Delhi.

Government of India. (2017). *Youth in India 2017*. New Delhi: Central Statistics Office, Ministry of Statistics and Programme Implementation, Government of India.

Greenberg, M. T., Weissberg, R. P., O'Brien, M. U., Zins, J. E., Fredericks, L., Resnik, H., et al. (2003). Enhancing school-based prevention and youth development through coordinated social, emotional, and academic learning. *American Psychologist, 58*(6–7), 466–474.

Guneya, S., Kalafatb, T., & Boysan, M. (2010). Dimensions of mental health: Life satisfaction, anxiety and depression: A preventive mental health study in Ankara University students population. *Precedia Social and Behavioral Sciences*, 1210–1213.

Hendren, R., Weisen, B. R., & Orley, J. (1994). *Mental health porgrammes in school*. Geneva: Division of Mental Health, World Health Organization.
Hindustan Times. (2017, May 30). 'Suicide city' Kota's new preventive tactic is ceiling fans with springs, sirens. *Hindustan Times*.
Huang, J.-Y., Wang, K.-Y., & Ringel-Kulka, T. (2014). Predictors of life satisfaction among Asian American adolescents—Analysis of add health data. *Springer Plus*.
Jaisoorya, T. S., Beena, K. V., Beena, M., Ellangovan, K., Jose, D. C., Thennarasu, K., et al. (2016). Prevalence and correlates of alcohol use among adolescents attending school in Kerala, India. *Drug and Alcohol Review, 35*(5), 523–529. https://doi.org/10.1111/dar.12358.
Jhala, J., & Sharma, R. (2017). Prevalence and nature of internet use among adolescents in Vadodara (Gujarat). *The International Journal of Indian Psychology, 4*(2), 28–42.
Jones, P. B. (2013). Adult mental health disorders and their age at onset. *The British Journal of Psychiatry*, s5–s10. https://doi.org/10.1192/bjp.bp.112.119164.
Lyon, A. R., Whitaker, K., French, W. P., Richardson, L. P., Wasse, J. K., & McCauley, E. (2016). Collaborative care in schools: Enhancing integration and impact in youth mental health. *Advances in School Mental Health Promotion, 7*(1). https://doi.org/10.1080/1754730x.2016.1215928.
McLeod, J. D., Uemura, R., & Rohrman, S. (2012). Adolescent mental health, behavior problems, and academic achievement. *Journal of Health and Social Behavior, 53*(4), 482–497. https://doi.org/10.1177/0022146512462888.
Meenakshi, & Narayana, L. (2013). Preventive mental healthcare in Indian education system. *Scholarly Research Journal for Interdisciplinary Studies*.
Mehta, M., Pattanayak, R., & Sagar, R. (2015). Adolescent psychiatry: An overview of the Indian research. In S. Malhotra & S. Chakrabarti (Eds.), *Developments in psychiatry in India* (pp. 313–341). India: Springer.
Meldrum, L., Venn, D., & Kutcher, S. (n.d.). Mental health in schools: How Teachers have the power to make a difference.
Mishra, A., & Sharma, A. (2001). A clinico-social study of psychiatric morbidity in 12 to 18 years school going girls in urban Delhi. *Indian Journal of Community Medicine, 26*(2).
Morrison, B. (2002). Bullying and victimisation in schools: A restorative justice approach. *Trends and Issues in Crime and Criminal Justice*.
Morrow, V., & Singh, R. (2014). Corporal punishment in schools in Andhra Pradesh, India children's and parents' views. *Young Lives*.
Mrazek, P. J., & Haggerty, R. J. eds (1994). Reducing risks for mental disorders: Frontiers for preventive intervention research. Washington, National Academy Press.
Mushtaq, U. (2016, August 12). Workshop held to offer psychological first aid to victims. *Kashmir Reader*. Retrieved from http://kashmirreader.com/2016/08/12/workshop-held-to-offer-psychological-first-aid-to-victims/.
National Sample Survey Organisation, Ministry of Statistics and Programme Implementation, Government of India. (2003). NSS 58th round (July–December 2002). Government of India.
National School Climate Council. (2007). *School climate*. Retrieved from National School Climate Center.
NCERT. (n.d.). *Education for values in schools—A framework*. Department of Educational Psychology and Foundations of Education, National Council of Educational Research and Training (NCERT).
NIMHANS. (2016). *National mental health survey of India 2015-16*. Bengaluru: National Institute of Mental Health and Neurosciences.
Nishida, A., Richards, M., & Stafford, M. (2016). Prospective associations between adolescent mental health problems and positive mental well-being in early old age. *Child and Adolescent Psychiatry and Mental Health*. https://doi.org/10.1186/s13034-016-0099-2.
Office of the Registrar General and Census Commissioner, Ministry of HomE Affairs, Government of India. (2011). Census of India. Retrieved August 2016, from Population Enumeration Data (Final Population): http://www.censusindia.gov.in/2011census/population_enumeration.html.

Our Story. (n.d.). Retrieved from All Kinds of Kinds. http://www.allkindsofkinds.org/index.php/curriculum/.

Patil, R. N., Nagaonkar, S. N., Shah, N. B., & Bhat, T. S. (2013). A cross-sectional study of common psychiatric morbidity in children aged 5–14 years in an urban slum. *Journal of Family Medicine and Primary Care,* 165–168.

Priess, H. A., Lindberg, S. M., & Hyde, J. S. (2009). Adolescent gender-role identity and mental health: Gender intensification revisited. *Child Development, 80*(5), 1531–1544. https://doi.org/10.1111/j.1467-8624.2009.01349.x.

Reddy, B. K., Biswas, A., & Rao, H. (2011). Assessment of mental health of Indian adolescents studying in urban schools. *Malaysian Journal of Paediatrics and Child Health Online Early.*

Rothon, C., Head, J., Clark, C., Klineberg, E., Cattell, V., & Stansfeld, S. (2009). The impact of psychological distress on the educational achievement of adolescents at the end of compulsory education. *Social Psychiatry and Psychiatric Epidemiology, 44*(5), 421–427. https://doi.org/10.1007/s00127-008-0452-8.

Rural Adversity Mental Health Program. (2015). The mental health wellness continuum, Australia. Retrieved from https://www.youtube.com/watch?v=sSvyPxcj7UM&t=2s.

Samanta, A., Mukherjee, S., Ghosh, S., & Dasgupta, A. (2012). Mental health, protective factors and violence among male adolescents: A comparison between urban and rural school students in West Bengal. *Indian Journal of Public Health, 56*(2), 155–158.

School Mental Health. (n.d.). Retrieved from Los Angeles Unified School District. https://achieve.lausd.net/Page/1316.

Sharma, M., & Chaudhary, M. (2016). A study of drugs and substance abuse among adolescents of slum dwellers. *The International Journal of Indian Psychology, 3*(3), 21–27.

Shidhaye, R., & Kermode, M. (2013). Stigma and discrimination as a barrier to mental health service utilization in India. *International Health, 5*(1), 6–8. https://doi.org/10.1093/inthealth/ihs011.

Singh, A. (2013). Size and sources of the private school premium in test scores in India. *Young Lives.*

Singh, S., & Gururaj, G. (2014). Health behaviours & problems among young people in India: Cause for concern & call for action. *Indian Journal of Medical Research, 140,* 185–208.

Singh, B. D., & Menon, R. (2015). Life skills in India an overview of evidence and current practices in our education system. *Central Square Foundation.*

Singh, R., & Sarkar, S. (2012). *Teaching quality counts: How student outcomes relate to quality of teaching in private and public schools in India.* Young Lives.

Srikala, B., & Kumar, K. (2010). Empowering adolescents with life skills education in schools—School mental health program: Does it work? *Indian Journal of Psychiatry,* 344–349.

Srinath, S., Girimaji, S. C., Gururaj, G., Seshadri, S., Subbakrishna, D., Bhola, P., et al. (2005). Epidemiological study of child & adolescent psychiatric disorders in urban and rural areas of Bangalore, India. *Indian Journal of Medical Research, 122,* 67–79.

Steinberg, L. (2010). Commentary: A behavioral scientist looks at the science of adolescent brain development. *Brain Cognition, 72*(1), 160–164. https://doi.org/10.1016/j.bandc.2009.11.003.

Steinberg, L. (2012). Should the science of adolescent brain development inform public policy. *Issues in Science and Technology, 28*(3), 67–78.

Sylva, K. (1994). School influences on children's development. *Journal of Child Psychology and Psychiatry, 35*(1), 135–170. Retrieved June 2017.

Tammana, S. (2016). The role of a school counsellor. In S. Sriram (Ed.), *Counselling in India: Reflections on the process* (pp. 163–181). Springer.

Taylor, R. D., Oberle, E., Durlak, J. A., & Weissberg, R. P. (2017). Promoting positive youth development through school-based social and emotional learning interventions: A meta-analysis of follow-up effects. *Child Development, 88*(4), 1156–1171.

The British Council. (2014). *Indian school education system an overview.* Mumbai: The British Council.

The Hindu. (2016, May). Only 3% private schools have counsellors. *The Hindu*. Retrieved from http://www.thehindu.com/todays-paper/tp-national/tp-newdelhi/only-3-private-schools-have-counsellors/article5607842.ece.
UNESCO. (2017). *Education for sustainable development goals learning objectives*. Paris: United Nations Educational, Scientific and Cultural Organization.
UNICEF. (2016). *Data on secondary education: Net attendance rate*. Data and Analytics Section, Division of Data, Research and Policy, UNICEF. Retrieved June 2017, from UNICEF. https://data.unicef.org/topic/education/secondary-education/.
University of Michigan. (2015). *The check-in*. Retrieved from Classroom Mental Health: A Teacher's Toolkit for High School. https://www.classroommentalhealth.org/mental-health-in-the-classroom/exercises.asp?url=the-check-in.
Weare, K., & Nind, M. (2011). Mental health promotion and problem prevention in schools: What does the evidence say? *Health Promotion International, 26*.
WHO. (2012). *Risks to mental health: An overview of vulnerabilities and risk factors*. World Health Organization.
WHO. (2014). *Social Determinants of mental health*. World Health Organization.
World Health Organization. (2016). Maternal, newborn, child and adolescent health. Retrieved September 2016, from World Health Organization: http://www.who.int/maternal_child_adolescent/topics/adolescence/dev/en/.
Wolke, D., & Lereya, S. T. (2015). Long-term effects of bullying. *Archives of Disease in Childhood*. https://doi.org/10.1136/archdischild-2014-306667.
Yadav, P., & Iqbal, N. (2009). Impact of life skill training on self-esteem, adjustment and empathy among adolescents. *Journal of the Indian Academy of Applied Psychology, 35*, 61–70.

Chapter 10
Efficacy of Reproductive and Sexual Health Education for School-Going Adolescents

Sibnath Deb

Abstract Adolescence is a transitional phase when an individual experiences a lot of psychological and physiological changes. During this phase, they require judicious guidance by parents and teachers. Curiosity about various issues during this phase is a normal phenomenon. Sometimes, some of them wish to experiment with their curiosity under the influence of the peer group members. Consciously or unconsciously, some of them get involved in high-risk behaviours, for which, they pay a heavy price in a conservative society like India where pre-marital sex is taboo. In addition, risk behaviour also adversely affects their concentration in studies and future career. Therefore, parents and teachers should discuss with them about all the developmental issues so that; they remain well informed and do not indulge in any high-risk behaviour. The objective of this chapter is to discuss the knowledge and perception of adolescents about various aspects of reproductive and sexual health, in addition to understanding their behaviour, based on the findings of an intervention programme. Further, the chapter suggests evidence-based measures for disseminating information among adolescents about various reproductive and sexual health-related issues, in a culture friendly and sensitive manner, so that they become receptive and may benefit from the intervention programmes. Empowerment with correct information is found to be very beneficial to relieve anxiety and make them psychologically competent to deal with the changing situations in life.

Keywords Adolescent · Reproductive health · Sexual health · School
Intervention programme

S. Deb (✉)
Department of Applied Psychology (A Central University), Pondicherry University, Puducherry, India
e-mail: sibnath23@gmail.com

S. Deb (ed.), *Positive Schooling and Child Development*,
https://doi.org/10.1007/978-981-13-0077-6_10

Introduction

The meaning of the term 'positive schooling' is very broad. It is not confined to safety and quality education only. It encompasses the holistic development of students in terms of good habit formation, disciplining students, guidance for studies, addressing their day-to-day challenges and ensuring non-risk behaviour through empowerment with correct information about various developmental issues, including reproductive and sexual health. During the transition phase from childhood to adulthood, especially at the ages of 12–13, they become very curious about physical changes. Unfortunately, India is a very conservative society where, in normal situations, parents and/or teachers hardly discuss reproductive health issues with adolescent children. As a result, when they first experience the same, some adolescents become nervous, while some feel ashamed to share anxieties with others. Let us have a look at the developmental characteristics of adolescent phase which would help us to understand the challenges of adolescent better.

The term 'adolescence' has been derived from the Latin word 'adolescere', which means 'to grow up' or 'to grow into maturity' (Muuss 1990). This phase in life may be regarded as a transition phase from childhood to adulthood.

Adolescence is generally considered to begin at puberty. The biological changes that signal the end of childhood, produce rapid growth in height and weight, changes in body proportions and form, and the attainment of sexual maturity. But adolescence is also a social and emotional process.

Adolescents may also start thinking that they are adults and wish to take independent decisions about various issues on their own. Their individual identity should be recognized by the parents and other adults, and should discuss their issues and concerns, and extend support as and when required. In some situations, their issues and concerns should be dealt with by the parents sensitively, instead of outright rejection of their views and concerns.

It is also relevant to mention here that during any transitional phase an individual becomes confused about the roles he/she is expected to play. The adolescent, at this stage, is neither a child nor an adult. If adolescents behave like children, they are told to 'act according to their age'. If they try to act like adults, they are often scolded and asked to stay within their limits. That is why this phase is also called as a period of 'identity crisis'. The change in identity which takes place in adolescence involves the first substantial reorganization and restructuring of the individual's sense of self at a time when she/he has the intellectual capacity to appreciate fully how significant the changes are. According to Piaget (1969, p. 22),

> Adolescence is the age when the individual becomes integrated into the society of adults, the age when the child no longer feels that he is below the level of his elders but equal, at least in rights. This integration into adult society has many affective aspects, more or less linked with puberty. It also includes very profound intellectual changes. These intellectual transitions enable him to achieve his/her integration into the social relationships of adults.

Physiological Changes During Adolescence

Puberty is derived from the Latin Word 'pubertas', which means 'adult'. Technically, the term refers to the period during which the individual becomes capable of sexual reproduction. Puberty refers to the physiological changes that the adolescent undergoes in order to reach sexual maturity. During the pubescent stage, the growth spurt begins to accelerate, males experience their first emission of semen usually in form of 'wet dreams,' and menarche occurs in females. The post-pubescent stage is characterized by the deceleration of the growth spurt, attainment of both primary and secondary sexual characteristics, and fertility.

The four chief physical manifestations of puberty as stated by Marshall (1978, p. 142) are: "(i) A rapid acceleration in growth, resulting in dramatic increases in both height and weight; (ii) The further development of the gonads, or the sex glands, which are testes in males and the ovaries in females; (iii) The development of secondary sex characteristics, which involves changes in genitals and breasts, and the growth of pubic, facial and axillaries (body hair) and the further development of the sex organs, changes in body composition, specifically, in the quantity and distribution of fat and muscle; and (v) Changes in the circulatory and respiratory systems, which lead to increased strength and tolerance for exercise."

Psychological Changes During Adolescence

There are marked psychological changes during adolescence. The main change is the development of an integrated and internalized sense of identity. During this phase, the adolescents become more interested in friendship with peer group members. Hence, there is a gradual move from involvement with groups of the same sex to mixed groups. Adolescents' thinking moves from the concrete to the abstract and young people begin to articulate independently. This is also teh time when they begin to explore new interests and influences, which can mould their thinking and their ideas and action. When the adolescent develops new ideas of their own about different areas of life like career, moral ethics and values, peer group and so on, there is evidence for clash or differences of opinion with their parents. Regarding career choice, there is a lot of parental pressure and the parents try to force the child to take up a particular stream of education/career. As a result, some adolescents suffer from frustration and irritation, which ultimately hampers their academic and social performance.

Need of Adolescents During This Phase

Adolescence is a period of rapid mental and physical changes when adolescents become more curious about different things, especially about sexuality. During this phase, they have a tendency to take risk, which sometimes results in early pregnancy, involvement in deviant social activities, and dependence on substance, and premarital sex, exposing adolescents to the risk of sexually transmitted diseases including HIV/AIDS.

For healthy psychological and/or emotional development, they need both moral and health education, and understanding from the parents. This does not always happen. Because of cultural taboos in India, issues relating to reproductive health are neither discussed in the family nor in the educational institutions. As a result, a significant number of adolescents become dependent on the peer group to fulfil the need of the curious mind and take risks under the influence of mass media. Availability of pornography and violent and adult movies are the main contributory factors to risk-taking behaviour of adolescents. Findings of a study speak in favour of including reproductive health and sex education in educational institutions and industries (Deb 2006). So far as nutrition is concerned, a good number of them do not have any clear idea about which food contains what food value, and which food items are not good for health. Therefore, dependence on fast food makes adolescents vulnerable to obesity. Interpersonal relationship matters a lot in maintaining a good social network which helps an individual during crisis. Adolescents need education about the value of good interpersonal relationships.

Emergence of the Concept of Reproductive and Child Health

In order to meet the challenges of various social and health problems like overpopulation, teenage pregnancy, infant mortality, maternal mortality, morbidity, and STDs—including HIV/AIDS—various measures have been undertaken by the government of India.

During the 8th Plan, an integrated Child Survival and Safe Motherhood (CSSM) programme was adopted by the Government of India. The International Conference on Population and Development held in 1994 in Cairo recommended that the countries should implement unified programmes for Reproductive and Child Health (RCH).

The RCH approach has been defined as

> People have the ability to reproduce and regulate their fertility, women are able to go through pregnancy and child birth safely, the outcome of pregnancies is successful in terms of maternal and infant survival and well-being and couples are able to have sexual relations free of fear of pregnancy and of contracting diseases.

During the 9th Plan, the RCH programme integrated all the related programmes of the 8th Plan. The concept of RCH is to provide to the beneficiaries, need-based, client-centred, demand-driven, high quality and integrated RCH services (Source: Reproductive and Child Health programme, Govt. of India 1997, p. 2). Components which are covered under the RCH include: adolescent care, antenatal, natal, post-natal care, respiratory tract infection, immunization and child care, family planning and STDs including HIV/AIDS.

Risk-Taking Behaviour Among Adolescents

Several factors make adolescents vulnerable to HIV infection and teenage pregnancy. Adolescence is an age of experimentation and risk-taking, consciously or unconsciously. Personal development, especially with regard to self-esteem and identity is hampered due to inadequate knowledge (Boyer and Kegeles 1991). In some cases, moreover, they may not be informed about the mode of transmission of HIV/AIDS and its preventive measures. Thus, their behavioural risk persists and many adolescents remain ignorant or confused about causes and prevention of HIV/AIDS and teenage pregnancy.

Suicide among school-going adolescents is increasing very fast in India, mainly because of academic pressure and failure. The figure has jumped from 18.23 students in 2012 to 24 students in 2015; that is, as per the 2015 reported data, every day, 24 students commit suicide in India because of academic pressure and failure (National Crime Records Bureau Report, the Ministry of Home Affairs, Government of India 2012 and 2015). Students committing suicide is also associated with poor body image. For example, in a study in Mississippi, the authors found the highest risk of adolescent suicide is for females with poor body image and a history of traumatic experiences (Mandracchia et al. 2016).

Yeh (2006) studied and evaluated the risk factors associated with alcohol consumption, problematic drinking, and related consequences among high-school students in Taiwan. The results showed that "alcohol consumption and problem drinking was 2.22–2.71-fold greater in the 10th grade male than in female adolescents. Parents and peer groups were the determinant influence in alcohol consumption, and these influences could be altered by the same group of people. The probability of developing adolescent problematic drinking was four-fold greater in students whose fathers had habits of drinking. The study suggests that a policy for the prevention of alcohol abuse among high school students should start by addressing the two major associated problems: a need to earn peer group recognition, and the lack of family support among high-risk students."

In a study in Iran, Mohammadi et al. (2006) found that "twenty-eight percent of the adolescents reported having engaged in sexual activity. Sexual experience was associated with older age, access to satellite television, alcohol consumption, and permissive attitudes toward sex. Substantial proportions of respondents held misconceptions regarding condoms, STIs, and reproductive physiology. Attitudes toward premarital sex were more permissive among respondents who were older, were not in school, had work experience, had access to the Internet or satellite television, lived separately from their parents, and reported having used alcohol, cigarettes, or drugs. The relatively high prevalence of sexual activity and the lack of knowledge regarding STIs and contraceptives pose a significant threat to the sexual and reproductive health of adolescent males in Iran. Programmes are needed to provide adolescents with the information and skills to make safe sexual decisions." In an earlier study, Blum et al. (2000) examined "the unique and combined contributions of race/ethnicity, income, and family structure to adolescent cigarette smoking, alcohol use, and involvement with violence, suicidal thoughts or attempts and sexual intercourse, covering the 7th to the 12th grade adolescents. Findings disclosed that White adolescents were more likely to smoke cigarettes, drink alcohol, and attempt suicide in younger years than the Negroid and Hispanic youths. Negroid youths were more likely to have had sexual intercourse and both Negroid and Hispanic youths were more likely than White teens to engage in violence."

In today's digitally driven society, adolescents are becoming more involved in the virtual world for faster communication with their friends, in the form of sending a text message and/or chatting. Though it is entertaining, the overall usage is wastage of valuable time, compromising with study hours. In this regard, Ohannessian (2015) found "gender differences in technology usage. Girls were found to be more engaged in texting, e-mailing/instant messaging and working on the computer more than boys, while boys were found to be playing more video games. Technology use also predicted later substance use for boys and girls. Nevertheless, technology use was observed to have both negative and positive effects on youth. Substance use also predicted later technology use for girls."

Need for Intervention

A series of studies speak in favour of reproductive and sexual health education for the adolescents so that they remain in the mainstream, study sincerely, and their potentials and skills are utilized for prosperity (Alekseeva et al. 2015; Bearinger et al. 2007; Deb 2005; Brieger et al. 2001). For example, Bearinger et al. (2007) were of the opinion that today's adolescents are at heightened risks from poor health outcomes. Therefore, all adolescents need access to quality youth-friendly services, provided by clinicians trained to work with this group. Sex education programmes should be made available for all adolescents, with a view to offering them accurate and comprehensive information about reproductive and sexual health, while building skills for negotiating sexual behaviours. Girls and boys also need equal access to youth development programmes that connect them with supportive adults and with educational and economic opportunities. In a study, Singh et al. (1999) covering 130 female students, aged 13–17 years in Haryana, found that "awareness about the process of menstruation was poor. Commonest reported the menstrual problem was dysmenorrheal (40.7%), followed by irregular menses (2.3%), of which only 5.3% consulted a doctor and 22.4% took over-the-counter medications from chemist shops. Knowledge about normal duration of pregnancy and need for extra food during pregnancy was poor. Most of the girls knew about the importance and duration of child spacing and need for three medical examinations during pregnancy. Major sources of information were television (73.1%), radio (37.1%) and parents (36.1%). Girls preferred to consult parents (49.2%) and doctors (44.6%) for help at times of having reproductive health problems. This study highlights the need for educating school girls about adolescent health, pregnancy, and reproductive health problems through schools and parents with the help of health professionals."

Broad Objective

The broad objective of the study was to understand the knowledge, perception, and behaviour of school-going adolescents about various aspects of reproductive and sexual health, and to develop feasible modules on the subject based on findings of an intervention programme. This was a multi-centric intervention study covering six centres in India. The findings of the present chapter are based on the data collected from the Kolkata study site only.

Method Adopted for Base-Line and End-Line Study and Intervention

This intervention programme was funded by the Indian Council of Medical Research (ICMR), New Delhi. In order to achieve the objective, first, a baseline study was conducted in four selected schools in Kolkata, three of which were located in the urban area while one was selected from the rural area.

One Structured Questionnaire was developed by a multidisciplinary group of professionals. It was pre-tested and used for collection of data from the students before and after the intervention. The Questionnaire consisted of eight broad sections.

Section I: Profile of Adolescents;
Section II Adolescents' Needs and Practices;
Section III: Knowledge and Practice; Section IV: Sexuality;
Section V: Interpersonal Relationship;
Section VI: Understanding RTIs, STIs and HIV/AIDS;
Section VII: Life Skill Development, Risk-Taking Behaviour and Substance Abuse; and
Section VIII: Efficacy of Intervention programme as Perceived by the adolescents.

In the baseline study, a group of 480 adolescent students from Grade IX, and 384 from Grade XI were selected following multi-stage cluster sampling method, and data was collected by using a Structured Questionnaire developed by the ICMR Task Force Team. Afterwards, inputs were provided to adolescent boys and girls following classroom lecture approach based on the six modules developed. The modules, which were developed based on baseline data and used, are as follows:

Module I: Growing Up Concerns and Nutrition
Module II: Reproductive and Sexual Health and Hygiene
Module Ill: Body Image, Sexuality, and Risk-Taking Behaviour
Module IV: Interpersonal and Gender Relationships
Module V: Understanding RTIs/STIs and HIV/AIDS
Module VI: Life Skill Development and Scholastic Achievement

The classroom lecture was followed by question-answer sessions. In addition, brief leaflets on all the modules were distributed among the adolescent boys and girls. Other approaches adopted for clarification of queries of adolescents included teen-clubs, question box, and exhibition.

After two rounds of intervention, end-line data were collected from the same group of adolescents, 401 from Grade IX students and 376 from Grade XI students, using the same questionnaire. It is of relevance to mention here that some additional information was collected during the end-line study in order to understand the views of the students about the method of implementation of the intervention programme, utility of educational materials and its efficacy. Most of the adolescents belonged to 13–15 and 16–18 year age groups.

Empirical Evidence

Adolescent Needs and Practices

When findings related to adolescent needs are concerned, it has been observed that the majority of them were curious about various aspects of reproductive health, especially: characteristics of puberty phase, pregnancy, family planning methods, abortion, sexual activities, career, and friendship with the opposite sex.

So far as the adolescent practices are concerned, for proper growth and development, baseline data indicates that more than 50% adolescents, irrespective of the gender and class, go for outings, and participate in various recreational activities, like games and sports, and also exercise. Findings also revealed that in 40–50% of the cases, children have inhibition in free communication with teachers, parents/ guardian, about various sensitive issues. Strangely, very few of them discussed or shared information about reproductive health issues. Some of them also indulged in sexual activities at an early age. At the same time, about one-third of them reported a discussion about career-related issues.

For studies, adolescents mostly consulted teachers, followed by parents, and then friends; while in case of general health, they mostly consulted parents and friends, followed by doctors. Regarding nutrition, they mostly consulted parents, followed by guardians, and parents. In case of reproductive health, a mixed response was found. The Grade IX students preferred to discuss it with friends, followed by doctors; Grade XI students preferred consulting doctors, followed by parents/ guardians, and friends. For sexual health, they mostly consulted doctors, followed by parents.

So far as the issue of friendship is concerned, for sharing personal issues, friends were the first choice, followed by parents and guardians and teachers. In real life, a good number of adolescents, ranging from 19 to 37%, never consulted anybody for sharing their personal issues. It may be because of their personality and/or the fact that they did not find anyone to trust and/or depend.

Knowledge and Practices Concerning Nutrition, Physical Changes, and Various Reproductive Health Issues

Balanced nutrition is very important for healthy physical and psychological development of adolescents. The baseline study demonstrates that the majority of the adolescents were aware as to what food items should be included in their balanced diet but were not quite sure as what nutrients are found in various food items. The intervention programme did help them to enhance their knowledge in this regard, but more efforts in this direction are needed.

During adolescence, a lot of bodily changes occur. From the findings of the baseline study, it has been observed that a majority of them observed rapid gain in height and weight, the growth of hair in under-arms and pubic areas, the appearance of facial hairs and change in voice (for boys). In this regard, the intervention programme had a positive effect on the adolescent boys and girls: significantly higher number of adolescents reported such changes during the end-line study

So far as reaction of adolescents after noticing the bodily changes is concerned, data indicates that 10–18% of them became worried, 1–13% felt embarrassed, 7–12% of them thought it to be natural, 2–6% became anxious, while the rest were happy and mature. Interestingly, after the intervention, anxiety among adolescents decreased significantly, in case of the Grade IX students. At the same time, after the intervention programme, a number of adolescent boys and girls of Grade IX and girls of Grade XI developed a feeling that they had matured psychologically, and thought it to be natural. About 50% boys shared the bodily changes with someone, while girls mostly preferred to share the same with their mothers.

Regarding health and hygiene, especially washing hands, cutting nails, uses of soap and shampoo, for cleaning genital or sexual parts, change of undergarments, and so on, the data highlights a positive picture: adolescent boys and girls were more conscious about the issues. Usage of water and shampoo had increased significantly after the intervention programme among Grade IX and XI students.

The knowledge of the adolescents was comparatively better about the male and female reproductive organs, as compared to their knowledge about the functions of the same. The intervention had a significant impact in increasing the knowledge level of adolescents about the male and female reproductive organs and their functions.

Regarding pregnancy—how a woman conceives a child—findings disclosed that a large number of adolescents had misconceptions. However, the majority of the respondents, ranging from one-third to two-third adolescents, had correct knowledge about the issue: women conceive children when the sperm of a man and the egg of woman fuse together inside the woman's body. After the intervention, the knowledge level had increased significantly only among adolescent girls.

A large number of women experience humiliation for delivering a girl child and it happens mostly because of lack of knowledge among males about the issue. Therefore, this issue was explored in the study, since today's adolescents are future parents and they should not experience the same situation. In the present study, adolescent boys and girls were found to have wrong perceptions about gender determination of a child. However, after the intervention, a significantly higher number of them reported that the father is responsible for determining the gender of the child.

Knowledge determines the behaviour and outlook of an individual. About half of the adolescents, with minor variations across gender and grade, reported that they read romance-related magazines. This was more common among girls of Grade IX (70%). In addition, they also frankly admitted that they watched adult films, visited adult internet sites, in addition to viewing pornographic materials. About 39–50% of them reported that they read educational materials on reproductive and sexual health, and/or bodily changes. After the intervention programme, 25% increased significantly.

The meaning of the term 'sex' has different connotations among different adolescents. The majority of the adolescents, irrespective of gender and class, stated that it means the distinction between male and female gender, followed by other understandings: intercourse, reproduction, hugging or kissing the opposite sex/boy or girl/man or woman, love between opposite sex and something pleasurable.

Allopathic doctors were the first choice, irrespective of the grade or gender—followed by mother, siblings, father, alternative medical practitioners—for discussion of sexual issues or related problems. Interestingly, consultation with the doctors regarding reproductive and sexual health had increased significantly after the intervention. Regarding health-seeking behaviour, Aura et al. (2016) undertook a study to identify and describe adolescent health-related behaviours from a socio-ecological perspective and found that "there was a complex set of relations connected to adolescent health behaviours, also encompassing socio-ecological factors. Although authors tentatively concluded that socio-ecological circumstances influence the adolescent's health-related behaviour, the issue needs further verification".

Most of the adolescents felt that a girl should become a mother between 22 and 25 years of age. The second majority of them stated that, a girl should become a mother after 26 years of age, since they will become more mature physically and mentally.

Regarding the prevention of pregnancy, almost an equal number of adolescent boys and girls, with minor variations, replied that abstinence and the use of family planning methods were the best options. In this regard, a significant difference is observed between the baseline and end line data. After the intervention, the number had increased significantly.

Further, an attempt was made to determine their knowledge about the kind of health care facilities available in the health centres. The areas of knowledge were about pregnancy, family planning contraceptives, STDs, HIV, MTP, and so on. Findings clearly indicate the efficacy of the intervention programme; that is, knowledge had increased after the intervention.

The knowledge of adolescent boys and girls, about both male and female family planning methods, was poor, except one male family welfare method; that is, using a condom. In this regard, intervention had a positive impact on adolescents in increasing their knowledge about the issue

Baseline data demonstrates that adolescents were also more curious to know as to who may use family planning methods, how to use the same, why to use it, its costs, the availability, and whether there were any side effects of the family planning methods.

For effective communication of information about the family planning methods and other reproductive health issues, adolescents were of the view that a lecture is the best approach, followed by booklet, TV, internet, documentary films, radio, and posters. After the intervention programme, a significant number of adolescents were of the opinion that documentary films could be the best approach, followed by a lecture.

Doctors were the first choice—followed by counsellor, teachers, peers, and parents—for the dissemination of information about reproductive and sexual health. A significant number of adolescents during the end-line study stated that teachers, doctors, and counsellors could be the best persons for disseminating formation about family planning methods among them

Although more than 65% of the adolescents stated that they were aware of the meaning of abortion, a large number of them openly admitted their limitation of knowledge about the issue. However, after the intervention programme, knowledge level among Grade XI girls had increased significantly.

More than 65% adolescents felt that abortion could be performed by a qualified and/or authorized doctor while the remaining 35% stated untrained individuals could perform an abortion. The majority of the adolescents had correct knowledge about the safe period for abortion; that is, it should be performed during early pregnancy (up to 12 weeks). However, a large number of them either had no knowledge or had misconceptions about this issue. Further, those who stated that they were aware of the safe period for abortion were asked as to what problems an unsafe abortion could cause. Fatal incidents, that is, death could occur in case of unsafe abortion as stated by the majority of the adolescents, followed by bleeding/haemorrhage, perforation of uterus, and sepsis, were reported by the adolescents. After the intervention, significant changes in knowledge had been observed as witnessed by end-line data.

Reproductive Health Issues Related to Girls

The knowledge of more than 85% of the girls was correct about the meaning of menstruation, although they were not sure of the cause of menstruation and intervention programmes also failed to enhance their knowledge in this regard, probably because girls believed in what their mothers had told them and were not ready to accept the knowledge provided to them easily. The majority of the adolescent girls either had misconceptions or no knowledge about the question of whether a woman can become pregnant if she has intercourse during menstruation. However, knowledge level had significantly improved among the girls after the intervention programme.

Between 11 and 14 years, most of the girls had first bleeding. However, in the case of a small number of girls, it happened even at 10 years of age or below. More than half of the adolescent girls stated that they were informed mostly by mothers about the onset of period or menses. The vast majority of the girls used napkins or sanitary pads during periods, while some of them used a clean cloth and/or ordinary cloth.

More than half of the girls faced problems during menstruation which included a headache followed by stomach ache/cramps, body ache, tiredness/weakness, laziness, pain in breast, and legs. So far as gynaecological problems are concerned, 2–8% girls reported thin watery discharges, while only 3% girls of Grade IX, during baseline study, reported having problems like discharge with a foul smell. So far as psychological problems are concerned, mostly they reported irritation, with minor variations among Grade IX and XI adolescent girls, followed by weakness, and mood variations, fear, anxiety, depression, incompleteness, embarrassment and so on.

Reproductive Health Issues Related to Boys

Regarding the perception of adolescent boys about semen discharge, mixed response was found. The most common response included semen discharge means: a sign of adulthood/masculinity; natural process; the effect of hormones; containing sperms which cause pregnancy; and weakness. So far as the perception of adolescent boys about masturbation is concerned, about one-fourth to half of them had a correct perception about the issue; that is, it is a natural practice during the adolescent period. However, a large number of the adolescent boys had a lot of misconception about masturbation: it reduces interest and attention in studies; it weakens the body; it is a dirty/messy act; it leads to impotence; it can cause dysfunction and/or deformity in sexual organs; it makes one sexually inactive; and it is an immoral act and/or sin.

Sexuality

Sexuality is another very sensitive issue, which is never discussed openly in the Indian society. Most of the adolescents stated that they want to be friendly and make friends with opposite gender, meet whom they like or love, and also want to watch movies with them since a large number of them feel lonely. About one-third to half of them, irrespective of gender, expressed some sexual desires like kissing and hugging and wanting to 'have fun' with the person they like most.

Replying to a question about what are the activities adolescent boys and girls like to do with their dream girl/boy, baseline data highlights a range of activities which they would like do with their dream boys/girls. Maintaining healthy friendship was the response received from most of the adolescent boys and girls, followed by holding hands, which was an equally prevalent desire in both boys and girls, watching a movie, and going for a picnic and to a restaurant. A large number of them, especially boys, expressed some sexual desires like hugging, kissing, and spending the night together. On the other hand, a good number of them shared opposite views: asking the opposite partner to wait for marriage till he/she completes studies or becomes independent.

Regarding the legal age of marriage for boys, more than 60% boys and girls (ranging from 61 to 94%) were of the opinion that boys should marry after 21 years of age. The knowledge level had increased significantly among both boys and girls after the intervention programme. Regarding the legal age of marriage for girls, a similar picture was found. Vast majority felt that a girl should marry after 18 years of age.

Regarding pre-marital sex, most of the adolescent boys and girls (ranging from 31 to 66%) stated that it is risky, while the second highest category, with minor variations, stated that it is bad or immoral. A small number of boys stated that it is all right or moral.

About 1–9% adolescent boys and girls reported having intimate relationship/ sexual intercourse mostly during 13–16 years age. In case of 8–44% adolescents, who reported having sexual intercourse, it happened within the same gender. Prevalence of sexual abuse and/or harassment among adolescent boys and girls ranged from 1 to 11%. The perpetrators included: an unknown person, own relatives, friends, a person whom they liked and others, mostly males, forced sexually, in case of girls, while in case of boys, males mostly forced sexually. Baxendale et al. (2015) found that "gender had significant associations with being a victim and perpetrator of violence-related behaviours. Males were significantly more likely than females to be a victim of threatening and physical violence at school and to be a perpetrator of physical violence at school and in the community. Further authors found that males were significantly more likely than females to watch violent media, with exposure to violent media associated with physically hurting someone at school."

Interpersonal Relationship

Good interpersonal relationship is very important for good mental health. Relationships between two individuals, irrespective of gender, age, and socio-economic background should be respectful as every individual deserves respect from another individual. It ensures positive thinking and enhances concentration in studies and/or activities. Although the interpersonal relationship of most of the adolescents with the parents was friendly and it improved significantly after the intervention, it was not strong for a good number of adolescents.

Evidence concerning parent–child communication about sexual and reproductive health indicates that it largely focused on assessing communication frequency, barriers, and who communicates with whom within the family. However, Manu et al. (2016) examined parental and family contextual factors that predict parental communication with young people about sexual and reproductive health following a cross-sectional interviewer-administered survey with 790 parents. Findings disclosed that nearly the same factors predicted the mother's and father's communication with young people about sexual and reproductive health matters. The predictors for both mothers and fathers included high socioeconomic status (SES), family religiosity, parent discipline, perceived parental sexual knowledge, and parent trustworthiness. Therefore, it might be stated that parental communication on sexual and reproductive health is influenced by high SES, family religiosity, parent sexual knowledge, parent discipline, and trustworthiness. Based on the findings, the authors suggested that interventional programmes on communication about sexual and reproductive health need to take cognizance of these factors to improve parent-child communication about sexual and reproductive health.

Sharing of feelings and views about various issues helps an individual to feel happy. The baseline data of the present intervention programme disclosed that the mother was the nearest person for sharing of feelings. However, during the end line, the adolescents stated that friends of the same gender and opposite gender were the first choices for sharing of personal feelings followed by mothers, fathers, good teachers, siblings, and relatives. End line data also indicates that more than one-fifth of the adolescents of Grade IX did not share their personal problems with anybody. This issue requires attention from teachers and parents so that they create an environment for encouraging the adolescents to come forward and share their feelings and views with somebody whom they trust the most.

As far as future aspirations of the adolescents were concerned, data indicate that a good number of them wanted to be teachers/doctors/engineers/executives. In addition, a large number of them expressed their desire to be involved in business.

But a large number of them had given a very realistic answer: that is, the situation in future will determine their occupation.

Adolescents are also affected by stress. Studies are the prime causes for stress for more than one-third of the adolescents, followed by poor academic performance, loneliness, strained relationship, physiological changes, and reproductive and sexual health. However, the stress reduced significantly after the intervention programme. These findings suggest the need for strengthening the mental health support services for the adolescent students in the schools.

Regarding knowledge of adolescents about sexually transmitted diseases, data indicates that more than 65% of them were aware of the diseases. However, one-fourth to one-third of them had known about the symptoms. Their knowledge and awareness about STDs and their symptoms had increased significantly after the intervention. The primary source of information about the disease was newspapers, followed by friends, teachers, and doctors. The majority of the respondents were aware of the mode of transmission of HIV/AIDS. The majority were aware of the four main established modes of transmission. At the same time, a good number of them had a lot of misconceptions and erroneous understanding about the mode of transmission and its prognosis. But it decreased significantly after the intervention. They were willing to receive more information about the issue. More than half of the adolescents felt that people with HIV/AIDS experience social discrimination.

Life Skill Development, Risk-Taking Behaviour, and Substance Abuse

Evidence suggests that a good number of adolescents occasionally take alcohol and smoke cigarettes out of curiosity under the influence of peer group members. A small number of them had also tried alcohol and narcotic drugs.

One-fourth to two-fifth adolescent boys and girls experienced a crisis in life. Failure in academic performance was the most common crisis faced by the adolescents, followed by the death of close family members, love affairs, accidents/injuries, financial crisis in the family, domestic violence, prolonged diseases, sexual and reproductive health, and some other problems. In order to deal with the crisis, they mostly adopted two strategies: discussion about the issue with someone close to them and speaking to a counsellor. During the crisis, they got mental support from parents followed by teachers. Some of them practiced meditation and did exercise while some studied literature/spiritual books. On the other hand, some became dependent on alcohol or drug or did something for which they felt scared and/or ashamed, later.

Adolescents Perception About the Intervention Programme

The overall perception of the adolescents about the intervention programme was very positive and that it was beneficial. This observation corroborates with other study findings (Peters et al. 2014; Rao et al. 2008). An overwhelming number of the adolescents stated that all the topics were covered in the intervention programme twice.

The vast majority of the adolescents remarked that the activities which were undertaken during the intervention phase included classroom lectures/presentation, question and answer sessions, exhibition, teen club, question box, and distribution of educational materials.

More than 80% adolescents stated that appropriate time was given to each topic in the intervention programme. The majority of the respondents stated that their doubts were resolved satisfactorily during the intervention. In fact, it may be stated that the adolescent boys and girls actively participated in the intervention programme. More than 55% of adolescent boys and girls did put up questions in the question box, more among adolescent boys of Grade IX.

Classmates were the persons with whom adolescents mostly shared issues, which they learned from the intervention programme. A few of them, especially boys, shared the same with other friends or parents. Distribution of educational materials developed on the basis of six educational modules, which was one of the activities of the project to disseminate correct information among adolescent boys and girls. The majority of the respondents expressed their happiness about the quality of educational materials.

Finally, two more questions were asked of the adolescents to know whether there was any change in knowledge and behaviour of the adolescents after the intervention programme with respect to various aspects of reproductive and sexual health. So far as enhancement of knowledge about different aspects of reproductive and sexual health was concerned, data clearly indicated that it had increased among the adolescents. So far as behavioural change was concerned, a lot of positive things were observed among adolescent boys and girls, like enhanced self-confidence, followed by more interest in studies, acceptance of bodily changes and making friends easily.

Conclusion and Recommendations

The present study revealed a host of interesting findings. The adolescent boys and girls were curious about a lot of issues related to the opposite sex. Although a common notion is that the girls are more vulnerable at this age, boys were found to be equally at risk. Adolescent boys were found to share fewer things with family members, and more with peers as compared to the girls. In general, the knowledge and awareness of adolescents concerning various reproductive and sexual health issues were found to be low in both Grade IX and XI students, thereby increasing their risk manifold. A good number of them also had misconceptions about some issues. The intervention programme was found to be very effective in most of the areas in the elevation of the knowledge level except in some areas of nutrition. The adolescents themselves felt that they needed knowledge regarding various aspects of reproductive and sexual health. In a nutshell, it may be stated that the current intervention programme yielded success in achieving the broad objective of the study: that is, understanding the knowledge and perception of adolescents about various aspects of reproductive and sexual health including their behaviour, and in developing six educational modules on various aspects of reproductive and sexual health, and ascertaining its efficacy on school-going adolescent boys and girls. The modules could be replicated in other schools. The findings of the present study corroborate the findings of an Indian study by Rao et al. (2008) which also says that "an educational intervention programme can bring about a desirable change in knowledge among adolescent girls regarding reproductive health" (2008). In another intervention study, Brieger et al. (2001) observed "significant differences over time and between intervention and control groups concerning reproductive health knowledge, use of contraceptives in the initial three months, willingness to buy contraceptives and self-efficacy in contraceptive use. The authors also observed that the intervention project provided evidence that peer education is most effective at improving knowledge and promoting attitudinal and behavioural change among young people in school settings" (2001). Another pilot study also speaks in favour of the benefit of reproductive health intervention programme. For example, Robinson et al. (2016) have "yielded important insights into requirements of a curriculum for young people with low English literacy levels and with variable school attendance patterns. It confirmed the need to adjust both pedagogical approach and curriculum content for the programme to have resonance with students from this linguistic and cultural background and with varying levels of exposure to multiple stressors in disadvantaged community settings."

Recommendations

On the basis of the findings of the present study, the followings steps are recommended for effective implementation of future intervention programmes

- Taking proper steps to ensure the full cooperation of the school authorities for effective implementation of the intervention programme so that they provide a minimum number of classes for disseminating information among the adolescents.
- Small handouts to be developed for the adolescent boys and girls describing the key information on various aspects of reproductive and sexual health.
- Pedagogical approach and content of the curriculum for the reproductive health programme should be taken into account keeping the emerging issues and local language in mind.
- Parents should be involved in the intervention programme for improving their skills in dealing with curiosities of adolescents and in developing a healthy parent-child relationship.

- During the Parent-Teachers meeting, problems faced by the adolescents on these issues should be dealt with sensitively by holding discussions regarding the same by professionals.
- So far as modules are concerned, much emphasis should be given on nutritional issues followed by sexuality and HIV/AIDS, if necessary third round of sharing of information must be done.

Implications of the Finding

The findings of the intervention programme have many implications. First, the findings are an eye opener for the school administrators and school education policy makers about the reality, that is, nature and extent of knowledge of adolescents about reproductive and sexual health-related issues. The knowledge-gap needs immediate attention of school authorities and school education policy makers for imparting correct knowledge to empower the adolescents for their healthy overall growth and development. Second, the findings provide evidence-based modules for imparting reproductive and sexual health education to school-going adolescents, which could be replicated to other schools across the country. Third, for validation of the efficacy of the modules, further investigation should be carried out by young researchers in other schools.

References

Alekseeva, E. G., Krasnopolskaya, I., & Skokova, Y. (2015). Introducing sexual education to Russian schools: Effects of dance4life programme on perceptions and behaviour of adolescents and teachers. *Health Education, 115*(1), 7–37. https://doi.org/10.1108/he-02-2014-0014.

Aura, A., Sormunen, M., & Tossavainen, K. (2016). The relation of socio-ecological factors to adolescents' health-related behaviour: A literature review. *Health Education, 116*(2), 177–201. https://doi.org/10.1108/he-03-2014-0029.

Baxendale, S., Lester, L., Johnston, R., & Cross, D. (2015). Risk factors in adolescents' involvement in violent behaviours. *Journal of Aggression, Conflict and Peace Research, 7*(1), 2–18. https://doi.org/10.1108/JACPR-09-2013-0025.

Bearinger, L. H., Sieving, R. E., Ferguson, J., & Sharma, V. (2007). Global perspectives on the sexual and reproductive health of adolescents: Patterns, prevention, and potential. *The Lancet, 369*(9568), 1220–1231.

Blum, R. W., Beuhring, T., Shew, M. L., Bearinger, L. H., Sieving, R. E., & Resnick, M. D. (2000). The effects of race/ethnicity, income, and family structure on adolescent risk behaviours. *American Journal of Public Health, 90*(12), 1879.

Boyer, C. B., & Kegeles, S. M. (1991). AIDS risk and prevention among adolescents. *Social Science and Medicine, 33*(1), 11–23. https://doi.org/10.1016/0277-9536(91)90446-j.

Brieger, W. R., Delano, G. E., Lane, C. G., Oladepo, O., & Oyediran, K. A. (2001). West African youth initiative: Outcome of a reproductive health education programme. *Journal of Adolescent Health, 29*(6), 436–446.

Deb, S. (2005). Knowledge, attitude and perception of adolescents about different aspects of reproductive health: A cross-sectional study. *Social Science International, 21*(l), 70–92.

Deb, S. (2006). *Report of a study on ICMR task force project titled a study on reproductive and sexual health education for adolescents—A multi centric study (2006).* New Delhi: Funded by the Indian Council of Social Science Research.

Mandracchia, J., To, Y., & Pichette, S. (2016). Suicidality in the Deep South: Risks for adolescent Mississippians. *Journal of Aggression, Conflict and Peace Research, 8*(1), 61–70. https://doi.org/10.1108/JACPR-10-2014-0141.

Manu, A., Manu, A., Kotoh, A. M., Kotoh, A. M., Asante, R. K. O., Asante, R. K. O., et al. (2016). Factors associated with parental communication with young people about sexual and reproductive health: A cross-sectional study from the BrongAhafo Region. *Ghana. Health Education, 116*(6), 595–610. https://doi.org/10.1108/he-09-2015-0025.

Marshall, W. (1978). Puberty. In F. Falkner & J. Tanner (Eds.), *Human growth* (Vol. 2), p. 142. New York: Plenum Press.

Mohammadi, M. R., Mohammad, K., Farahani, F. K., Alikhani, S., Zare, M., Tehrani, F. R., ... & Alaeddini, F. (2006). Reproductive knowledge, attitudes and behaviour among adolescent males in Tehran, Iran. *International Family Planning Perspectives*, 35–44.

Muuss, R. É. (1990). *Adolescent behaviour and society: A book of readings* (4th ed.). New York: McGraw-Hill.

National Crime Records Bureau Report, the Ministry of Home Affairs, Government of India, 2012 & 2015.

Ohannessian, C. M. (2015). A longitudinal examination of the relationship between technology use and substance use during adolescence. *Technology and Youth: Growing Up in a Digital World, 19*, 293À313. https://doi.org/10.1108/s1537-466120150000019010.

Peters, I. A., Schölmerich, V. L., Van Veen, D. W., Steegers, E. A., & Denktaş, S. (2014). Reproductive health peer education for multicultural target groups. *Journal for Multicultural Education, 8*(3), 162–178. https://doi.org/10.1108/JME-02-2014-0013.

Piaget, J. (1969). The intellectual development of the adolescent. In G. Caplan & S. Lebovici (Eds.), *Adolescence: Psychological perspectives* (pp. 22–26). New York: Basic Books.

Rao, R. S., Lena, A., Nair, N. S., Kamath, V., & Kamath, A. (2008). Effectiveness of reproductive health education among rural adolescent girls: A school based intervention study in Udupi Taluk, Karnataka. *Indian Journal of Medical Sciences, 62*(11), 439–443. https://doi.org/10.4103/0019-5359.48455.

Robinson, G., Leckning, B., Midford, R., Harper, H., Silburn, S., Gannaway, J., et al. (2016). Developing a school-based preventive life skills programme for youth in a remote Indigenous community in North Australia. *Health Education, 116*(5), 510–523. https://doi.org/10.1108/he-09-2015-0026.

Singh, M. M., Devi, R., & Gupta, S. S. (1999). Awareness and health seeking behaviour of rural adolescent school girls on menstrual and reproductive health problems. *Indian Journal of Medical Sciences, 53*(10), 439–443.

Yeh, M. Y. (2006). Factors associated with alcohol consumption, problem drinking, and related consequences among high school students in Taiwan. *Psychiatry and clinical neurosciences, 60*(1), 46–54. https://doi.org/10.1111/j.1440-1819.2006.01459.x.

Chapter 11
Life Skills Education (LSE) in a Volatile Context for Promotion of Peace and Harmony: A Model from Gujarat, India

Subhasis Bhadra

Abstract Life Skills Education (LSE) is one of the most accepted preventive, promotional models for dealing with various challenges, and for reinforcing positive behaviour among children and adolescents. Use of LSE in after disasters is still limited, and LSE is mostly used to enhance resiliency among students in school as part of routine activities. The age group of 6–16 years is the ideal time for inculcating life skills, in various simulated situations by following participatory exercises, to facilitate experiential learning among the participants. The purpose of LSE activities is to help the students develop their internal psychosocial resources, and thus, to manage the situational demands in favour of the self. This chapter explains the use of life skills education for the promotion of communal harmony among students in the post-riot context of 2002. The communal rift in Gujarat had torn apart the basic social fabric and human relationships, deeply affecting the minds of the young and adolescent who were caught in the hostility, fear, mistrust, myths, stereotypes, prejudices, and the environment of hatred between the majority (Hindu) and minority (Muslim) communities. There were two prominent peace-building initiatives driven by the NGOs and other civil society organizations: 'Aman Samudaya' and 'Gujarat harmony project'. Working with students in schools was a priority like any other disaster, as establishing normal routine of functioning was quite crucial. Similarly, reopening schools and getting the students back in a protective learning atmosphere was initiated. The students and their families, being the survivors of the communal rift, were suffering the psychological effect of the riots, along with multiple losses in the socio-economic sphere. The situation posed a major challenge for continuing with the regular functioning in the school and classroom. The students' interactions were reflecting the hostile community relationships in the school. In this context, LSE was designed to work with ten identified Government-aided schools, located in the most communally-sensitive

S. Bhadra (✉)
Department of Social Work, School of Social Science, Central University of Rajasthan,
Ajmer 305817, Rajasthan, India
e-mail: bhadrasubhasis@gmail.com

S. Deb (ed.), *Positive Schooling and Child Development*,
https://doi.org/10.1007/978-981-13-0077-6_11

areas. It was also realized that a large number of students belonging to Muslim religious education system (*Madarasa*) were deprived of any psychosocial interventions though they were equal suffers of the situation. Thus, life skills education was also promoted in these religious schools. In both these interventions, model teachers were the key functionaries who were trained, and who worked with the students through designing a module on communal harmony promotion, and psychosocial resiliency building. This produced a major change in the interaction pattern and understanding among the students, which helped them to deal with prejudices and develop a perspective towards teh values of acceptance and pluralism.

Keywords Life skills education · Promotion · Peace · Gujarat India

Introduction

Life skills Education (LSE), is one of the most widely used approaches for the promotion of positive coping, and for facilitating healthy development, for the children and adolescents across cultures and regions. Contextualization of the concept, based on standard methodology and pedagogy, is key for implementation of LSE in different social settings, such as classroom in school, youth groups in informal learning centres, groups of girls or boys in playgrounds, and in various special institutional set-up, such as treatment centres, homes for rehabilitation of juvenile delinquents, residential facilities for orphans, differently-abled children and adolescents. The inception of the concept of life skills is a culmination of different projects and programmes conducted over the years in different parts of the globe for personality development, various soft skills development and leadership development programmes, rehabilitation training, capacity building of the young learners, and various preventive programmes, such as, prevention of use of addictive substances, smoking, adolescent pregnancy, bullying, peer conflict and violence. Scientific studies conducted with control groups invariably showed that LSE can bring positive desirable changes in behaviour of the intervention (experimental) group (Bharath and Kumar 2010; Maryam et al. 2011). LSE is, therefore, an accepted and widely used methodology for inculcating positive desirable changes, such as developing study habits, school attendance, performance in examination, strengthening positive peer relationships, and in the prevention of HIV/AIDS, sexual violence, onset of drug addiction and other negative practices that often threaten the healthy progress of the children and adolescents surrounded by the harsh realities of poverty, ethnic conflict, political instability, racial tensions, family and community disturbances. While the applicability of LSE is beyond doubt, its appropriate use is pivotal for a successful outcome. In this chapter, the use of LSE for the promotion of communal harmony among the pupils of schools in Ahmedabad, after the city was torn apart due to communal violence between the majority Hindu and minority Muslim community in 2002, following the Godhra train burning incident. The author was part of two major peace building programmes for the promotion of harmony: 'Aman Samudaya' (Community of peace) and 'Gujarat Harmony project' (GHP). The former programme emerged as a consortium of a few prominent NGOs under the leadership of Action Aid (India Programme) in the aftermath of the communal rift which caused displacement of the people in the city of Ahmedabad and in other districts of Gujarat, whereas the latter one emerged at the end of 2002, with the financial support of CARE (India Programme), an international organization. The Life skill approach was used effectively in various formal and informal institutional and community settings in GHP.

Life skills are abilities for adaptive and positive behaviour that enable individuals to deal effectively with the demands and challenges of everyday life (WHO 1997, 2005a, b; Bharath and Kumar 2010, 2002). The school is an important primary agent of socialization in any society, which shapes the ideas, characters, and behaviour of the pupil. The contribution of the school in nation building is often equated with the future potential of development and progress of a nation. Therefore, positive school experience becomes crucial to creating a healthy responsible adult who contributes towards protecting nature, democracy, and the nation. Educational institutions have an unparalleled opportunity to improve the lives of young people. One of the recommendations of the WHO expert committee on comprehensive school health education and promotion mentioned that "comprehensive, integrated life skills education that can enable children to make healthy choices and adopt healthy behaviour throughout their lives; health education that enables young people to promote the well-being of the families for which they will eventually become responsible and the communities in which they reside" (WHO 1993). LSE is based on a cooperative, experiential, participatory learning methodology, and there are various successful life skills intervention models in the schools to deal with academic stress, health issues, understanding changes in body during adolescence, and developing efficiency among the adolescent students. For dealing with such daily events of stress, life skill training is most crucial as the student develops important skills through designed sessions on decision making, problem solving, creative and critical thinking, coping with emotions and stress, self-awareness, empathy, interpersonal relations, and effective communication. With the traditional approach of value education that often encountered limitations, life skills education, as a pattern of actively engaged teaching pedagogy, effects wider skill development among students (Bharath and Kumar 2010; Bhadra 2011).

Through life skills education, children and adolescents develop psychosocial competencies. Psychosocial competencies are individual resources that need to be inculcated and tuned for effective use in personal, academic, and familial life. Psychosocial competence has an important role to play in the promotion of health in its broadest sense, in terms of physical, mental, and social well-being. In particular, in areas where health problems are related to behaviour, and where the behaviour is related to an inability to deal effectively with stresses and pressures in life, the enhancement of psychosocial competence could make an important contribution.

The development of psychosocial resources makes the adolescent student resilient and effective in dealing with the demands of the situation. The individual perspective of resiliency has two important dimensions: exposure to adversity and ability, quality of adoption positively (Masten 2001). In an adverse situation, the student will be able to deal with it based on his/her capacity and the resources available. The resources include both material and non-material resources. The material resources may come from the family, parental, and school support and the non-material support is derived from the student's own psychosocial competencies. Therefore, students need to develop their psychosocial resources to eventually make themselves more resilient in dealing with demands and challenges. In the aftermath of the human-made disaster (riots), the social situation was characterized by feelings of hostility, hatred, mistrust, apprehension, and threat, which had almost destroyed the social fabric of human relationships within the city of Ahmadabad (in the context of this chapter). The school, as an integrated unit of the social system, was not insulated from this social pandemonium. In this context, developing life skills for the students in the school to promote communal harmony was a crucial requirement of the time.

LSE for Pupil in Schools

Life skills programmes are developed considering the principles of social learning theory of Bandura (1977). According to this theory, learning happens by observation, imitation, and performing the role. Thus, learning is considered as an active acquisition, processing, and structuring of various experiences. In LSE, the participants are actively engaged in the dynamic process of teaching, learning, reflection, and practice. LSE plays an important role in improving the emotional intelligence of the adolescent. The outcome of emotional intelligence is significantly linked with the relationship that one is able to develop with others and the self. Mayer and Salovey (1993) explained emotional intelligence as the ability to monitor the feelings and emotions of the self and others, to distinguish between them, and use this information to guide one's own thinking process and action thereof. Emotions are involved in very action, decision, and judgment. People with higher emotional intelligence are better able to use their mind to manage their emotions, rather than allowing their decisions to be controlled by emotion. Emotional intelligence entails both interpersonal and intrapersonal skills. Interpersonal skills consist of: the ability to understand other's feelings, empathy, ability to develop and nurture positive mutual relationships, and thus develop a sense of responsibility in the social context. Intrapersonal relationship is about understanding and managing one's own emotions, and motivations, and responding to the situation effectively. This is a crucial component for developing and establishing peaceful, harmonious, coexistence in social situations, which is formed from the interaction of multiple religions, languages, cultures, and practices. The riots and communal conflict caused a severe disruption in the social relationship.

Thus, developing adequate logical thinking through LSE, which could promote a positive relationship was designed and implemented for the students in secondary schools of Ahmadabad.

To initiate the work of conflict resolution and peace building among school students, the intervention was designed to focus on health-promotional models to deal with the regular problems of the students in schools related to academics, attendance, motivation, communicable disease, ill-health, and such other issues. Further, communal harmony and peace building were incorporated with the module, and were mostly focused on during implementation. Thus, life skills become a major tool to work with the students in formal, informal, and religious schools. In the life of the adolescent students, parents, teachers, and peer groups play important influencing roles and shape their belief system. For the implementation of life skills, assessing and ascribing the social milieu was crucial. The health promotional model looked at the critical post-disaster context where the students in school was caught between reality and rumours, religious identity and nationalism, identity of self and community, and the disturbances in the family, community, and city. Some of them had suffered losses and displacement, while some had been stuck at home, due to the ongoing curfew and disturbances. Ultimately, the fear was deep rooted, and needed time, as well as designed intervention, to heal. Such a disturbed social milieu deeply impacted the social and psychological condition of the students. Along with widespread fear, anger, frustration, and personal experiences of trauma, the school students also missed attending school, had fears about examinations, and mostly felt de-motivated to study, complained about the inability to remember, lack of interest, and deep-seated confusion. Such a social and psychological context often pushed the students to adopt negative coping strategies, like smoking, consuming alcohol, and some even engaged in high risk or violent behaviour, showing a tendency to disobey elders, and developed deep-rooted hatred against other religious communities. Such negative coping, resulting in negative life style choices, caused ill-health as an outcome. LSE can be practically seen as a health promotional model that develops abilities for adaptive and positive behaviour. Health is seen as a combined state of well-being of physical, psychological, social, and spiritual sphere of an individual, enabling the individual to contribute positively and effectively to society.

The sessions for life skills are designed by the trainer keeping in mind a few specific learning outcomes and skill developments for the participants. Thus, in each session, the participants are put through an activity. The activity is based on a problem that needs to be resolved by discussion, reflection, participation, sharing, and exchanging views in a group situation. Through this activity, participatory learning takes place in a cooperative, supportive atmosphere. The activity itself provides an experience for the participants. Through the process of joining in the activity and by resolving or reflecting on the issue the participants derives the solution. Definitely, there can't be only one solution; rather through group activities, the participants derive multiple solutions to a problem. Thus, multiple options become available to the participants. Here, the skills used are focused and discussed by the facilitator to strengthen skill building. Further, the facilitator connects the

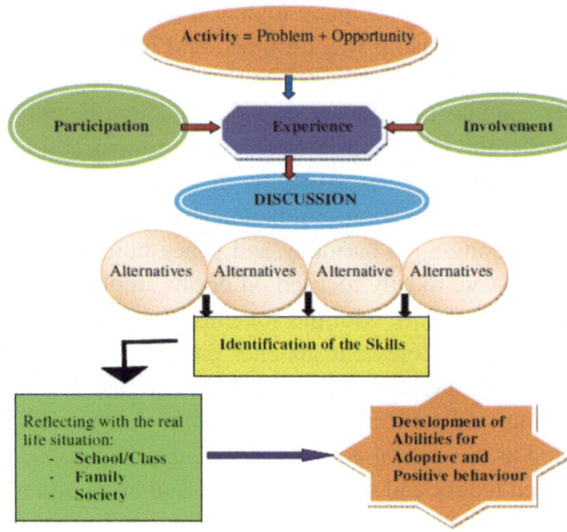

Fig. 11.1 Process of life skills session for implementation

situation with the real life context, that the participants become better capable to choose the best option by using his/her skills. Such sessions are repeated with different methodologies and themes and also needs regular follow-up with the participants. In life-skills training, the facilitator has a major role to calculate skill building in its true spirit among the students. Figure 11.1 represents the process engaged in life skills session as discussed above.

LSE and Research Findings

Life skills, as defined by the World Health Organization are cognitive, emotional, interpersonal, and social skills that work on enabling an individual to strengthen coping mechanisms and deal efficiently with problem situations and challenges of life (WHO 1998). Life skills modules have been widely accepted; formally, various national and state level education implementation bodies have given instruction to schools, and started conducting sessions on life skills for the students in high school. CBSE (Central Board of Secondary Education) has published various teachers' manuals and students' session for the teachers, to be practiced in the school (CBSE 2013). Different schools have also started promoting life skills. Working in the school through the teachers, mental health workers, and professionals by using life skills education is considered as an important strategy by DMHP (District Mental Health Programme) (Roy and Rasheed 2015). Mental health promotion among adolescents in schools using life skills education (LSE) and teachers as life skill educators are practices being developed and advocated widely and found to have positive impact in the life of adolescents (Bharath and Kumar 2010; Bhadra 2011; Vranda 2015). In a report of the State Planning Commission of Tamil Nadu about the role of SCERT

(State Council of Educational Research and Training) mentioned "the CCE (Continuous and Comprehensive Evaluation) introduced by the Government has an inbuilt life skill component giving an opportunity to the young children in the schools to attain valuable life skills from an early age" (State Planning Commission 2014, 18). While LSE has been a part of various social science programmes in college and university level, a post graduate course in LSE also has been introduced by an Indian university that focuses on different implications of life skills in different social settings.

LSE has been considered one of the best intervention modules for prevention of HIV/AIDS and other sexually transmitted diseases, as well as issues of sexual relationship among adolescents. A review of such programmes around the world has shown that LSE-based intervention programmes worked best to positively influence knowledge, attitude, intensions, skills and abilities (Yankah and Aggleton 2008). School-based LSE is very important to communicate information about sexual disease and to improve behaviour (Magnani et al. 2005). Similarly, LSE has been found important for decreasing onset of smoking behaviour among adolescent students (Botvin et al. 1980). LSE training with high-school students reported significant level of increase in self-esteem among the participants. "The students, who had participated in life skills training programme, could be successful in social communications using assertive behaviours" (Maryam et al. 2011). School behaviour, and bonding in the school has been significantly improved through LSE programmes and it has also helped in prevention of alcohol and substance misuse. Trained teachers are always a crucial link for the implementation of such programmes (Wenzel et al. 2009). Life skills training can improve emotional intelligence of the participants. LSE training is equally important for the improvement of mental health and other social skills (Lolaty et al. 2012).

The outcome of LSE is well documented in violence and aggression prevention programmes. A report by WHO (2009) on violence prevention provided evidence of successful interventions, based on LSE. It focused on five types of programmes:

- Preschool enrichment programmes aim to enhance a child's preparedness for new social surroundings of school and helps the children improve their academic and social skills at an early stage.
- Social development programmes designed to improve children's social and emotional problem solving skills in order to help them channelize their energies and work productively without being frustrated.
- Academic enrichment programmes focused on improving academic achievement of a child. It aims at developing a support structure for the child outside school.
- Incentives for youths to complete education provided financial assistance to young people to complete their studies and pursue higher education.
- Vocational training for underprivileged youths helped underprivileged children and youngsters to find employment and prevent them from becoming vulnerable to adult criminality and delinquency.

Prevention of violence and aggression is always a major challenge and LSE programmes have a very high potential to deal with these, and were thus used for peace building initiatives in Ahmedabad. A study with school-going children of early adolescence showed that LSE can act as an excellent medium to generate awareness and address problems like increasing aggressive behaviours in school children, through its active learning methods and interesting format (Khanam and Bhadra 2015). Life skills education has been consistently used with different kinds of vulnerable youth populations, especially with juvenile delinquents. Research studies indicate the change in the behaviour, relationship, anger outburst, and ideas about the future among them (Singh and Bhadra 2014; Naseri and Babakhani 2014).

Therefore, LSE is a model that can bring change in different kind of social issues for dealing with problem behaviour or to inculcate positive behaviour, thereby socially desired positive social interactions, and relationships. Importantly, the impact of LSE among adolescent students for improving mental well-being and building resiliency are reflected in all studies that have considered life skills, and development of various soft skills among the students in the schools or in other institutional set-ups.

Conflict and Peace in Gujarat Context

Conflict is a product of differential interest, attitude of groups or individuals, manifested in personal, family, or community life. Often, aggregated conflict takes the form of violence, which becomes more detrimental. It is unanimous that any kind of conflict creates stress in life and also produces an unfavourable effect on the life of the young. Conflict and violence are major threats to leading a peaceful life in society. Major outbreaks of conflict deprive the young of fulfilment of their basic rights as the tense socio-political condition jeopardizes the facilities of civic society. The situation affects psychological and physical growth and development, and deprives children of adequate standards of living, facilities for school, education, and games.

Education for peace and conflict resolution for children and adolescents is a logical outgrowth of this situation. Through life skills, education (LSE) inculcation of peace among the students in the schools was an important programme to support the positive school atmosphere in a volatile situation. The LSE programme in Gujarat was designed with three primary objectives.

- Skills orientation for reconciliation as the students can take part to bridge the gaps between the communities by developing more shared identity and vision.
- Enhancement of skills for developing the preventive role among the new generation, in the process of peace making.

- Skills development for promotion of peace and tolerance through mutual respect and understanding in a multi-religious, multi-cultural, multi-lingual diverse unique Indian society.

Learning to resolve conflict peacefully is not only about understanding conflicts and gathering information; rather it has more to do with changing the attitude and behaviour, and learning new skills for developing cohesive living through the promotion of interpersonal skills, communication, and being empathetic to other's situations. There are conflicts at the interpersonal level as well, as there are broader contexts of socially and politically charged issues. As life skills education is aimed at developing individual ability, it also impacts society at large. Developing a parallel between interpersonal and social conflict resolution processes for peace making, is essential to enhance positive peace and inculcate values of pluralism and inclusion among the young generation. Positive peace can be defined as not only the absence of conflict or violence, but the presence of factors that reduce the likelihood of conflict and promote better quality of life for all (Pieper 2008). These factors include: social economic justice, inter-group understanding, ecological balance, and opportunity for democratic participation in decision-making. Negative peace denotes the absence of conflict or violence, and any other significant relations. In such situations, the undercurrent of tension exists and is often controlled by power, by authorities or powerful communities, which dominate the powerless (Pieper 2008). In India there are six main sources of conflict; patriarchy, inequality, sectorality, peripherality, externality, and hierarchy; all of which adversely affect the democratic ethos (Oommen 2005, 64). The communal rift, in a complex reflection of these situations, stems largely from sectorality, peripherality, and externality. Lack of internal relations, connectivity, and communication, cause divisions between different sectors of society. In the case of cultural heterogeneity, due to difference in food habits, faith, rituals, and practices, the peripherality emerges in spatial or cultural locations. Externality features violate the cultural of pluralism and causes conflict as one group considers the other external. Considering specific religious, ethnic, castes or linguistic group as external, evoked a significant amount of conflict between the groups. Such features dominated the post-communal riot situation in the city of Ahmedabad. In helping the young generation to think and act independently, towards development of inclusive ideals, practice, and society, LSE was an important component in peace-building initiatives.

Life skills education aims to inculcate positive peace on a sustainable basis in the schools for the young generation. Stanford Siver (2006) emphasized some principles (Box 11.1), which were followed for developing and sustainable peace making process and initiatives:

Box 11.1: Principles for Sustainable Peace Making Process

1. *Relationship*: building strong interpersonal and inert group relations throughout the fabric of society.
2. *Long-term Commitment*: making an ongoing commitment to people and to processes, which may take years to come to fruition.
3. *Cultural Synergy*: Respecting the cultural wisdom of all parties and welcoming the creative interaction of different cultural ways.
4. *Partnership*: modelling collaborative process by partnering with local parties and institutions and coalitions.
5. *Multiple Technologies*: Utilizing a variety of technologies, as appropriate and creating new methods, as needed, to meet the unique the needs of each situation.
6. *Facilitation*: Assessing parties in taking responsibility of their own dream and destiny.
7. *Empowerment*: Helping people become empowered agents of change and transformation within their societies.
8. *Action Research*: Learning from all that we do and sharing that learning with others.
9. *Invitation*: Entering the system where there is an invitation, an open door.
10. *Trust*: Building relationships of mutual trust caring within the system.
11. *Engagement*: Acknowledging that once we enter a system, we become a unique part of it, an engaged, caring, and accountable partners.
12. *Transformation*: Catalyzing changes at the deepest level of beliefs, assumption, and values, as well as behaviour and structure.

Source Siver (2006).

It is important to understand that some amount of conflict is unavoidable in life, but conflict does not mean the outbreak of violence in a destructive form. The resolution of conflict is a way of looking at the situation where a harmonious coexistence of difference can be developed by ensuring a certain amount of commonality in the whole scenario. Conflict is not the same as violence; therefore, it is possible to avoid violence by acquiring certain skills and through application of the same. It is an essential task of education to teach younger generations about choosing peaceful ways of resolving conflict. Teaching skills in conflict resolution is different from just taking about peace. Children and adolescents need to learn the skills and put them into practice. Education for conflict resolution through LSE is an active and participatory process through experiential learning methodologies, which was implemented in a sustainable frame of practice for the students in schools in Ahmedabad.

Communal Rift and Its Impact on School and Students

Children and adolescents were one of the worst victims of the social turmoil that destroyed the stable coexistence of Hindus and Muslims, who had lived in proximity or had functional dependency for generations together (Engineer 2003a, b). Incidents of riots and violence continued for months, and almost every day there were incidents of violence in some or the other area (Roy 2008; Christophe 2007). Riots are a threat to democratic values and human rights that spill over to every social institution, relations, and other sectors such as political, economic, cultural, and social. School is a unique institution and primary agent of socialization that transmits knowledge, values, and heritage for the purpose of development and growth of future generations. When school and education system cease to function effectively, it also threatens the stability and progress of the nation. Therefore, strengthening the education system becomes extremely important for rebuilding of nation and community. The aftermath of the communal rift deeply divided society, and impacted the school atmosphere and the psyche of the learners. Due to riots for almost three months (PTI 2002) the schools were closed and even after they reopened, students took time to come back and rejoin. Some of the parents were worried about the safety of their children on the way to school, as the social situation was volatile and unpredictable. Even a small incident could cause tensions and often curfew was imposed in some of the areas of the town. Thus, there was an atmosphere of apprehension and restriction of movement, free expression, and gathering. While many children and adolescent students did not face any loss or displacement, they were deeply affected by the news, and by negative influences in the community and surroundings. Some of them shifted to Mumbai, Pune, or other cities of Gujarat by their parents for months together, and they were very anxious when they returned to thei home and came back to school. There were some school students who were direct survivors of the communal conflict and faced personal losses, as they had lost their books, school bag, uniform, and other personal belonging. Many of them stayed for months in relief camps or at the home of their relatives. Some of them lost their close family members and were shifted to new housing colonies under rehabilitation programmes. While most of the students returned to school, some of the students had to change their school and a few could not return for studies any more (Engineer 2003a, b).

Psychological trauma due to communal conflict was quite high, like any other such human-made disaster where children and adolescents have witnessed and survived such experiences (Gooder 1996). Children and adolescents bear the scars for long periods of time and the situation raised confusions and questions that impacted their social attitudes and behaviours—consciously or unconsciously. "Incidents of riots created a perceived threat and fear in the mind of the children and adolescents. They were highly sensitive to and aware of events that were happening around the city. The perceived threat raised lot of questions and doubts about their identity and religion and suspicions about each other. This behaviour greatly hampered their study habits and discipline in the family, school, and community.

The communal conflict had a wide and detrimental effect in terms of their development, life opportunities, and ability to become a free and independent individual and impacted their capacity to think and act independently" (Bhadra 2012). The children also experienced psychological and biological reactions to stress (Yule 2002).

Following riots, the school atmosphere, and interaction among peers in the classroom changed and caused a negative atmosphere. The teachers reported that, following the riots, students preferred to have friends from their own religion only and they favoured segregation according to their religious identity. Often, they formed their own peer groups during recess or had other interactions inside and outside the classroom. At times, students made offensive comments about each other's religion, food habits, differences in rituals, and so on, which fuelled tensions and generated an unfriendly atmosphere within the school. In some cases, students identified the teachers by their religious affiliations or vice versa (Bhadra 2012). This was a problem that required serious attention.

As the schools reopened and the students began their school life, teachers observed a wide difference in behaviour and social interactions among the students. The children were highly sensitive to noise and sound and were generally very much disturbed in the classroom. Lack of concentration, creating noise, and talking about different incidents of riots, was very common among the students. There was a drastic reduction in performance for most students. The students who were enrolled in new schools and those who stayed in relief camps for prolonged periods also had multiple adjustment issues. At times they felt inferior; marked by other students as victim or riots with derogatory statements: "he lost everything in riots"; "he became poor after the riots"; "now she has only one set of school dress". Teachers reported that some of the students also became aggressive or timid. Some of the teachers felt that students were overly conscious of their religious background, as they started identifying religious issues in classwork or the religious affiliation of writers, scientists, and historical characters from their textbooks" (Bhadra 2012).

Another group of school students were highly affected by riots but they received very little focused attention and support following the communal conflicts. These were the students of Muslim religious institutions (*madrasas*) widely perceived to be the bastions of Muslim religiosity and conservatism (Oommen 2005, 247). These institutions train students who are expected to become religious teachers and follow religious principles in their life. These institutes were located in the cities and in the far off districts. A large number of students in these residential schools were mostly from a poor socio-economic background. The teachers (*mufti*s and *moulavi*s) of these schools expressed the need to talk about the psychological sufferings of the students who have faced such difficulties; their families were affected, and the students were equally disturbed with persistent fear and rumours. The teachers felt the need to help the students understand the changing situation and to take-up positive roles in peace-building for the betterment of their community.

Considering these wider impacts in the school life of the children and adolescent the LSE programme was implemented in 10 selected schools of Ahmedabad city and 4 *madrasas* in different districts of Gujarat during 2002–2004. The programme of LSE was conducted under the Gujarat Harmony Project of CARE India (Ahmed 2004) with active partnership of two implementing organizations: SAATH and GSWT (Gujarat Sarvajanik Welfare Trust). "The Gujarat Harmony Project was with a strong commitment to promote peace and harmony at a moment when the communities were torn apart with tension, mistrust and misleading information, worries, and insecurity. GHP with an aim to promote value of pluralism, tolerance and acceptance ensured that every programme it funds has to be directed for ensuring communal harmony by engaging people in the community by common dialogue, sharing ideas, exchanging support and mutual cooperation" (Bhadra and Dyer 2011). The peace building programme was '*Aman Samudaya*' (a campaign for peace and justice) that was mainly supported by Action Aid India as well as other professionals and NGOs (Chachra 2004, 156). This forum started in the aftermath of communal violence. Under the banner of '*AmanSamudaya*', peace and justice, psychosocial support started immediately by identifying and training local community level workers (CLW) through the NGOs. In this programme, LSE was used in informal schools and community level.

Process of LSE in Formal Schools and Minority Religious School

The LSE programme was initiated as a model with a few schools, on health promotion coupled with conflict resolution. For this reason, ten schools were selected from the middle socio-economic background (both Government aided and private trust managed) from different areas of Ahmedabad. During selection of the schools, the affected population and a good mixture of the religious background was kept in mind. Therefore, four Muslim managed institutions, two Christian managed schools and four Hindu majority schools were selected. Approximately 12,000 children are covered in this programme. For understanding the situation, a systematic needs assessment was done by visiting the schools, discussion was held with the teachers, principals, and managements; a FGD (focused group discussion) was also organized with representatives from all the selected schools. It was seen that there were problems with study habits and motivation, as well as with discipline, along with many other issues. The schools also reported the two sequential disasters—earthquake and the riots—had made a very deep impact on the students and the performance had decreased to some extent. Some of the other important issues discussed were: (a) over-sensitivity about religion and the gap between Hindu and Muslim communities had widened creating a number of prejudices and stereotypes; (b) confusion about religious identity and its meaning; (c) change in school behaviour and school interaction; (d) adjustment issues among peers and feeling of being unsafe. Some other common issues were: dropouts due to poverty among the students was common; after eighth or tenth grades it was difficult for girls to continue education as marriage become priority; parents engaged in low-income jobs often had less focus on education of their children (Oommen 2005, 222–223). These issues are discussed in detail in the section above.

Considering the situation, LSE was prioritized as one of the important institution-based interventions in the formal schools and *madrasas*. The teachers as facilitators were the agents for transmission of knowledge and skills to the students and thereby also to the parents and larger community. Thus, LSE was intended to remove religious prejudices and stereotypes that were causing tension in the school atmosphere. Building bridges between the communities was crucial for establishing sustainable peace that could support a safe nurturing school atmosphere. Helping the teachers to recognize the situation, and developing skills for handling the same, was important to support and strengthen the learning atmosphere in the schools. Therefore, health promotion, focusing on psychological and physical well-being, was coupled with peace building and conflict resolution in the LSE programme. The programme objectives were:

- Promote the skills for upholding the spirit of democracy and citizenship, by inculcation of values of tolerance and pluralism which are part of Indian culture and social structure.
- Infusing changes among the teachers about their perception of the problems and solutions, and thus, making them responsible for working on skill building for the students who can work as change agents in the family and community at large.
- Promoting well-being of the children and adolescent and educational atmosphere for the students in the formal schools and in religious school.
- Promoting atmosphere of religious empathy and values of harmonious social existence among the students.

To attain these programme objectives for the purpose of ensuring a positive school atmosphere, the sequential action plan was designed.

- Intensive training for all the teachers on LSE in the formal schools and in religious schools.
- Facilitating the process of implementation of the LSE classes for health promotion and conflict resolution for the students in the schools on regular basis.
- Providing support to the teachers in the schools to conduct sessions on LSE through visit to the school by experts (Author and team who are LSE trainers)
- Developing manuals and support materials for conducting LSE sessions by the teachers
- Assessing the outcome of LSE programme and establishing suitability of the programme.

Peace building is a long process but a good start always depends on effective capacity building of the key role players in the right direction. Teachers were the key players in this programme. An intensive capacity building methodology was designed that started with two days of sensitization of the teachers with fifteen hours of engagements in two days, in batches of 25–30 teachers. Subsequently, the teachers started conducting sessions in the school and it was expected that the teachers would facilitate an empowering atmosphere in the classroom interaction rather than just being suggestive or instructive in every case. The teachers were expected to incorporate the participative teaching methodology as pedagogy in teaching the courses and spend one specific period (of at least 45 min) in a week on the designed life skills session. The teachers were engaged further in discussion by the experts while visiting the schools and some common coordination meeting were organized with all the ten schools of Ahmedabad. It was suggested that the students could develop various group initiatives in the school and better engage in school environment beyond academic engagement. The programme outlay was same for the residential *madrasas*. After the sensitization and regular sessions through visits in schools and focused group discussion with the teachers from each of the 10 schools, three teachers from each school were selected—a total of 30 teachers—and were trained as Master Trainers in a residential mode for five days. This second capacity-building programme was very intensive and teachers were engaged in a manner that, on return to Ahmedabad they could develop a support group and also advocate the LSE programme in other schools and to the Government also. Development of Master Trainers was also important to ensure suitability in the practice. The major focus of the training programme was the subject matters covered, considering the issues identified, and developing the most participatory methodology for experiential learning of the participants that could be replicated for implementation with students in the school and classroom.

The available manual of LSE developed by NIMHANS for health promotion (Bharath and Kumar 2002) was adopted and translated into the local language for use in the schools. The health promotional sessions were on various issues: developing adequate food habits, knowledge about communicable diseases, practicing personal health hygiene, keeping the school campus and surrounding areas clean, understanding change in the body and mind during adolescent stage. There were sessions particularly to support betterment in academics. These were on developing memory, focusing on study habits, preparation of lessons and doing home task, developing routines, and preparation for examination. Further, sessions on conflict resolution and peace building were introduced that could support creation sustainable positive peace in the schools and community.

The declaration on ‘Culture of Peace’ was adopted by the UN General Assembly on 13 September 1999 (United Nations 1999) and this was one of the key guiding sources for peace education through the LSE programme. The LSE session for conflict resolution dealt with harmonious living, power of peace, establishing communal harmony, and establishing mechanisms for positive peace building. There were four to six sessions under each section. Further, teachers were encouraged to design sessions for the promotion of peace considering the situation of their school and students. There were different facts sheets developed under the theme of promotion of peace. The sessions were designed by taking help of already available sessions on peace building by different organizations like, ‘Play For Peace’, UNICEF (Fountain 1999), UNESCO (1998, 2001), Peace Corps (2001) and others. Three such important sessions are given here to explain the process. For peace building in the community, it is also pertinent to have peace at personal and family level. Internal peace is equally important for the promotion and to advocate peace in the school and community. Therefore, the students need to understand the interpersonal issues that raise conflict and widen the gap between people.

LSE Session of Harmonious Living

Here in this activity module (Box 11.2) the main focus was interpersonal issues, which are common and take the shape of conflict in a student's life. For example, conflict may arise from lack of understanding about each other's needs and requirements. It may also rise due to lack of empathy; lack of open discussion between the parties; looking at each other with 'feelings of hostility' rather 'fellow feelings'. Once the child learns to manage conflicts in his/her life, he/she is also able to contribute in the peace building process in the society. Conflict resolution is not only an issue in the societal context; it is also important at the personal level to reduce the stress and strain of everyday life. The students need to understand situations which are conflict prone or which are more problematic, for identifying the conflict, as well as for looking for the alternative solutions. So, before reaching the conflict, the mechanisms to understand the conflict situation as well as to deal with it in a manner which promotes co-existence, are important for conflict resolution. Developing capacity among adolescents certainly helps them to deal with the various conflicts in their life and also to develop harmonious living. In the adolescent stage, due to the change in the social expectations and status, relationships in the peer group become more important. Family relations also start changing where the adolescent becomes very vulnerable and prone to different kinds of interpersonal conflicts. To resolve these issues, identifying one\s own emotions as well as learning positive coping and handling the anger become crucial. There are various emotional expressions which are detrimental to health as well as for developing healthy relationships. Therefore, positive expressions of emotion help to deal with many of the problems. Inclusive ideas and thoughts are two important aspects in developing healthy relationships as well as dealing with conflict situations. As in many of the cases, the idea of exclusion becomes very complex. Developing personal boundaries creates divisions in the mind, which starts excluding others based on some or other criteria. Harmonious living denotes a way of living where harmony can be ensured even at personal level in practice and belief, which includes people within the relations, or thoughts based on similarities rather than those focusing on differences. This was essential; for the students belong to different religious faiths to accept each other based on their similarities in student-hood, future aspirations, and academic demands, rather than looking at differences based on food habits or religious practice.

Box 11.2: Activity Module for Addressing Interpersonal Issues

Name of the Activity: *Happiness—The positive expression*

Emotions are essential components of behaviour. People express their emotions in different ways.

Positive expressions help to look at the situation assertively and express feelings more constructively. Usually, being happy helps to maintain good mental health and a stress-free life. Happy living and positive mental health are very closely connected. To be happy, it is essential to find out and understand the source of happiness. 'Well-adjusted people', 'subjective well-being', 'progressive outlook' are allied aspect of happiness. Positive expression of feelings is very essential to maintain happiness and resolve the conflicting situations.

Objective of the activity:

- Facilitate the identification of emotions within self and understand the expressions which are essential for harmonious living.
- Identifying appropriate ways of expression of certain emotions

Outcome of the activity:

- Students understand that inappropriate expression cause a lot of conflicts in life.
- In personal life, expressing feelings positively is very essential to maintain a harmonious living.

Process:The session is conducted through group activity and role play.

1. Identify different emotions by brain storming and make a list on the black board and also write on a card. One emotion to be written in one card.
2. Distribute the emotion card among the students randomly and ask them to come in around and start moving in the room with the expression as it is written in the card without making any sound.
3. Ask them to observe each other very closely and identify the emotions. Student sit in-group and make two lists, the first indicates the ways in which they feel it is appropriate to express the emotion, either verbally on non-verbally; the second indicates ways they feel it is not appropriate to express the emotions; then they present it in front of others.

Facilitative questions:

- How was it to do the activity?
- Was any difference raised in the group as to what are the appropriate and inappropriate ways of expression emotions?
- To what do you attribute these differences? Individual difference, family background, cultural difference, gender?
- How can negative ways of expression of emotions contribute to conflict?
- How can the way we express our emotions help to prevent conflict?

Summarize:

- Various conflicts start due to inappropriate expression of emotions. Therefore, expressing emotions in right manner, which are not hurtful to others should be practiced and entertained.
- Developing effective ways of expressing emotions helps to live in a harmonious way and much interpersonal conflict can be avoided.
- Developing effective strategies of expressing emotions will help to build relations also help to handle the negative emotions in a more positive manner.
- Anywhere, at any time, resolving conflict is the responsibility of each one of us.

Reflection for the student:

- How do I express my emotions, is it appropriate or sometimes goes inappropriate.
- How can I resolve the conflicts, which I come across by showing positive expressions of emotions?

Source Adopted and modified from: Bharath and Kumar (2002).

LSE Session for Communal Harmony

In this module (Box 11.3) the purpose is to make the students aware about the need of maintaining communal peace in the society as well as their responsibilities for ensuring peace in the society. There are various culture beliefs and practices in different religion, but maintaining peace is the basic human need, which is at the core of every religion. Simultaneously, there are various divisions in society, but there are many connecting factors also present. So, strengthening the connecting factors is essential to building harmony and promoting peace in the society.

Harmony is one of the most important survival needs of any community. Peace can be established only when communities live together in a harmonious atmosphere. Harmony is an equation, which is based on various factors in the community. Cultural faith, belief, stereotypes, practices, ways of interaction, interdependency, all are important for ensuring peace and harmony. But community members are active partners in maintaining peace in the community. In the world scenario, it has been seen many times in different parts of the world, that countries and communities are torn apart due to conflict and violence. Efforts have been made by different organizations, NGOs, UN agencies to make people aware about the loss due to conflict, various programmes have been organized to combat conflict, but still, in many situations, peace is yet to be achieved. Gujarat also has experienced the same many times and in the recent past. Thus, competence building of the young generation for peace building is one of most urgent requirements for promoting peace and harmony as well as in preventing conflict. The most important loss due to riot were the divisions which were created in the minds of people. There were lots of reasons for co-existence between the communities but one division in the mind—in the form of lack of understanding and misconception about each other's culture, as stereotypes and prejudice—can devastate an entire community and society. Addressing the issue of communal harmony is based on building individual and community competencies and confidence to practice and inculcate peace.

Developing relationships is most important for increasing connections among people. It may happen by increasing interaction between the conflicting communities or we need to cultivate social connectors for bringing the people together and to heal the scars of the mind. Once skills are built up among the younger generation to increase the social connections between conflicting communities, it is possible to bring large-scale change in future. There are many factors present in society which keep communities together, that are considered as connectors: inter-dependency, co-existence, festival for all, some institutional set-ups where both communities come together are considered as connectors. Many of these connectors get disrupted or weakened due to conflict but many others may still survive which are essential to understand and strengthen the work towards peace and harmony. There are, similarly, some factors, which are considered as dividers of society, which creates tension among people, and may cause or instigate conflict or create a disharmonious atmosphere. Therefore, finding out the matters which are causing disharmony, is equally important for sustaining peace. People also have to try to work on the divisions as those factors gets weakened or eroded. As life skills operate at an individual level to increase the capability of the younger generation, the purpose of involving the students in school is to make them active partners in the peace making process.

Box 11.3: Activity Module for Addressing Communal Harmony

Name of the Activity: *Trust And Faith—Connecting Us All.*

Objectives of the Activity:

- To help the students to understand that developing trustworthy relationships is every one's responsibility.

Expected outcome:

1. The students realize that trust and faith develop the connectivity in a relationship, which we have to keep alive.
2. The students also learn to take responsibilities for developing harmonious relationships.

Situation 1:

Rafi and Ranjan are very close friends. Both of them are studying in Grade IX in a school. Rafi is good in science subjects and Ranjan in language and social science. So, they help each other in preparing notes on different subjects. They have a feeling that they will be friends for all their lives. Rafi wants to choose a medical course and Ranjan is intent on going for administrative services. Both of them are very hard-working and support each other all the time. During their Board exam (final exam of Grade 10) both of them had to go to a school which was far from their school. In the meantime, there was some tension in some areas and it becomes problematic to travel every day up to the examination centre. So, they decided to stay together with Rafi's uncle, who lives near the examination centre. Though both their parents were happy about their friendship and Rafi's uncle was also happy to host them, the neighbours of Rafi's uncle, as well as the neighbours of Ranjan, started saying it was risky to bring people from other communities into their houses or to go to another community's area. But they continued to stay in Rafi's uncle's house and completed the examination very well. Both their parents and uncle developed family friendships with each other.

In this situation, Rafi and Ranjan were very upset to see the reactions of their respective neighbours. They decided to make more friends, started celebrating friendship day, and established a friendship club in the school. Their teacher helped them to develop the idea and also to work on this matter.

Facilitative question:

- In this situation is common like Rafi and Ranjan?
- What are the factors that kept Rafi and Ranjan together?
- What are the factors, which were creating doubts and imposing restrictions on Rafi and Ranjan?
- How did the parents react to the situation?
- Why were the neighbours not happy? What was lacking in their understanding?
- How a friendship club can promote harmony among the people, young generations?

Summarize:

1. The most important thing in any relation is 'fellow feeling' for each other and building a trusting bond.
2. Building a trusting relationship is very essential among all of us to maintain a strong bond of relationship.
3. Friendship is the most important matter, which kept them together and they helped each other in every aspect of their study.
4. The parents' attitude also is very important to make a friendship strong and accepted by others. A friendship based on trust and good faith is always beneficial.

5. In society, many people who are not close related to others, have various wrong notions about others, which have to be corrected by talking and showing good practices.
6. We have to remove the divisions from our minds to build a society and also help others to remove the divisions from their minds.

Reflection for the student:

- Do I have a relationship with a friend whom I trust and who belongs to other community?
- If yes, what are all the good things we share between us?
- If not, how can I develop this kind of relationship?

Source: Bhadra (2012). Psychosocial Support for the Children Affected by Communal Violence in Gujarat, India, *International Journal of Applied Psychoanalytic Studies,* 9(3), 212–232, p. 228. (The author designed this activity while working)

LSE Session for Peace Building

Peace building is the process and a harmonious society is the outcome of the whole exercise. Therefore, peace is a long-term goal, which society attempts to achieve by modifying and altering many existing thoughts and practices. The effort for the peace building has been initiated by different countries as one of the most important promotional tasks for ensuring a happy and secure life for citizens. The work on this front may take generations to achieve a final result but initiating the process itself can show the new directions for change. In the process of peace building, though all factors which cause tension in society need to be addressed, many times it is found that it is not possible to deal with all factors. Therefore, implementing such a change is not an easy task but the effort of peace building will ensure a better atmosphere. Considering the situation, the effort of positive peace building is not only for controlling violence or conflict, but rather involves building trust, faith, and mutual understanding between people, groups, and communities. The LSE sessions (Box 11.4) on peace building are intended to deal with developing inclusive identity, building hope for the future of the nation collectively, dealing with prejudices and stereotypes, and so on. LSE as a peace building measure works at three levels: first, learning the skills and acquiring for application in day to day life in different occasion; second, application of life skills for dealing with broader social issues; and third, use of skills for challenging the restrictive forces towards developing sustainable peace. The students, as messengers of peace in the community, are expected to deal with restrictive forces and work towards peace making.

Box 11.4: Activity Module for Addressing Peace Building

Name of the Activity: *Inclusion and Identity.*

Objective of the activity:

- It is a tendency to identify an in-group based on some identity and make others out-groups
- Establishing and emphasizing the identity which many people can share, as common identity rather developing narrow identifications.

Expected outcome:

- There are some identity criteria, which are personal and need to be personal.
- There are identities which are shared, and developing more shared identities strengthens the social fabric.

Procedure:

Step 1:

Ask all the students come in the same group. Then instruct them to be separated and form different groups as per the instruction by the teacher.

- Ask the students to get separated on the basis of 'can drive' and 'can't drive'. So there will be two groups.
- Ask them to be separate on the basis of Grade. So there will be one group.
- Ask them to come together and then form separate groups as per their preference of tea, coffee, milk, or others, so there will be four groups.
- Ask them to come together and then to form separate groups according to birth order, i.e., elder, younger, middle. So, there will be three groups.
- Ask them to form groups on the basis of who can speak Gujarati. So there will be one group.
- Ask them to come together and get separated as per the month of birth. So there will be 12 groups.

Step 2:

Then ask again them to come together and then separate into groups on the basis of:

- Those who want to be successful and those who do not want to be successful in life.
- Those who want to get good marks and those who do not want good marks.
- Those all belong to India and those who do not
- Those who wants to be in a peaceful state and those who do not?

It will be seen that all are in the same group.

Step 3:

Teacher explains that there are lots of identities which are very personal but there are lots of identities which are broad and which hold us together. In those cases people feel together as same group and can support each other,

Step 4:

Ask them to get divided in four groups and make a list in the groups about the identities which hold us together and the identity which are personal with fewer boundaries.

Facilitating questions:

- How did you like joining in this activity?
- Do you think we can make a more sharable and inclusive identity?
- How can we identify ourselves more with the shared identity rather the personal identity to resolve the divisions and conflict?

Summarize:

- We have to inculcate more sharable identity to hold our country together.
- The emphasis on segregated identity divides people.
- More identification with caste, class, and religion, poor, rich divides society.
- By emphasizing on the sharable identity, we can inculcate the value of inclusion and maintain pluralism.

Reflection at home by the students:

- Do I maintain the shared identity?
- How do I make myself more inclusive with others?

Source Developed by Author while implementing the programme.

Many such sessions were conducted by the teachers in the classroom with the students of Grades 5–12 on different occasions and the outcome was extended in the school life and also in their personal and social interactions.

Outcome of LSE Interventions and Recommendations

The review of the LSE programme saw very specific and significant outcomes which were encouraging and also showed the possibility of replication of such LSE models for students in schools that contribute to positive changes in the attitude, behaviour, interaction among the students and can also ensure sustainable peace. Importantly, the teachers also observed multiple changes and reflected a wide difference in their understanding, and appreciated the issues with the students. There were few key changes identified in the review process. The review was done through FGD with the teachers, students and with a few parents in the schools and *madrassa*.

(a) Teachers identified changes in their outlook and interactions with the students. One of the teachers mentioned that she almost stopped scolding on the occasion of not doing homework by some of the students. Rather, she asked what prevented them from completing the task. She also asked students who completed their homework, how they managed. The exercise influenced the students a lot; they realized that they could make efforts to improve. Similarly, another teacher asked the students to make questions and allowed the students to think seriously about their preparation. Teachers mentioned that the session on harmony was initially a bit difficult to conduct as some students would be quiet, but gradually participation was almost hundred percent. At times, it was difficult to stop them from giving their opinion and complete the session on time. The teachers explained that LSE sessions were very alive and students enjoyed and talked quite openly in a non-threatening atmosphere.

(b) The discipline improved and students were far more regular as the LSE sessions were conducted in the classroom. The teachers reported development of a sense of responsibility among the students. Senior students were more active and responsive than the junior students in the sessions dealing with conflict resolution and peace building. Conducting sessions on health and well-being and communicating the same with the students was easier as there was no perception of threat. Students also mentioned that they were initially hesitant to talk about the issues of peace building, but gradually felt quite interested in contributing opinions and participating as the issues of communal conflict were always unanswered and these were bothering them a lot.

(c) Students took various steps on their own to improve the school atmosphere. Teachers had suggested making friendship clubs, organizing school clean-ups, making school beautification plans, developing posters on communal harmony and peace building. The students took active interest in the same. The students reflected that they were quite happy to see their teachers talking and conducting sessions, something beyond the syllabus and that motivated them also to take active part in such activities beyond the limits of the syllabus. Students took extracurricular activities seriously and enjoyed them. Many of the senior classes in the schools produced wall magazines with poems, pictures, and stories of peace building.

(d) Interaction among the students belonging to different religious groups changed from moderate to high and often parents reported changes in the behaviour of their wards in the parent teacher meetings. In some of the schools, majority of the students were Muslim or majority were Hindu students and with very few numbers of students from other religious groups. In such situations, when session were conducted on peace building, it was difficult to elicit views of minority groups, but the sessions were very neutral about religious identity; therefore, talking about peace as every one's responsibility was easier.

(e) The school management was quite supportive in the whole process of project implementation and also appreciated the active role of the teachers in LSE activities. The trustees of the school committee felt that the LSE is very much a need of the time and such initiatives should be continued with active support from the government.

(f) In *Madrasas*, the religious teachers were equally appreciative about the sessions and felt that they could also look at the developmental issues of the children actively and there was a need to talk about the psychological issues of development with the students. The sessions were a kind of 'fresh air' and established a new milestone in *madrasas*. Many of the *muftis* (senior religious teachers) were of the opinion that in coming days life skills would be part of the regular curriculum and they would also advocate the same (Oommen 2005, 152, 247).

The programme was largely successful in developing a positive school atmosphere, but, at times, less number of teachers, academic pressures, and too large a number of students in the classroom restricted the outcome of the LSE sessions.

LSE for peace education is now accepted as one of the important ways to prepare the younger generation as the peace keeper all around the globe. UNICEF mentions: "Life Skills Based Education for Violence Prevention and Peace Building promotes the development of knowledge, skills, attitudes and values needed to bring about behavioural change that will enable children, youth and adults to prevent conflict and violence, both overt and structural; resolve conflict peacefully; and create the conditions conducive to peace, whether at an intrapersonal, interpersonal, intergroup, national or international level" (UNICEF 2012). Therefore, applicability of LSE showed the need for wider use of it for students through regular curriculum in the Indian context to promote peace education and to ensure violence prevention. In different parts of India, participation of school and college youths in violence is now a major concern. There are incidents of youths participating in hostility during political rallies, protests, in communal conflicts, or in violent attacks on others based on religious, caste, or regional identities. Such events often threaten the democratic values and secular structure of India and cause a major imbalance in the regional, societal, and human relationships. Thus, it is high time to consider peace education through LSE for children, adolescents, and youths through educational institutes, to inculcate skills and values for nurturing a 'culture of peace' at personal, groups, community, and societal levels. Capacity building of teachers and educationists is a crucial step in this direction. Though LSE has been adopted in various educational initiatives for health promotion, vocational training, prevention of diseases, use of LSE for peace education has not been prioritized.

Conclusion

As a whole, peace building is an individual, community, and institutional process, and LSE is an important model for institutional engagement for restoring justice and preparing the new generation for maintaining harmonious living, and being actively engaged in conflict resolution and peace making process. LSE was a successful model for engaging the school community— teachers, religious teachers, students, and parents—actively for transforming the conflict, and restoring justice that supports human rights principles and fulfils the requirements for advocating for an inclusive society in school, the stepping stone for the next generation to grow into responsible citizens.

References

Ahmed, S. (2004). Sustaining peace, re-building livelihoods: The Gujarat harmony project. *Gender and Development, 12*(3), 94–102.

Bandura, A. (1977). *Social learning theory*. New York: General Learning Press.

Bhadra, S. (2011). *Life skills for children and adolescents: Teacher trainees' perception*. Saarbucken: LAP LAMBERT Academic Publishing.

Bhadra, S. (2012). Psychosocial support for the children affected by communal violence in Gujarat, India. *International Journal of Applied Psychoanalytic Studies, 9*(3), 212–232.

Bhadra, S., & Dyer, A. R. (2011). Psychosocial support for harmony and peace building: Rebuilding community in Gujarat. In H. U. Peacebuilding (Ed.), *Peace from disasters—Indigenous Initiatives across communities, countries and continents* (pp. 97–104). Hiroshima: Hiroshima University.

Bharath, S., & Kumar, K. K. (2002). *Activity manual for teachers on health promotion using life skills approach*. Bangalore: NIMHANS.

Bharath, S., & Kumar, K. K. (2010). Empowering adolescents with life skills education in schools —School mental health programme me: Dies it works? *Indian Journal of Psychiatry, 42*(4), 344–349.

Bharath, S., Kumar, K. K., & Vranda, M. (2002). *Activity manual for the teachers on health promotion using life skills approach: 8th Standard life skills manuals*. Bangalore, India: National Institute of Mental Health and Neuro Sciences.

Botvin, G. J., Eng, A., & Williams, C. L. (1980). Preventing the onset of cigarette smoking through life skills training. *Preventive Medicine, 9*(1), 135–143.

CBSE. (2013). *Teacher's manual—Life skills for class—VI*. New Delhi: Central Board of Secondary Education.

Chachra, S. (2004). Disasters and mental health in India: An institutional response: Action Aid India. In J. O. Diaz, R. S. Murthy, & R. Lakshminarayana (Eds.), *Disaster mental health in India* (pp. 151–160). New Delhi: Indian Red Cross Society.

Christophe, J. (2007). The 2002 pogrom in Gujarat: The post 9/11 face of Hindu nationalist anti-Muslim violence. In H. R. John, R. King, H. R. John, & R. King (Eds.), *Religion and violence in South Asia: Theory and practice* (pp. 164–180). New York: Routladge.

Corps, Peace. (2001). *Life skills manual*. Washington: Office of Overseas Programming and Training Support. Peace Corps.

Engineer, A. A. (2003a). Communal riots in 2002: A survey. *Economic and Political Weekly, 38* (4), 280–282.

Engineer, A. A. (2003b). *The Gujarat carnage*. New Delhi: Orient Longman Private Limited.

Fountain, S. (1999). *Peace education in UNICEF*. New York: UNICEF.

Gooder, I. M. (1996). Recent undesirable life events: Their influence on subsequent psychopathology. *European Child and Adolescent Psychiatry, 5*(Suppl 1), 33–37.

Khanam, A., & Bhadra, S. (2015). Prevention of early childhood aggression through life skills education training—An experimental study. In N. Kumar & Z. Meenai (Eds.), *Early childhood development, knowledge series-I*. New Delhi: Global Books organization, Centre for Early Childhood Development and Research, Jamia Millia Islamia.

Lolaty, H. A., Ghahari, S., Tirgari, A., & Fard, J. H. (2012). The effect of life skills training on emotional intelligence of the medical sciences students in Iran. *Indian Journal of Psychological Medicine, 30*(4), 350–354.

Magnani, R., MacIntyre, K., Karim, M. A., Brown, L., & Hutchinson, P. (2005). The impact of life skills education on adolescent sexual risk behaviours in KwaZulu-Natal, South Africa. *Journal of Adolescent Health, 36*(4), 289–304.

Maryam, E., Davoud, M. M., Zahra, G., & Somayeh, B. (2011). Effectiveness of life skills training on increasing self-esteem of high school students. *Procedia—Social and Behavioral Sciences*, 1043–1047.

Masten, A. S. (2001). Ordinary magic: Resilience processes in development. *American Psychologist, 56*(3), 227–238.

Mayer, J. D., & Salovey, P. (1993). The intelligence of emotional intelligence. *Intelligence, 17*(4), 433–442.

Naseri, A., & Babakhani, N. (2014). The effect of life skills training on physical and verbal aggression male delinquent adolescents marginalized in Karaj. *Procedia—Social and Behavioral Sciences, 116*, 4875–4879.

Oommen, T. K. (2005). *Crisis and contention in Indian society*. New Delhi: Sage.

Pieper, C. (2008). Peace, Definitions and concepts of. In L. Kurtz (Ed.), *Encyclopedia of violence, peace, & conflict* (pp. 1548–1557). New York: Academic Press.

PTI (2002, April). *Nine killed in Gujarat on eve of PM's visit.* Retrieved Nov 8, 2010, from Rediff News: http://www.rediff.com/news/2002/apr/03train1.htm.

Roy, A. (2008, February). Listening to gras: Genocide, denial and celebration. *Outlook*, pp. 50–60.

Roy, S., & Rasheed, N. (2015). The national mental health programme me of India. *International Journal of Current Medical and Applied Sciences, 7*(1), 7–15.

Singh, A., & Bhadra, S. (2014). Life skills education (LSE) for juvenile delinquent: Developing a behaviour health promotional model. *Artha—Journal of Social Sciences, 13*(2), 21–32.

Siver, S. (2006). *Process work and the facilitation of conflict.* Michigan, Ohio: UMI Dissertation Publication.

State Planning Commission. (2014). *Role of state council of educational research & training (SCERT) on educational reforms in Tamil Nadu*. Chennai: State Planning Commission.

UNESCO. (1998). *Learning to live together in peace and harmony*. Bangkok: UNESCO Principal Regional Office for Asia and the Pacific.

UNESCO. (2001). *Learning the way of peace—A teachers' guide to peace education*. New Delhi: United Nations Educationa, l Scientific and Cultural Organization.

UNICEF. (2012, May). *Life skills: Violence prevention and peace building*. Retrieved June 2017, 23, from UNICEF-LIfe Skills: https://www.unicef.org/lifeskills/index_violence_peace.html.

United Nations. (1999, September). *53/243 A declaration on a culture of peace, fifty-third session, Agenda item 31. Resolution adopted by the General Assembly*. Geneva, Switzerland: United Nations, General Assembly.

Vranda, M. (2015). Promotion of mental health and well-being of adolescents in schools—A NIMHANS model. *Journal of Psychiatry, 18*(5), 2–5.

Wenzel, V., Weichold, K., & Silbereisen, R. K. (2009). The life skills programme IPSY: Positive influences on school bonding and prevention of substance misuse. *Journal of Adolescence, 32* (6), 1391–1401.

WHO (1993). *Mental Health programme me in schools, WHO/MNH/PSF/93.3 Rev. 1.* Geneva: Division of Mental Health, WHO.

WHO. (1997). *Life skills education for children and adolescent in schools; programme on mental health*. Geneva: World Health Organization, Mental Health Division.

WHO. (1998). *Partners in life skills Education: Conclusions from inter-agency meeting*. Geneva: WHO, Department of Mental health.

WHO. (2005a). *Child and adolescent mental health policies and plan. Mental health policy and service guidance packages*. Geneva: WHO.

WHO. (2005b). *The physical school environment, as essential component of health—promoting school*. Geneva: World Health Organization.

World Health Organization (2009, August). *Preventing violence by developing life skills in children and adolescents, Series of briefings on violence prevention.* Retrieved from http://www.who.int/violence_injury_prevention/violence/life_skills.pdf.

Yankah, E., & Aggleton, P. (2008). Effects and effectiveness of life skills education for HIV prevention in young people. AIDS Education and Prevention. *AIDS Education and Prevention, 20*(6), 465–485.

Yule, W. (2002). Alleviating the effects of war and displacement on children. *Traumatology, 8*(3), 160–180.

Chapter 12
Child Friendly Schools: Challenges and Issues in Creating a Positive and Protective School Environment

Shinto Thomas, K. Alphonsa Jose and P. Aneesh Kumar

Abstract Schools are considered to be one of the safest places where children are seen on a daily basis and are under the supervision of teachers who are trained and equipped caregivers. Children are victims of all forms of abuse, punishment, neglect, discrimination, and ill-treatment within the school setting. Though there are various policies and programmes at international and national levels, addressing child protection has been a serious challenge for every community. Children need to be protected and any acts that hamper their well-being and safety need to be curbed. The objective of this chapter is to critically evaluate school-based child-protection programmes and suggest a model of child protection through positive schooling. Positive schooling is an approach to create a healthier and safer school environment. Positive schooling emphasises inclusiveness, strength-based education, developing character strengths, creating least restrictive environments, and fostering well-being among the school community, including students and teachers. It aims at creating a positive culture where every learner gets equal opportunities to learn and develop. It gives value to overall well-being of the individual and happiness within the learning environment. It promotes positive teaching strategies without the use of punishment and pressure. The positive culture within the school environment would promote peer support and collaboration, preventing bullying and abuse. Learners and facilitators would respect and support each other, focusing on strengths rather than weakness, which would, in turn, create an inclusive environment accommodating everyone. The chapter also highlights the

S. Thomas (✉)
Department of Psychology, Kristu Jayanthi College (Autonomous), Bengaluru, India
e-mail: sthadathil@gmail.com

K. Alphonsa Jose
Department of Applied Psychology, Pondicherry University, Puducherry, India

P. Aneesh Kumar
Department of Psychology, Christ University, Bengaluru, India

S. Deb (ed.), *Positive Schooling and Child Development*,
https://doi.org/10.1007/978-981-13-0077-6_12

need for: trained professionals, like counsellors, in school settings; stronger school-based polices; and the need for collaboration among school administrators, counsellors, teachers, and parents.

Keywords Child protection · Positive schooling · Students · Maltreatment

Introduction

Schools and educational settings are key platforms for development in children and adolescents. School climate and connectedness, relationship with peers and teachers, and the overall schooling experience, foster a child's development. Most of the research in development psychology focuses on issues and maladaptive development. It is equally important to address the role of protective factors and positive development. Since students spend half of their waking life in schools, it is quite essential to study their development and impact of schooling on students. The levels of stress are rising and, as schools are a major part of the child's life, it is important to keep a check on the intensity of the stressors. Research demonstrates that a supportive learning environment assumes a vital part in expanding students' motivation, their self-efficacy, and their engagement in the educational process. Longitudinal research notes a causal relationship between school connectedness and a decrease in health-risk behaviour. Focus on interpersonal relationships, as a central part of academic motivation, raises questions about the need for change in the outlook of current models in school communities. Connectedness to school has been associated with increased positive results in academic achievement and mental health of high-school students (Waters et al. 2009).

Schooling is an important period involving the beginning, growth, and maturation of one's community life. Schooling requires special attention and an atmosphere of care, trust, and safety. Obviously, teachers play a major role in one's school life. But it is not just the teachers who are involved in making the schools safer and secure. It requires a collective action of teachers, parents, school authorities, local society, administration in the local and national level and, to an extent, the geographical location of the school and available resources. A safe and supportive school, according to the National Safe School Frame Work of Australia (2011), is defined as follows: "In a safe and supportive school, the risk from all types of harm is minimized, diversity is valued and all members of the school community feel respected and included and can be confident that they will receive support in the face of any threats to their safety or well-being". This definition emphasizes a strong association between student safety, well-being, and learning. Safety is enhanced in a school set-up where students feel connected and identified to their institution, classmates, and teachers, and competent enough in emotional, social skills, and learning outcomes. Children who lack an identification and positive feeling with the school are reported to be vulnerable to juvenile delinquency;

indicating the crucial role the school climate plays in the formation of its students (Varma 2014). This chapter deals in detail with the factors that make school a safer place, the policies and programmes available and strategies make schools better, safer places.

School as Protective Environment

School as a protective environment is a concept in debt to the UNICEF's safe schooling policy. Following the recommendation of UNICEF, many countries came up with their own manuals and policies to make the schools safer places for children to grow up. Now, the safe school is of utmost importance, especially since climate change is at its strongest, and the scientific community is certain that the severity and prevalence of natural disasters are gaining momentum across the globe, and many buildings which are not strong enough to handle the effects of natural disasters are serving the role of school buildings. History is filled with many stories, and it is important to have policies in place to prevent and reduce the hazards of many foreseen and unforeseen catastrophes. School as a protective environment is not just about the physical safety and strength of the physical structures to deal with the natural hazards, but it is also about making the environments safer and growth promoting.

There are cases of children being physically and psychologically abused both in schools and on their way to school (Pednekar and Makwana 2017; Sharma 2017; Special Correspondent 2014; Khan and Balakrishnan 2017). There are news reports of children being kidnapped or held for ransom, killed in schools during wars, or internal conflicts, or even in a terrorist attack, as happened recently in Pakistan (Lewis 2014; Correspondent 2017). Sexual, physical, and psychological abuse at the hands of teachers (Khan 2017), school bus drivers, and other non-teaching staff, are also not very rare these days. Many school children are at the risk of drug abuse and many are engaged in crimes to raise funds for their abuse of drugs. Gang violence, corporal punishment, and bullying, also make schools unsafe, along with the threat of natural hazards. "The UN Study on Violence against Children reveals that children worldwide are at risk of violence in and around the school. The threats range from rape, sexual abuse, sexual harassment and physical beatings to verbal abuse, bullying, taunting, stereotyping and other forms of humiliation. At times, teachers, school authorities and peers are the perpetrators of such abuse" (UNICEF 2009).

Safety in Schools

According to UNICEF (2009), three things—Prediction, Prevention, and Preparation—are the must-do things to ensure that the schools are safe. Prediction involves foreseeing the possible risks in and around schools that can harm the children; prevention involves the precautions taken to prevent these occurrences; and finally, the schools should be prepared to deal swiftly and effectively with safety-threatening situations. There should be enough materials—first aid kits, fire extinguishers—as well as trained professionals, mock training sessions arranged for the students to make them prepared. It should not just be the school authorities and teachers who take part in this endeavour; the whole student community, parents, school neighbourhoods, and local law enforcers, should also take part in the safe school programme.

Why are the systems at the macro level also important? In a Child-Friendly School, everyone participates in prediction, prevention, and preparation. The practices of safety mapping and developing a risk index are important in the safe school programme. When a mapping exercise is conducted, all the students are given a chance to locate places in and around the school where they feel safe and the places where they feel unsafe. Not just students, but teachers, adults, parents, police, and other stakeholders, are also required to identify the places in a similar fashion and, at the end, a map of safe and unsafe places is completed; intermittent reviewing is also required to update the map. This approach of every one participating in the procedure is called a zoom lens approach (AISA 2017); a similar approach is required in indexing risks and in responding to these indexed possible risks in the physical, and psychological realms. The maps, as well as the indices, are used in order to further develop plans for prevention and preparation.

The UN Convention on the Rights of the Child (UNCRC) (UNICEF 1989), which is the ultimate reference of child rights, spells out the obligations of governments to facilitate children's right to learn in a safe and secure environment. UNCRC specifies the governmental duty in developing appropriate child protection measures against all forms of violence, injury, abuse, and neglect, to ensure that school discipline is administered in a manner consistent with the dignity of the child, and to ensure children's right to the best possible health care. UNCRC also takes special note of making the school infrastructure and surroundings healthy, safe, and child-friendly (Miske 2010).

The minimum required standards of safety provision (WHO 2003, 2007) are as follows:

- Ensuring the availability of fresh potable water, with proper and hygienic facility to dispense it to the students
- Hygiene facility areas for washing hands using cleaning agent or soaps
- Separate toilets, maintaining cleanliness and privacy for both boys and girls
- Classrooms with proper lighting (avoid glare and reflection), air circulation, not located in excessively polluted or noisy surroundings
- Buildings and learning spaces should be coloured using light, natural finishes, whereas bright colours can be used for play corners, and corridors
- Power for proper lighting, communication, and other equipment using either electricity or alternative sources should be incorporated in the school design.

Health Care

Many girls prefer to skip breakfast since their school does not have adequate toilet facility (Corder 2013; Kesztyüs et al. 2017); and many fail to respond to nature's call, or even try to control it by not taking water and food in the required amount. Both of these habits are detrimental to physical health, and the failure to keep genital area clean during menstruation may even result in health risks such as infections (United States Department of Health and Human Services 1991). School Sanitation and Hygiene Education (SSHE) component of Total Sanitation Campaign (TSC), *Nirmal Gram Puraskar* for ensuring separate toilets in upper primary schools for girls and boys, Global WASH programme for ensuring sanitation and safe water facilities in schools, also ensures that the effectiveness of the school nutrition programme is supported via the simple act of washing hands before meals. This practice will ensure that the disease transmission routes are broken; and, as the children learn new healthy habits, can act as change agents in the larger society. The *Swachh Bharat: Swachh Vidyalaya* national campaign recently launched by the Prime Minister of India also mandates the need of functioning and well-maintained water, sanitation, and hygiene facilities in schools.

Other criteria are the provisions of emergency evacuation and fire prevention plans in the design, health provisions such as first aid kit, and the proximity of medical facilities. A strategically located reading room, with enough materials and an environment promoting reading for enhancing learning, and reading in general, should be provided to the students. School yards should be landscaped with trees as a natural filter against dust, light, and noise; it will also effectively beautify the campus and provide a calm environment for the learners. Schools with excellent indoor and outdoor air quality, adequate protection from Ultra Violet (UV) radiation, proper disposal of solid and non-solid wastes, and control in using chemicals, pesticides, and the like, are also considered to be important.

Open spaces should be provided allowing the children to be in contact with nature. It should be arranged as play area, sports area, or open learning and performance area. Kitchen space promoting healthy preparation and safe-keeping of food is mandatory. Protection elements of child-friendly school designs take care of both physical and psychological abuses. Parents and teachers should be trained in non-violent discipline strategies, instead of corporal punishment; class rooms and other areas can be designed such that the activities are under the surveillance of teachers, to deter bullying or other forms of child abuse. Boundaries to keep children safe within the campus are also required.

Drivers of the school buses and their assistants, who bring the children to schools, should be selected with proper care and attention; reports abound of incidents of road accidents and related death, and sexual abuse of children at the hands of these persons (Mendonca 2015; Shaikh 2017). Weight reduction of school bags is also an important procedure to make schools a safer place. Children who continuously carry heavy bags on their back, are at the risk of developing back pain, shoulder pain and many other difficulties.

The reports of abuse, violence, and school becoming an unsafe environment need to be an eye opener for policy and programme makers. These reports should act as a reality check, and ensure the creation of a platform to assess and evaluate the efficiency and effectiveness of the programmes introduced.

Student Well-Being in School

Corporal Punishment and Abuse

Many cultures consider corporal punishment or physical abuse of children at the hands of teachers as a very normal and positive practice. However, many children are victims of physical and mental abuse in the name of corporal punishment, and teachers are the culprits behind it. Most of the time punishments are so severe that the psychological well-being of the children is at risk, and they start finding the school as a difficult place to belong to. A few of them, who begin to fear the teachers, somatise the fear and anxiety, and start falling sick. Either way, the practice of corporal punishment becomes a hindrance to the child's growth and development. It is important for a safe school to develop and practice many positive teaching practices. In many cases teachers, authorities, management, non-teaching staff, school drivers and their assistants, have been reported as perpetrators of sexual abuse of school children (Special Correspondent 2018); these issues related to the use of corporal punishment, abuses are alarming and requires special attention from the service providers to prevent them (Ba-Saddik and Hattab 2012).

Peers, teachers, sometimes even the authorities, consider name calling, scolding, and the like, as presenting no risk, but the reality is different. Verbal abuse can undermine the well-being of the student population. There are many reports of cases where students were affected negatively due to verbally abusive behaviours. Teachers have power over their student's present and future; considering this factor, many students and even parents will not consider reporting the bullying behaviour of the teacher, which is actually emotional abuse. This practice has the same effect as physical or verbal abuse (UNICEF 2009). The manifestations of this kind of abuse are varied: berating, harassing, giving tasks which are beyond the student's capability, showing disgust or lack of interest through expressions, and even neglecting students in the class room.

Bullying and Peer Pressure

According to United Nations (2006), "Bullying refers to the repeated negative actions of one or more students against another. It can include taunting, teasing and other forms of verbal abuse, physical violence and other harmful actions, and can also be expressed through new technologies—cyberbullying, for example. While some forms of gang violence may also be categorized as bullying, the main differences between the two are the structural features of organized gangs and their use of weapons. Gangs and gang conflict may be located within a school or between schools, or they may exist outside schools but have a major impact on what happens inside schools by way of drug use, drug trafficking, extortion, gang rape and so on." (United Nations, UN Study on Violence against Children, New York 2006). A school environment where some students bully other students, or spread the use of addictive substances is a real threat to a positive and safe school. Bullying or victimization has many physical consequences, such as injuries, fractures, or even death in severe cases, and disciplinary punishments such as expulsion from school, suspension for a period of time as a punishment; or it can lead to the experience of psychological consequence such as poor psychological well being, depression and anxiety, increased feelings of sadness and loneliness, changes in sleep and eating patterns, and loss of interest in activities they used to enjoy (Rigby 2003).

Presence of truant peers, and frequent interaction or affiliation with bully gangs will also result in truant behaviours in adolescents, and make them vulnerable to future antisocial activities. Cyber security is a major concern of the time; children are at the risk of online exploitation either as sexual abuse, or exposure to violent or suicide-provoking games such as blue whale Correspondent (2017a, b). Schools should ensure that their e-safety procedures are robust and that pupils are taught online safety skills so they know about online risks, how to recognize unsafe online contact, and to be confident to report any such issues.

Academic pressure, stress, and anxiety due to academic pressure both from school and family, is also a hindrance to creating a safe school. A school situation, where children face a lot of pressure—as well as the expectation from their teachers—to be the class topper, or a nine-pointer, is not a safe school. At times, knowingly or unknowingly, parents also become part of this stress, and they may even push students very hard to be toppers. Academic pressure and fear of failure in exams, experiences of rejection from family and teachers, and similar stresses, are found to be causal factors in many adolescent suicides in India (Saha 2017; Jayanthi et al. 2015; Arun et al. 2017).

National Policies and Programmes for Child Safety

The Indian Constitution lays the foundation for all the child protection laws and policies in India (The Constitution of India 2017). Some of these are: guarantee of free and compulsory education to all the children through Article 21A; prohibition of human trafficking of all kinds including children (Article 23); and prohibition of child labour, especially in hazardous and dangerous conditions. In line with the Constitution, many laws and national policies have been formed: National Policy for Children (1974), National Charter for Children (2004), National Plan of Action for Children in India (2005), National Commission for Protection of Child Rights (2006); and Right of Children to Free and Compulsory Education (RTE) Act

(2009). In addition to ensuring free and compulsory education, the RTE act also requires the provision of drinking water and sanitation facility in every school. Other specifications—like pupil teacher ratio, criteria for buildings and infrastructure, appointment of appropriately trained and qualified teachers, prohibition of mental harassment and physical punishment, and addressing malpractices such as capitation fee, schools running without recognition—are detailed; it has also provided a curriculum revision in consonance with the values preserved in the Constitution, and which would ensure the all-round development of the child. Further, the Act also advocated child-friendly and child-centred learning.

Juvenile Justice (Care And Protection) Act, 2000, established a framework for taking care of children who are in need of care and protection, and who are in conflict with law. Other existing laws are the Prohibition of Child Marriage Act (2006), and the Child Labour Prohibition and Regulation Act (1986). The Integrated Child Protection Scheme (ICPS), established in 2009 by the Ministry of Women and Child Development, is aimed at preventing violence against children and to provide a protective environment for children, especially children who fall within the provisions of Juvenile Justice (care and protection) Act. It raises public awareness, and strengthens child protection at the family and community level.

National Commission for Protection of Child Rights (NCPCR) is another step by the Government of India to look into child right issues. It was established in March 2007 by an Act of Parliament, with a wide mandate and considerable powers. State-wise commissions for protection of child rights and telephonic help line—1098—and child welfare committee (CWC) that investigates reports of child abuse, are part of the NCPCR.

Prevention of children from Sexual Offences (POCSO Act 2012) deals with the issue of sexual offences against children. It prevents the disclosure of a child's name in public and media, punishes the convict according to the gravity of the crime; in addition, many child-friendly judicial practices, including special courts to complete trial within a one-year period, are also covered in this act.

The Everywhere Child Project, released by CHILDLINE in the year 2011, communicates the standards of child protection in various spaces such as school. Nationwide assessment shows that, despite the laws and policies, many places are still unsafe for children. The National Policy for Children (2013), clarifies that children are any person below the age of eighteen years and that childhood is an integral part of life; each child has unique needs, vulnerabilities, and circumstances. The overall harmonious development and protection of children, an important national asset, requires a long-term, sustainable, multi-sectoral, integrated, and inclusive approach.

School-Based Programmes

Other programmes especially developed and practiced in the school education system are introduced in this section. District Primary Education Programme (DPEP) launched in 1994, universalized primary education, Mid-Day Meal scheme (1995) took care of nutrition for all elementary school children. The scheme of *Sarva Shiksha Abhiyaan* (SSA), launched in 2001, also served a similar purpose, and helped in widening the compulsory and free education to the under-served sections of the community in a time-bound manner, ensured required infrastructure facility for water, sanitation, and hygiene facilities in all new schools. *Rashtriya Madhyamik Shiksha Abhiyan* (RMSA), launched by MHRD in 2009, enhanced the children's access to secondary education and prompted schools to follow the instructions regarding quality physical infrastructure for class rooms, toilet and safe water provisions, and keeping the schools disabled-friendly. *Kasturba Gandhi Balika Vidyalaya* (KGBV 2004) takes care of the specialized needs of girl children from the under-served social categories of SC and ST population, by providing special residential schools at upper primary level. School Sanitation and Hygiene Education (SSHE) component of Total Sanitation Campaign (TSC), *Nirmal Gram Puraskar* for ensuring separate toilets in upper primary schools for girls and boys, Global WASH programme for ensuring the sanitation and safe water facilities in schools, also ensure the effectiveness of school nutrition programme via the simple act of washing the hands before meals. This ensures the availability of drinking water, hand washing, toilet, and soap facilities in the school compound for use by children and teachers.

Positive Schooling: The Way Forward

The mission of building schools as places that support all parts of the development of students is addressed by an increasing number of projects and innovations that endeavour to overcome barriers to students' learning. However, the present effect of these activities is limited as a result of lack of coordination among the components of the school group, and limited mechanisms for implementation and evaluation of these shared projects. Research on school change attempts to identify the key elements of school that contribute to creating a strong learning environment and generating a feeling of connectedness for all individuals within the school.

Waters et al. (2009), proposed a theoretical model that assists with a better understanding of the complex relationship between school environment and adolescents' connectedness (Sugar 2012). The model has four stages. The first stage defines school ecology that incorporates organizational factors—for instance, school structure and work—and interpersonal factors, such as peers, teachers, and family. The second stage focuses on creating association with the school through autonomy, competence, and relatedness. In this perspective, connectedness to class is "The degree to which students feel independent yet supported, competent in all they endeavour and identified with adults and peers" (Waters et al. 2009). The third stage represents a person–environment fit, which, for adolescents is described by a declining need of parent and teacher support, and expanding dependence on companions and friends. In this stage, building a school environment that furnishes young people with a feeling of respect and appreciation by others is most useful. The presence of these three phases leads to establishing connectedness within a school community, which is the purpose of the whole system. The fourth phase represents health and academic outcomes as results of the effective functioning of a learning community.

Further, according to the PERMA Model proposed by Seligman, there are five core elements that help achieve happiness as he defines it, PERMA: Positive emotion, engagement, relationships, meaning, and accomplishments (Pascha 2015). 'Positive emotion' deals with the ability to be optimistic in any given situation, and the ability to focus on the positive aspects. 'Engagement' refers to the concept of flow wherein every individual is able to be fully engaged in a particular activity deriving enjoyment from it. Such an experience is said to increase emotional capabilities, aptitude for skills, and stretch intelligence and creativity. 'Relationships' is the third component in this model, which throws light on the importance of social relationships—family, friends, and siblings, and peers—in maintaining individual well-being. Recent research also concurs with this stand that Seligman takes. The fourth component, 'Meaning', refers to living a purposeful life. Seligman proposes that higher is the sense of purpose in life greater is life satisfaction, and therefore higher is the chances of the individual achieve happiness. The last component in this model is 'Accomplishment', which refers to activities that provide a sense of fulfilment once the task is completed. Setting realistic goals is an important step to feeling accomplished (Pascha 2015).

According to another theory, the way to achieve happiness lies within a developmental character; that is, if one chooses to progress by development, he will develop the skills that empower him to become a holistic being, standing at par with other human beings, and forming loving and supportive relationships, thus directing himself with a clear sense of self.

Recommendations

Recommendations for making a school safe and protected, as well as child-friendly are well-documented, and many policies already ensuring exist, but still the situation is alarming as many of our institutions fall below expected standards. This section discusses possible ways to make schools safer places. Initially, it is important for governmental or other agencies to ensure that the schools are working appropriately under the prescribed child-friendly and protective policies. The United Nations Children's Fund (UNICEF) defines child protection as the "strengthening of country environments, capacities, and responses to prevent and protect children from violence, exploitation, abuse, neglect, and the effects of conflict." It advocates the need for schools to create and implement a Child Protection Policy, supportive curriculum, and staff recruitment (Osher et al. 2009). Bringing in the concept of child protection in education systems can lead to essential changes in the ways schools function, in children's behaviour when attending school, and the method in which teachers or school authorities interact with children. Recommendations regarding school policy and implementation are provided below.

Developing a School Policy

Schools should develop their own policies keeping international safe-school policies, local facilities, and the vision of the school, in mind. Principal, teachers, non-teaching staff, parents and local society and children themselves should be part of the school level policy. All the staff should be provided with a code of conduct, defining expectations from the staff, clarity in the mechanisms to report misconduct or abuse. Staff and parents should be kept aware about the consequences of child abuse and corporal punishment, as well as alternative effective child-centred measures to correct unacceptable behaviour from students. Clarity should be provided in the measures against bullying, gang fights, ragging and other forms of violence and substance abuse among the students.

Safety in School Yards

The physical environment should also be carefully designed with security systems, surveillance measures for visitors and students, open design for the school buildings to prevent unwanted entry of outsiders in the school premise.

Other policies can be an open door policy for staff, half doors on toilets for nursery children, clearly bounded areas around schools; expansive school yards require extra security measures such as additional staff or surveillance facilities or emergency notification or alarm systems that can alert students and teachers to an ongoing emergency. It is also important to constitute 'crisis teams' which include parents, teachers, and school personnel to communicate immediately and appropriately with the rest of the school community about the crisis (Child Line India Foundation 2008).

Circulation of Child Protection Policies

Schools should have their own published child-protection policy, circulated among the students, school personnel, teachers, and parents. Training should be provided regularly to identify and voice concerns, and for the parents and children to inquire about and confirm them with the staff. Schools can seek additional suggestions from law enforcers, local authorities, psychologists, social workers, and other professionals regarding safety concerns, and can conduct awareness classes for a safer school. Schools should work with parents in the interest of protecting children.

Procedures to Support the Policy

Support procedures are important in the implementation of policies. Curriculum in support of child safety policy with age appropriate definitions of child maltreatment, most frequent offenders, and body awareness lessons will give them a voice to report abuses. It should also clearly mention that the offender is responsible for the maltreatment, not the victim, and available support systems and possible ways to obtain support should be clear.

Skill Training

Additional training to enhance assertiveness, the ability to question confusing behaviours, support- or help-seeking skills, self-defence skills, recognizing abusive situations, behaviours, is very meaningful. Role plays and other training activities will strengthen capacity to recognize possible abuse, possible sources of support, and provide a way for appropriate reporting of the offence. Awareness programmes and classes to make students, parents, and teachers aware of the risks associated with schools are another important step to make schools safer. Without knowledge and awareness, it is difficult for someone to identify the risks. Availing the assistance of competent professionals in school is also very important. Many schools in India presently employ nurses, school psychologists, and other professionals to make schools a much safer place for young minds to grow up in and enhance themselves. These actions should be given publicity, to provide a good model for others to follow.

Training for the Service Providers

Teachers, student counsellors, doctors, and other professionals, who provide support and help to the children, should also be provided with proper training. Teachers should be comfortable in dealing with situations and syllabus regarding abuse especially sexual abuse. If the teachers and help providers consider abuse to be an embarrassing topic to discuss, students will also find it as difficult and uncomfortable to do so. Specialized training to identify the abused children, to familiarize students and staff with reporting procedures and available treatment procedures is also important. Involving parents in the training is also vital in maximizing the result. School should follow its own means to respond to child abuse in congruence with the country's laws. Sufficient records regarding child abuse reportings should be prepared and kept in every school. Policies and supporting procedures should be reviewed and revised thoroughly at proper intervals.

Recruitment and Selection

Recruitment and selection also requires a lot of scrutiny; every applicant should be scrutinized before their appointment. In all cases with previous employment, previous employer should be contacted. Child protection awareness, pleasant personality, proper identity, presentation of original certificates, and checking medical and psychological fitness of the candidate should be ensured during the appointment of every candidate. School authority should also verify the background and criminal history of contractors, vendors, drivers, goods and service providers, security people, and others who may come in contact with the students on the school property and on the way to the school.

School-Based Child Protection Team

A team with trained professionals to monitor the functioning of child-protection policies and supportive procedures should be formulated. Every team member should be clear about their role and responsibility. Formal networks with neighbouring schools, and care and service providers should be formed. Listing of available medical, legal, and psychological resources related to child protection, and making them available for public use to the children, staff, and parents should be undertaken. Coordinator for the monitoring should be chosen officially and he/she should be responsible for conducting proper evaluation and reporting of child-protection programmes and for conducting meetings with relevant personnel. Proper funding and other technical support should be provided to every school from the government and other agencies. MPs, MLAs, other public servants should work in coordination with the schools and provide them with enough funding and facilities.

Conclusion

School is a primary context for social interaction, cultivation of interpersonal skills, and formation of peer groups, self-expression, and development of self. Several studies have demonstrated that school-related variables have important implications for determining the likelihood that an adolescent will follow a pro-social path through adolescence, as opposed to becoming involved in delinquent behaviours such as truancy. In this chapter, several risk and protective factors that describe the school environment and/or a student's experience at school were found to be associated with truancy. Most importantly, the two most robust predictors were school performance and involvement with delinquent peers.

Child-friendly schools need to work with parents and local communities to prevent violence. There must be clear, transparently enforced policies and procedures, as firm interventions to protect children from physical harm and verbal, physical, emotional, and sexual abuse. Schools must educate parents and local communities in order to eliminate acquiescence to or tolerance of violence against children. Child protection and safety can be extended to homes and communities, reinforcing the accepted codes of conduct adopted by schools.

References

Arun, P., Garg, R., & Chavan, B. S. (2017). Stress and suicidal ideation among adolescents having academic difficulty. *Industrial Psychiatry Journal, 2*(1), 64.

Association of International Schools in Africa (AISA). (2017). Child protection handbook. Retrieved from www.aisa.or.ke/images/CP_Handbook_Appendicies_March_2017.pdf.

Ba-Saddik, A. S., & Hattab, A. S. (2012). Emotional abuse towards children by schoolteachers in Aden Governorate, Yemen: A cross-sectional study. *BMC Public Health, 12*(1), 647.

Child Line India Foundation. (2008). The essentials of child protection a handbook for beginners. Retrieved from https://www.childlineindia.org.in/pdf/Essentials-of-child-protection-Oct%2008.pdf.

Correspondent. (BBC NEWS, 2017, 1 December). Pakistan attack: Gunmen storm Peshawar training college. Retrieved from http://www.bbc.com/news/world-asia-42191487.

Correspondent. (2017a, August). Manipur teen death: Blue Whale game to blame? *Times of India*. Delhi News, Retrieved from http://timesofindia.indiatimes.com/city/delhi/blue-whale-game-to-blame-for-eatery-death-cops-probe/articleshow/60066022.cms.

Correspondent. (2017b, August). Another suspected suicide due to Blue Whale challenge reported from Kerala. *Hindustan Times*, Thiruvananthapuram, India. Retrieved from http://www.hindustantimes.com/india-news/another-suspected-suicide-due-to-blue-whale-challenge-reported-from-kerala/story-IpcMkzvGiWVSvqCv1Exs8M.html.

Corder, K., van Sluijs, E. M., Ridgway, C. L., Steele, R. M., Prynne, C. J., Stephen, A. M., ... & Ekelund, U. (2013). Breakfast consumption and physical activity in adolescents: Daily associations and hourly patterns. *The American Journal of Clinical Nutrition, 99*(2), 361–368.

District Primary Education Programme (DPEP). (1994). Govt. of India.

Integrated Child Protection Scheme (ICPS). (2009). Ministry of Women and Child Development, Govt. of India.

Jayanthi, P., Thirunavukarasu, M., & Rajkumar, R. (2015). Academic stress and depression among adolescents: A cross-sectional study. *Indian Pediatrics, 52*(3), 217–219.

Kasturba Gandhi Balika Vidyalaya (KGBV). (2004). Govt. of India.

Kesztyüs, D., Traub, M., Lauer, R., Kesztyüs, T., & Steinacker, J. M. (2017). Skipping breakfast is detrimental for primary school children: Cross-sectional analysis of determinants for targeted prevention. *BMC Public Health, 17*(1), 258.

Khan, I. (2017). Pre-school principal booked under POCSO, after more complaints pour in. *CNN-News18*. Retrieved from http://www.news18.com/news/india/pre-school-principal-booked-under-pocso-after-more-complaints-pour-in-1352656.html.

Khan, I., & Balakrishnan, D. (2017, April). French diplomat Pascal Mazurier acquitted in child abuse case. *CNN-News18*. Retrieved from http://www.news18.com/news/india/french-diplomat-pascal-mazurier-acquitted-in-child-abuse-case-1377837.html.

Lewis, R. (2014). Peshawar school massacre terrorist attack. *Peshawar*, Pakistan. Retrieved from https://www.britannica.com/event/Peshawar-school-massacre.

Mendonca, G. (2015, 16 December). School bus driver held for sexually abusing girl. *The Times of India*, Mumbai. Retrieved from https://timesofindia.indiatimes.com/city/mumbai/School-bus-driver-held-for-sexually-abusing-girl/articleshow/50193998.cms.

Mid-Day Meal Scheme. (1995). Govt. of India.

Miske, S. J. (2010). Child-friendly schools—Safe schools, (Keynote Speech). In *Second International Symposium on Children at Risk and in Need of Protection*. Ankara, Turkey. Retrieved from miskewitt.com/assets/2.-final_cfs-safe_schools_050810.pdf.

National Charter for Children. (2004). Govt. of India.

National Commission for Protection of Child Rights. (2006). Govt. of India.

National Plan of Action for Children in India. (2005). Govt. of India.

National Policy for Children. (1974). Govt. of India.

National Safe Schools Framework. (2011). Department of education, employment and workplace relations, Australian government. Retrieved from https://docs.education.gov.au/system/files/doc/other/national_safe_schools_framework.pdf.

Osher, D., Kelly, D., Tolani-Brown, N., Shors, L., & Chen, C.-S. (2009). *UNICEF child friendly schools programming: Global evaluation final report*. Washington, DC: American Institutes for Research.

Pascha, M. (2015). *The PERMA model: Your scientific theory of happiness*. The University of Queensland. Retrieved from https://www.uq.edu.au/wellness-program/health-and-wellbeing/focus-wellness/perma-model.

Pednekar, P., & Makwana, B. (2017, June). Andheri school abuse case: Child rights panel to look into police investigation. *Hindustan Times*, Mumbai city.

Prohibition of Child Marriage Act. (2006). Govt. of India.

Rashtriya Madhyamik Shiksha Abhiyan (RMSA). (2009). MHRD, Govt. of India. Retrieved from http://unicef.in/Story/190/Child-Protection-In-India, http://www.childlineindia.org.in/Child-Protection-Policy-in-all-schools.htm, http://www.hindustantimes.com/mumbai-news/andheri-school-abuse-case-child-rights-panel-to-look-into-police-investigation/story-ihjOBSMlhYNPufPwctprXK.html.

Rigby, K. (2003). Consequences of bullying in schools. *The Canadian Journal of Psychiatry, 48*(9), 583–590.

Right of Children to Free and Compulsory Education (RTE) Act. (2009). Govt. of India.

Saha, D. (2017, 8 May). Every hour, one student commits suicide in India. *Hindustan Times*, New Delhi. Retrieved from https://www.hindustantimes.com/health-and-fitness/every-hour-one-student-commits-suicide-in-india/story-7UFFhSs6h1HNgrNO60FZ2O.html.

Sarva Shiksha Abhiyaan (SSA). (2001). Govt. of India.

Shaikh, A. (2017, 5 February). 4-year-old sexually assaulted in school bus, driver arrested. *The Times of India*, Pune. Retrieved from https://timesofindia.indiatimes.com/city/pune/4-year-old-sexually-assaulted-in-school-bus-driver-arrested/articleshow/56979383.cms.

Sharma, M. (2017, February). Horror unfolds in Bengaluru school as more children claim sexual abuse. *NDTV*. Bengaluru. Retrieved from http://www.ndtv.com/bangalore-news/horror-unfolds-in-bengaluru-school-as-more-children-claim-sexual-abuse-1662487.

Special Correspondent. (2014, August). Here are five cases of child molestation in Indian schools, *IndiaToday.in* New Delhi. Retrieved from http://indiatoday.intoday.in/education/story/top-10-cases-of-school-molestation-in-india/1/375447.html.

Special Correspondent. (2018, 6 April). Sex abuse case in school: Principal, 9 teachers quit. *The Times of India*, Mumbai. Retrieved from https://timesofindia.indiatimes.com/city/mumbai/sex-abuse-case-in-school-principal-9-teachers-quit/articleshow/63635299.cms.

Sugar, I. (2012). *Measurement of School Connectedness (MOSC) modified connectedness questionnaire for secondary schools*. University of Southern California.

The Child Labour Prohibition and Regulation Act. (1986). Govt. of India.

The Constitution of India. (2017). Government of India, Ministry of Law and Justice, (Legislative Department), New Delhi. Retrieved from http://lawmin.nic.in/olwing/coi/coi-english/coi-indexenglish.htm.

UNICEF. (1989). Convention on the rights of the child. Retrieved from http://www.ohchr.org/EN/ProfessionalInterest/Pages/CRC.aspx.

United Nations Children's Fund (UNICEF). (2009). Child protection from violence, exploitation and abuse. New York, NY: USA. Retrieved from https://www.unicef.org/protection/files/2009_Global_Thematic_Report_FINAL.pdf.

United Nations. (2006). UN study on violence against children. New York. Retrieved from http://www.ohchr.org/EN/HRBodies/CRC/Study/Pages/StudyViolenceChildren.aspx.

United States Department of Health and Human Services. (1991, October). Preventing lead poisoning in young children. Retrieved from http://aepo-xdvwww.epo.cdc.gov/wonder/prevguid/p0000029/p0000029.asp.

Varma, M. V. M. (2014). Right to Education Act, 2009—History and salient features. *International Journal of Multidisciplinary Advanced Research trends, 1*(2), 160–167.

Waters, S. K., Cross, D. S., & Runions, K. (2009). Social and ecological structures supporting adolescent connectedness to school: A theoretical model. *Journal of School Health, 79*(11), 516–524.

WHO. (2003). Sun protection and schools: How to make a difference. Retrieved from http://www.who.int/uv/publications/en/sunprotschools.pdf.

WHO. (2007). The physical school environment: An essential component of a health-promoting school. The World Health Organization's Information Series on School Health, Document 2. Retrieved from http://www.who.int/school_youth_health/media/en/physical_sch_environment.pdf.

Chapter 13
Mental Health Promotion at Schools: Need, Challenges and Role of Teachers and Counsellors

M. Manjula

Abstract The need for mental health promotion in order to prevent mental illnesses and to promote mental health has been increasingly endorsed and encouraged in the recent times across the globe. Early interventions in children and adolescents largely happens in the school setting due to the accessibility of the youth, amount of time spent by youth in school as well as ease of implementation. The focus of such programmes range from skills training, sensitization to specific problems/issues, to targeted interventions addressing specific problems. The time duration also ranges from few months to years. The effect sizes of such programmes are small to moderate at the maximum. A combination of universal and targeted interventions is often recommended to promote mental health. Methodological rigour of school based intervention is limited, questioning the reliability of these studies. Also, the question of who should be implementing these programmes, and the willingness and training of the stakeholders, is a challenge in the developing countries. While there is growing evidence on the effectiveness of these programmes, there is no agreement on what programmes are needed, how much inputs are required, the uniformity of these programmes and the training of the persons involved. In India, though scattered attempts towards this are made by governmental and nongovernmental organizations, uniform implementation of the same is lacking. There is a lot of difference between the private and government schools in terms of the inputs and implementation of the programmes. Also, the motivation and the attitude of the school authorities, teachers, and counsellors vary across setting, based on socio-economic and cultural backgrounds. Against this background, it becomes important to formulate programmes on the basis of some generic models applicable to all, and some specific models to address the unique needs of the youth in their settings.

Keywords Mental health · Schools · Challenges · Teachers · Counsellors

---

M. Manjula (✉)
Department of Clinical Psychology, National Institute of Mental Health and Neuro Sciences, Bengaluru 560029, India
e-mail: drmanjula71@gmail.com

S. Deb (ed.), *Positive Schooling and Child Development*,
https://doi.org/10.1007/978-981-13-0077-6_13

Introduction: Need for Mental Health Promotion at Schools

About 20–25% of children and adolescents experience mental health problems in the form of behavioural and emotional difficulties, of whom 10% fulfil the criteria for mental health disorder (Harden et al. 2001). Srinath et al. (2005) found 12.5% of children and adolescents suffering from Mental and Behavioural Disorders. The prevalence of psychiatric disorders varies with age. In school age children (4–10 years), disruptive behaviour and anxiety disorders are commonly seen, whereas generalized anxiety, conduct disorder, eating disorders, and depression are more common in secondary school students (aged 11–18 years). Mental health problems increase the likelihood of academic underachievement, difficulties in personal, familial, school and social functioning, risk of suicide, and impact negatively on the quality of a child's life (Rothy and Leavey 2006). Attention Deficit Hyperactivity Disorder (ADHD) and Autism Spectrum Disorders pose particular difficulties for children (Costello et al. 2005). Disruptive or challenging behaviours, developmental disorders, learning difficulties, bullying, and school violence are the most common challenges reported by teachers.

Common mental health problems among adolescents are largely understood as 'internalizing' disorders, where they feel distressed inside themselves, and 'externalizing' disorders, which create difficulties for the child's external world. Children with externalising disorders fail to control their behaviour according to the expectations of parents, peers, teachers, and/or legal authorities. They may violate age-appropriate social rules and norms. Commonly, internalizing and externalizing disorders are referred to as Emotional and Behavioural disorders. Among behavioural and emotional disorders, Anxiety disorders are the most common conditions (31.9%), followed by behaviour disorders (19.1%), mood disorders (14.3%), and substance use disorders (11.4%) (n = 10,123 adolescents aged 13–18) (Merikangas et al. 2010). The lifetime prevalence of Anxiety disorders is 10%, which increases with age (Costello et al. 2003; Meltzer et al. 2003). In the 12–13 years age group, the prevalence is 14.7% and in the 16–17 years age group, it is 22.0% (Essau et al. 2000). Anxiety and depressive disorders are commoner in females, in the 2:1 ratio. Annual rate of major depression in children is 2.8% whereas that of adolescents is 8.3% (Birmaher et al. 1996; Costello et al. 2006; Essau et al. 2010), and upto 70% of them will have a further depressive episode within 5 years (Lewinsohn et al. 2000; Fombonne 2001) and 20% will suffer at least one clinically depressive episode by the age of 18 (Birmaher et al. 1996). Suicides, though less during childhood (0.5–1.0 per lakh in the 5–14 years age group), increases during adolescence and adulthood (12–16 per lakh in the 15–24 years age group). While major depression increases the suicide risk, even the 'Sub-threshold' depressive symptoms confer a similar risk of suicide and depression in adulthood (Fergusson et al. 2005).

The prevalence of externalizing disorders generally declines with age, although it declines at much earlier ages for girls than for boys. Externalizing symptoms in childhood predict disruptive behaviours, anxiety, mood, and substance use disorders in adulthood (Reef et al. 2011). Most commonly seen externalizing disorders are Attention-deficit/hyperactivity disorder (ADHD), Oppositional Defiant Disorder (ODD) and Conduct disorder (CD). Anxiety, depression, conduct disorder, and substance use often co-occur. The majority of youth do not receive assistance (75%) (Essau et al. 2000; Sawyer et al. 2001).

Childhood psychiatric disorders persist into adulthood. Children with psychiatric disorders are 3 times more likely to have a disorder in adulthood (Costello et al. 2003). However, early interventions shorten the duration of episodes of mental illness and prevent substantial morbidity in later life (Patton et al. 2014).

The percentage of children requiring counselling ranges from 3 to 25% (Kauffman and Landrum 2013; Simpson and Mundschenk 2012). It is an established fact that unaddressed mental health problems can push children into an unhealthy, personal, academic, social and mental health trajectory. They may acquire inappropriate behaviours such as dropping out of school, drug abuse, enter the criminal justice system, and may fail to retain healthy relationships with peers and adults (Kim-Cohen et al. 2003; Whear et al. 2014).

Extremely challenging behaviours, which teachers are not able to manage, usually result in conflicting situations and inappropriate practice, trapping them in a vicious cycle of negative and ineffective reactions with the "problem" students (Kourkoutas 2012). The burnout cascade can negatively affect teacher–pupil relationships and the classroom environment, and might damage both teacher and child mental health (Jennings et al. 2013). Poor relationship between teacher and pupils are a predictor of childhood onset psychiatric disorders and low academic attainment (Lang et al. 2013; Cadima et al. 2010). However, supportive teacher and early mental health intervention can reduce this risk and prevent dropout and facilitate student teacher relationship (Kauffman and Landrum 2013).

Often the students' emotional and/or behavioural problems are manifestations of trauma/difficulties experienced in the context of dysfunctional family backgrounds. However, these get played out in the school context; which is true both in western and Indian contexts. Adolescents identified family problems as the second most important source of stress in studies carried out in Indian schools (Manjula et al. 2015; Singh and Manjula 2010). Against the background of lack of training for teachers to understand and handle such situations, it becomes all the more difficult to help the child as well as the unsupportive parents (Anagnostopoulos and Soumaki 2012). Also, often teachers have poor understanding about the nature of mental health problems, the causes, and treatments. This may include the specific learning disabilities which becomes very obvious in their academic performance compared to other psychological problems.

Schools are considered apt and appropriate locations to promote and deliver health care including mental health, as most children and adolescents attend schools at some time in their lives. They spend most of their waking time in schools and colleges. Teachers play the role of surrogate parents and influence development in children and adolescents. The educational system is well-established in all countries. In studies carried out with Indian school-going adolescents, on suggestions of helping them with coping with psychological problems, they recommended classroom-based, universal interventions addressing common problems faced by them as an important requirement. They also reported stigma issues to be not important if the interventions are delivered in groups, rather than counselling individual children (Singhal et al. 2015).

School-Based Interventions

School based interventions can be classified as universal and targeted programmes. A Universal Programme is promotional in nature and targets all the children and adolescents with the goal of enhancing their potentials and psychosocial competence. Targeted Programmes focus on children and adolescents requiring specific inputs from child mental health specialists or specifically trained personnel—like special children with mental retardation, autism, attention deficit disorder, specific learning disabilities, and psychiatric conditions including emotional and behavioural problems. The targeted programmes can be divided into selective interventions and indicated interventions. While selective interventions address children at risk due to adverse socio cultural and individual factors, indicated interventions address children who have sub-syndromal problems.

A systematic review of the intervention studies carried out in school settings showed a wide range of beneficial effects on students, families, communities and on a range of mental health, social, emotional, and educational outcomes. Most of these effective interventions addressed enhancing positive mental health. Balanced universal and targeted approaches started with the youngest children and continued till they completed school, adopted a whole school approach, liaisoned with teachers, parents, and outside agencies, and were implemented accurately (Weare and Nind 2011). School-based universal interventions are known to create resilience, and help children to thrive in adverse conditions. Especially for the children who come from less optimum home backgrounds, interventions at school can be the turning point (Gross 2008). Outcomes of interventions for internalizing problems, such as anxiety and depression, carried out in schools showed small to large effects. The impact was higher for children with higher severity (Horowitz and Garber 2006; Payton et al. 2008; Manjula et al. 2015). Implementation of such ongoing, long-drawn, combined interventions would definitely need the support and help of teachers. Thus, more than counsellors, teachers may have to play a critical role in being sensitive and knowledgeable in identifying and providing ongoing support to students.

Social and emotional learning (SEL) programmes implemented as universal and longitudinal interventions showed impact on social and emotional skills, self-esteem and confidence, and reduction in depression, anxiety, bullying, violence and anger (Blank et al. 2009; Catalano et al. 2002; Berkowitz and Bier 2007; Gansle 2005; Waddell et al. 2007). Review of universal interventions in externalizing problems has shown positive impact, especially for high risk, older students (Farrington and Ttofi 2009; Adi et al. 2007b). However, the universal interventions did not show significant impact on students without mental health problems.

Overall, methods using multilevel interventions (including universal and indicated), with multiple modalities (groups, level of intervention, length of intervention, one-to-one and whole class work), involving a wide range of people, agencies, seem to be more effective, single interventions carried out by only few people (Adi et al. 2007a; Browne et al. 2004). Interventions which are at least 9 months to one year long are found to be more effective (Horowitz and Garber 2006; Wells et al. 2003). What seems to be effective in mental health promotion is a balance of targeted interventions while continuing to embed and integrate them with robust universal approach. For such embedded ongoing interventions to be effective the cooperation as well as involvement of teachers in the program implementation becomes integral.

Role of Teachers

Parents do recognize the signs of mental health problems in their children. However, they may not seek help because of many reasons: having a poor understanding of mental health, available services, or sources of help; parenting difficulties; culture, religion, and beliefs held by the wider community; stigma; and inadequate help-seeking strategies (Rothy and Leavey 2006). Sometimes, the problems are reported to the teachers in the context of academic difficulties of their children. Most often consultation is related to behaviour or developmental problems. Identification of psychological problems by teachers also has been found to be higher for children with behavioural disorders as compared to emotional disorders (Meltzer et al. 2003; Loades and Mastroyannopoulou 2010). Teacher behaviour such as being strict, and poor relationship with students is reported to result in mental health/behavioural problems in children (Soyingbe et al. 2013). Thus, seeking help for a child depends on teachers' awareness and perception of their problems (Sayal et al. 2006). Teachers are often not trained to identify mental health problems and feel confused; for example, they may be unable to differentiate between normal and ADHD-related problem behaviours. Also, teachers often respond differently depending on the gender of the child, with inflated ratings for girls as compared to boys on some kinds of problems and vice versa for other kind of problems. However, when the students perceive the teacher as supportive, it significantly predicted improvement in self-esteem and depression and behavioural difficulties in children (Reddy et al. 2003; Jennings and Greenberg 2009). Also, a supportive and non-conflicting relationship with the teacher is found to help students to recover from academic difficulties and establish cordial relationships with peers (Rohner and Khaleque 2010). Teachers play a significant role in preventing students from developing psychological problems.

There are critical views about the capacity of teachers to deliver mental health interventions. In addition, when they are not supported by the school administration, they may not be able to shoulder the additional burden of add-on programmes and participate effectively due to the general inadequate prospects for their professional advancement in such contexts (Fazel et al. 2014).

How Can They Help?

Teachers spend a substantial amount of time with students and hence can provide vital information regarding the behaviour and functioning and help professionals to design appropriate interventions (Kauffman and Landrum 2013). In order for teachers to be sensitive, it becomes imperative that they are aware of psychological problems of children as well as aware of their own emotional processes and behaviours which affect the students. So teachers' emotional competence plays an important role in helping students as well as protecting themselves from burnout (Jennings and Greenberg 2009). Further implementation of any programme is dependent on the teachers' awareness of the programme, their belief in applicability and utility, and knowledge about nature of psychological problems and also implementation skills. So, they act as a bridge between the students, mental health professionals, parents, and the school administration.

Addressing Stigma in Students

For adequately addressing stigma in students and parents, teachers need to educate themselves in order to address their own misconceptions. Being culturally sensitive, aware of one's own attitudes and behaviours towards others with problems and, if necessary, working on changing the way one thinks, becomes crucial. For facilitating discussion on topics related to mental health, teachers can organize reviews on mental illness and Mental Health. Choosing words carefully in describing mental health problems is important, as colloquial words used for mental health problems, treatments, and hospitals, can be quite stigmatizing. Such labels can also make students hesitant towards seeking help. Diagnostic labels may also lead to stigma. Treating students with mental health issues with compassion, and as equal to others would help them in coping with academics and adjusting with peers and school.

Educating the Parents

It is easy for teachers to access parents; often communication with them is about academics. However, these opportunities can be used to educate them about mental health problems. The first objective of such attempts should be de-stigmatization of mental health problems and treatment seeking. Often parents seek help for severe mental health problems, but fail to identify and seek help for emotional and behavioural problems as these are not considered mental health problems. Parents play an important role in the management of a child with mental health problems in terms of facilitating improvement and also working on family and interpersonal factors contributing/maintaining the problems.

Addressing Bullying and Academic Difficulties

Children who are perceived as weak by their peers often become victims of those who are dominating and have psychological problems. However, this often goes unnoticed by the teachers. The effects of bullying and teasing are multifaceted and have long-term consequences. Teachers have a critical role to play in addressing the issue of both bullies and the victims. However, often the teachers are not aware of effective ways of addressing the problem. Adopting a whole school anti-bullying intervention is suggested to be useful (Fekkes et al. 2005). Academic problems are considered as one of the main stressors by most students (Manjula 2016). Teachers have a big role to play here because they are the best persons identify the nature of difficulty in each student and teach study skills.

Identifying and Addressing Special Needs

Teachers are the first persons to notice if any child has special needs with respect to studies, as well as when a child is generally slow in learning due to intellectual disability. When there is a lack of awareness, the problem may go unnoticed resulting in undue pressure and stress on the child and distress on part of parents and teacher. Such unnoticed needs may put the child in a vulnerable position to develop long-lasting psychological problems.

What Kind of Programmes Can Teachers Implement?

Socio-emotional programmes and interventions in which teachers are involved both at academic and interpersonal level, are said to have a preventive effect on development of psychological problems in future.

School-Based Help: General Strategies

Some children need individual classroom support and an assessment of learning difficulties. Once confirmed to have learning difficulties/disability the teacher need to facilitate the learning through various accommodations based on the nature of the difficulty. Here again, the knowledge about learning disabilities and ways of helping them becomes important. When the problems are severe, they may have to be moved to special educational placements or schools where their behavioural problems can be managed.

Social and Emotional Learning Skills (SEL)

SEL programmes are largely used as preventive interventions. These programmes involve components such as recognizing and managing emotions, developing care and concern for others, establishing positive relationships, making responsible decisions, and handling challenging situations constructively and ethically. They help children to calm themselves when angry, make friends, resolve conflicts respectfully, and make ethical and safe choices. For teachers to effectively deliver these components, they need to have an understanding of the principles of child and adolescent development (Kimberly et al. 2016).

Behavioural Problems

It is important to assess both problem and positive behaviours. Use of reinforcers abundantly is a must while dealing with children (both primary and secondary is essential with young children). Positive reinforcement to increase the behaviour, and social reinforcement to increase attention, are most effective. However for the reinforcement to be effective, it has to be delivered immediately, it should be clear and unequivocal. Children with Attention deficit hypearctivity disorder (ADHD) have difficulty in perceiving other's rights, and subtle rules in social situations, so the rules should be clear and simple, and have clear consequences. As children with ADHD have difficulty in sustaining attention, teachers should create a relaxed atmosphere, have short training phases, avoid distraction, provide alternative material, help to discover mistakes, not criticize, use praise, and facilitate self-talk.

Children with ADHD have significant academic difficulties as well. They require individual assistance and lower pupil-teacher ratio in the classroom for monitoring to be possible. The time has to be reduced to situations leading to problem behaviour; and increased to situations leading to positive behaviours. They should be seated in the front row, closer to the teacher to reduce distractions, increase eye contact, and ensure attention to teacher's instructions (Barkley 1990).

Conduct Disorder and Aggression

Children and adolescents with conduct disorders show behaviours deviating from generally accepted social norms, impulsivity, low frustration tolerance, and lack of empathy. Generally, punishment results in negative consequences, such as increased negative attitudes toward school and school personnel leading to more behavioural problems, anti-social acts, dropping out of school, and various mental health problems. So, stopping misbehaviour must be accomplished along with re-engaging of the student in positive learning. The first step in assessment would be to understand whether the misbehaviour is unintentional or intentional, and if it is intentional, to see if it is reactive (reaction to threat) or proactive (achieve satisfaction with deviant behaviours). Intervention might focus on helping these youngsters identify and follow through on a range of valued, socially appropriate alternatives to deviant activity, setting clear expectations and procedures for non-class room behaviours, for example, in the playground, cafeteria, and so on. Structural changes for places where the crowding happens also helps; for example, keeping the cafeteria in the centre rather than towards a corner where supervision is not possible. There should be consistent consequences for violations. Provisions for social skills training would be beneficial as well. The curriculum should be matched to their interests. Usually, early interventions are useful and if it is not controlled by 8 years, it becomes a chronic problem. It is better to have common agreed-upon approaches to discipline and, procedures for monitoring and evaluation of the effectiveness of the discipline system (Doll and Cummings 2008).

Addressing Emotional Problems

Children with anxiety problems are sensitive to criticism, think negatively, and avoid situations. Thus, teachers should help them in building self-confidence through teaching healthy self-talk, thinking and problem solving skills. Gradual exposure to feared situations, through participation in group activities, classroom activities, modelling calm responses by peers and teachers would be helpful. Through all these, it is important to provide reinforcements for small efforts.

For children with depression, a supportive classroom has to be fostered; unconditional support has to be provided, and singling out of the student for criticism has to be avoided. The feedback has to be specific and the tone while giving the feedback has to be positive. As children with depression are not interested in engaging in any activity, they have to be encouraged to involve themselves in pleasurable activities, such as drawing, writing, or practicing music in their downtime. The homework has to be lowered, they need to be given more breaks throughout the day, larger assignments have to be broken into smaller assignments, and extra time has to be provided. Reassurance by teachers that they can catch up, helps them to continue the school work. Expectations of the teachers have to be lowered. The teachers should help students use positive statements about their performance and encourage positive and realistic goal setting, and physical activity. The teachers should be sensitive to pick up the students feelings', and foster peer support.

Often, depression is precipitated by difficulties in academics. The reasons may be real difficulties in studies, or due to lack of study skills. In addition to teaching subjects, teaching the study strategies would be of help. The students benefit from skills such as ways to organize, plan, and execute tasks on short term and long term basis; goal setting, stress management, conceptual mapping of the work, and self-monitoring and self-reinforcement.

Making a Referral

The teacher should demonstrate a positive attitude towards psychological help seeking. However, a mutual decision is best. The teacher should not force the issue if the student takes a defensive posture. In such situations, it is important to simply restore one's concern and recommendations. It is also important to explain about whom to visit, when and where to go.

Guidelines for Interaction

The teacher has to be careful and adopt certain skills while interacting with children having mental health issues. Some of the general guidelines are as follows:

- Openly acknowledge to the student that you are aware of their distress and are concerned about their welfare (for example, Recently, I have noticed some difference in you and wondered how you are doing, I wanted to check with you because you have seemed pretty down lately).
- See the student in private
- Listen carefully to what the student is troubled about and try to see the issue from his/her point of view, without necessarily agreeing or disagreeing
- Be yourself and be prepared to listen
- Be non-judgmental, patient, calm, and accepting
- If you feel out of your depth, do not to try to deal with the situation alone; take help.

Role of Counsellors

School counsellors are better able to understand the needs of the students in the context and collaborate with teachers and parents; thus they can serve better than professionals working in the hospital set up (Adelman and Taylor 2010; Kauffman and Landrum 2013). Professionals outside may be able help only individual students and may not often have access to teachers and the set-up issues, and the intervention may not be holistic. More so, in case of students who are not severely disturbed (Harwood and Allan 2014; Schmidt 2010; Simpson and Mundschenk

2012). In order to function effectively in the school set-up, it is necessary for the counsellors to work with collaboratively with school authorities and teachers. In addition to helping children with severe problems, they may have to deal with difficult children and children with mild problems, children with family issues, as well as enhance overall resilience of children. Thus, they have to adopt holistic-systemic, flexible, resilience-based approach in counselling (Cohen 2013; Doll 2013; Tol et al. 2011). Furthermore, it is also the role of counsellors to support the teachers, and enhance their awareness and skills to help children such that they are able to adequately respond to students' needs. Teachers also may require guidance with respect to their own personal and professional issues contributing to their stress levels (Harwood and Allan 2014).

One such inclusive model is called inclusive partnership model which emphasizes working in partnership with families and teachers in order to enhance parenting as well as the pedagogical skills for helping at risk/vulnerable children. Most important in such cases is attitudinal change in teachers and parents towards the problems in the child (difficult/problematic) such that their prejudice does not jeopardize the psychosocial and emotional development of the children (Kourkoutas 2012). Sometimes, teachers may have to improve their own emotional and educational skills in order to facilitate learning and support the students. The role of the school authorities in facilitating communication between the counsellor and teacher is crucial to reduce the gap between them. Often teachers do not understand the role of the counsellors mainly due to lack of knowledge; this leads to teachers maintaining distance from the counsellor, or not cooperating in implementing the instructions of the counsellors (Billington 2006; Neven 2010).

Helping Teachers

While training teachers it is most important to promote insight into emotional and family-social, or interpersonal factors of children's problematic functioning. It helps in enhancing teachers' overall knowledge and competence to support their students at risk, social and school inclusion, and avoid further mental health problems. In addition, specific guidelines in handling difficult, or at risk students, and supervising the application of interventions, is found to be useful in making them more confident in discussing, evaluating, and handling difficult children. In order to achieve the above, a working relationship/alliance with teachers is important. It helps in sharing their own difficulties in dealing with difficult children, their negative feelings towards these children, and also feel acknowledged, respected, and rationally explained. Once they are aware of the causes and sources of these negative emotional interactions, they become more able to emotionally step back, develop more empathic involvement with the child and understand the child's academic failures and problematic behaviour (Espelage and Poteat 2012; Rendall and Stuart 2005; Schmidt 2010).

Understanding and addressing sources of stress in teachers helps in modifying their classroom attitudes and strategies, thus preventing a toxic environment in the classroom set-up (Hanko 2001; Kourkoutas 2012). However, teachers who work with difficult or challenging students are exposed to many stressful situations and emotional risks, and are prone to developing inappropriate emotional and pedagogical reactions as a consequence (Hanko 2001). In such cases, they need more support and acknowledgement of their difficulties, and a non-blaming stance from counsellors.

Sometimes the teachers' attitude towards counsellors itself may create hindrance in reflecting on their maladaptive methods. Some of the factors which can create hindrance are as follows: (a) overestimation of their learning and experience; (b) pride in one's own method or fears of being exposed or criticized about one's teaching methods and tactics; (d) lack of previous positive professional experience with school psychologists; (e) strong resistance due to personal difficulties/problems (Kourkoutas 2008). In such instances, counsellors should recognize and respect the experience of teachers, recognize the difficulties they experience with respect to 'problem' children, and be aware of their own negative feelings and tendency to become competitive when interacting with educational staff. Counsellors should take a non-critical position towards teachers' stereotypes and provide them with concise theoretical frameworks relating to specific case-formulation. Resistance in teachers may be addressed by discussing alternative approaches to dealing with problem child and rationally explaining the strategies which work and which does not. It is also helpful to make them aware of the contribution of dysfunctional families in the classroom behaviour of children (Brooks et al. 2012; Monsen and Graham 2002).

Intervention programmes focusing on enhancing teachers' emotional intelligence have showed an increase in self-introspection, emotional awareness, emotional regulation, and understanding others (Hen and Sharabi 2014). Mindfulness skills training of teachers help them in handling 'problem' students and facilitate enhancing these students' academic and emotional resilience (Cohen 2013; Doll 2013). Counsellors and educational psychologists may have to work with teachers who reject challenging students and are very hostile towards them. In this case, counsellors should use their professional skills to gain the teachers' trust, collaborate constructively with them.

Researchers in India do acknowledge the need of delivery of therapeutic services through school, as it is likely to benefit children and adolescents who cannot afford the expensive private consultations offered at the specialized clinics that exist in cities. Considering the mental health needs of our country, population size, and the paucity of trained professionals, there is an urgent need to establish a school mental health delivery system headed by psychologists that would work in close collaboration with the educational system and health care system.

Armbruster (2002) recommended that delivering child and adolescent mental health care through the school system, could lead to: (1) access to services for disadvantaged and under-served youth; (2) system-wide collaboration; (3) prevention of acute psychiatric disorders; (4) fulfil a gate-keeper role for more acute or specialized care; (5) systematic programme evaluation in a 'naturalistic' setting; (6) professional training in working with a range of systems and cultures; and (7) outreach and community-based care.

In an intervention study conducted in a rural area in Chennai, it was found that the students reported academic problems and behavioural problems; in addition, they also reported several family related factors, like parental conflict, absence of father, parental alcoholism, and poverty. While providing services, the students were found to be less motivated to study and to participate in the intervention programmes (Manickam et al. 2005). The findings again emphasize the need for providing training to teachers, to help them understand and identify the problems in children including the family and social context. There is also a need for better co-ordination between mental health service providers and the schoolteachers in order to help identify more children who could benefit from psychological intervention. Adopting student-friendly and flexible strategies in approaching the children may result in better outcome of the programmes.

School Mental Health Programmes in India

Mental health policies for children in the country such as National Mental Health Programme (1982) and National Policy for persons with disabilities (2006) recognize the need for addressing some child mental health issues like epilepsy, mental retardation, and behavioural problems in children. Personnel at Primary Health Centres are trained to actively liaise with schools and *anganwadis* for identification and intervention aspects of child mental health issues. Similarly, special schools and rehabilitation, and formation of self-help groups are emphasized. However, lack of clear focused policies on child mental health, and uncoordinated efforts of the various sectors are the reasons for failure to have uniform programmes across public and private schools (Murthy 1993). Since the late 1970s, there have been initiatives by child psychiatrists and psychologists towards a School Mental Health Programme. However, such programmes are largely carried out in major metropolitan cities and, recently, even some town and rural schools have been covered. Most initiatives have focused on increasing the awareness of the teachers, and/or parents, about child mental health issues. It was also evident in these programmes that teachers could be trained effectively in basic mental health aspects and problems of children and adolescents; they could be provided with skills to identify psychological problems in their students and handle them effectively.

Over the years, most mental health institutes have carried out programmes to orient teachers and parents about mental health needs of children. The orientation programmes often were modified to suit the need of the school, age of the students and the programme under which the mental health orientation was done. No continuing programme has been instituted in any of the trained schools, exclusively for mental health. Some programmes trained the teachers in counselling techniques and they were expected to identify and intervene at the school level where possible and refer to a child mental health unit in other cases (Kapur and Cariappa 1979; Kapur 1997; Bharat et al. 2008).

The Department of Psychiatry, NIMHANS Bangalore, developed a Cascade Model of Life Skills Education after extensive need assessments and focus group discussions with adolescents in secondary schools, secondary school teachers, parents, NGOs, social scientists, bureaucrats, and policy makers working with adolescents. A programme of Life Skills Education for adolescents was developed by using this model as a project over the last 4–5 years (Bharath and Kumar 2007). The Impact of the programme was assessed at the end of one year in the state run government schools. It was found that students in the LSE programme had better adjustment at school and with teachers; they had better self-esteem, perceived coping, and prosocial behaviours, compared to students not in the programme (Bharath and Kumar 2010).

Expressions: A comprehensive Model of School Mental Health is an innovative movement set up in the last decade by Dr. Nagpal in Delhi with the technical support of the Ministry of Human Resources and Development, and NCERT. The programme focuses on Life Skills Education and Mental Health Awareness involving teachers, parents, and students. A Cascade Strategy for disseminating Life Skills Education is used in the adolescent population. Interested teachers are trained as Life Skills Educators who initiate the programme in schools and run it. Interested and competent students are identified as 'Peer Educators' and trained in life skills training, to impart Life Skills to other students (Nagpal 2011). Most of these programmes were carried out as projects and not as co-curricular programmes integrated into the school system.

In Kerala state, in recent years, there are many school-based interventions specifically focusing on mental health and wellbeing of children are implemented. These services are provided by multiple agencies such as governmental (Education department, Social justice department, Department of health, Kerala police, Home department and District panchayats), non-governmental and private sectors (NGOs). The nature of the programmes are parallel with the developments happening in mental health scenario in schools of high income countries (Ramkumar 2015). The interventions broadly can be divided into universal, selective, and indicated. The universal interventions were implemented as ongoing programmes involving children from primary school to Grade 12. The major components of these programmes are life skills education, sensitization and awareness programmes for children and parents, guidance for children, empowerment programmes for parents, teachers and students, stress management, and leadership programmes. Selective and indicated interventions included scrutiny of high-risk children for drug abuse using shadow police, SMS alerts to parents, online counselling by counsellors, interventions for ADHD by specialists, telephonic support for exam anxiety, and early identification of children with problems though drop box activities. Many programmes have utilized teachers as counsellors and coordinators, especially because of non-availability of qualified counsellors, and to ensure coverage, continuity, and cost-effectiveness. Indicated interventions currently are being delivered by minimally trained personnel, with inadequate specialist support.

There is a call now for greater attention to evaluation of programmes. There is a lack of rigor in the stated objectives and lack of clarity on the mechanisms for their delivery. This would include measuring fidelity to the declared interventions of the particular programme, process evaluation, and assessment of cost effectiveness of the interventions. However, it has been identified that these remain as research gaps (Fazel et al. 2014).

Issues like non-cooperation from teachers towards counsellors posted from a different department, counsellor-related issues like poor job prospects, lack of experience, and systematic training, and lack of formal process for referral to psychiatrists were reported, across the school based interventions using the teachers. Similarly, in a long term programme carried out in colleges by teachers trained in counselling by faculty from NIMHANS (Chandrashekhar 2002), the programme was reported to be useful. However, it was stopped because of the difficulties in implementing, and the administrative problems in continuing the programme. In this programme, about 1091 teachers were trained in 44 batches starting from 1975 to 2010.

According to a report on the strengthening of counselling in schools, the presence of multiple agencies from different funding streams doing the same and overlapping work, without any cross talk, is the norm now. In Kerala, though lacunae in training programmes for Resource Teachers were identified (SAA 2014), they are not being adequately addressed. Minimally trained personnel are currently delivering the interventions in most of the programmes/schools. There are ongoing attempts to improve aspects of quality of the counselling services and accreditation of service personnel. Also, attempts are being made to equip schools with counselling centres, and have protected teachers as counsellors after providing them with training in student counselling (Ramkumar 2015).

Conclusion

Though the mental health needs of school children are accepted in most countries including India, there is a glaring lack of coordination between programmes, which leads to limitations in their efficiency. Even when some programmes are funded and encouraged by the Government itself, the uniform implementation is lacking across the States in India. This may be addressed by the creation of a nodal agency with mandate for coordination and quality assurance. The DMHP could focus more on facilitating and coordinating selective and indicated prevention programmes in schools. Also, there is lack of evaluation of programme processes and outcome, and so on, limiting the scope for choosing a particular programme for uniform implementation. The programme planning and implementation has to happen at national level. School mental health should become a part of the National Mental Health programme. For such programmes to be effective, promotive and preventive mental health services should be run as ongoing collaborative programmes wherein health and education departments work together. It should ideally start from primary school and continue throughout their schooling. For the programmes to be successful, the role of school administrators and teachers is very important.

Who needs to be trained and the role of teachers and counsellors would become the next important point to be contemplated. In India, where there is limited number of well-(adequately-)trained counsellors, teachers definitely need to do more than their share. However, there is severe lack of training opportunities for them. Similarly, the roles of teachers as mental health professionals and the role of counsellors often overlap and clarity is lacking. The training of teachers should include a mental health component as well as exposure to training in identifying mental health problems, basics of interventions and ethics of providing support and care. They should also be equipped with information of referral procedure, contact of professionals as well as special services. The school and teachers should facilitate and cooperate in the treatment of children identified to have mental health problems, such as anxiety, depression, ADHD, learning disability, and the like. They should not be stigmatized or isolated. Mental health referrals—within the school system as well as to community-based professionals and agencies—should be coordinated by using written protocols, should be monitored for adherence, and should be evaluated for effectiveness. There should be opportunities for students to have consultations outside the school campus (Bharat et al. 2008). Similarly, there should be specific training for counsellors to work in the school setting. Their training should include understanding and interventions in mental health issues as well as methods of addressing issues in academics and also skills of managing people in the school administrative setting. There should be clear guidelines to be followed by administrators, teachers, and counsellors in the school set up. The referral systems also need to be in place.

Overall, though there is fair understanding of the importance of school mental health, there is a long way to go in achieving coordinated, objectively established, uniformly implemented interventions to take off.

References

Adelman, H. S., & Taylor, L. (2010). Creating successful school systems requires addressing barriers to learning and teaching. *The F. M. Duffy Reports,15*(3).

Adi, Y., Killoran, A., Janmohamed, K., & Stewart-Brown, S. (2007a). *Systematic review of the effectiveness of interventions to promote mental wellbeing in primary schools: Universal approaches which do not focus on violence or bullying*. London: National Institute for Clinical Excellence.

Adi, Y., Schrader McMillan, A., Kiloran, A., & Stewart-Brown, S. (2007b). *Systematic review of the effectiveness of interventions to promote mental wellbeing in primary schools: Universal approaches with focus on prevention of violence and bullying*. London: National Institute for Clinical Excellence.

Anagnostopoulos, D. C., & Soumaki, E. (2012). The impact of socioeconomic crisis on mental health of children and adolescents. *Psychiatric, 23*(1), 15–16.

Armbruster, P. (2002). The administration of school-based mental health services. *Child and Adolescent Psychiatric Clinics of North America, 1,* 23–41.

Barkley, R. A. (1990). *Attention deficit hyperactivity disorder: A handbook for diagnosis and treatment*. New York: Guilford Press.
Berkowitz, M. W., & Bier, M. C. (2007). What works in character education. *Journal of Research in Character Education, 5*, 29–48.
Bharat, S., Kumar, K. V. K., & Mukesh, Y. P. (2008). Clinical practice guidelines for school mental health programme. *Indian Journal of Psychiatry*, 307–321.
Bharath, S., & Kumar, K. V. K. (2007). Health promotion using life skills approach for adolescents in schools: A district model—NIMHANS. *DSERT Collaboration—A Report*, NIMHANS.
Bharath, S., & Kumar, K. K. (2010). Empowering adolescents with life skills education in schools —School mental health programme: does it work? *Indian Journal of Psychiatry, 52*, 344–349.
Billington, T. (2006). *Working with children*. London, United Kingdom: Heinemann.
Birmaher, B., Ryan, N. D., Williamson, D. E., Brent, D. A., Kaufman, J., Dahl, R. E., et al. (1996). Childhood and adolescent depression: A review of the past 10 years. Part I. *Journal of the American Academy of Child & Adolescent Psychiatry, 35*(11), 1427–1439.
Blank, L., Baxter, S., Goyder, E., Guillaume, L., Wilkinson, A., Hummel, S., et al. (2009). Systematic review of the effectiveness of universal interventions which aim to promote emotional and social wellbeing in secondary schools. *Interventions, 56*(4.5), 1.
Brooks, R., Brooks, S., & Goldstein, S. (2012). The power of mindsets: Nurturing student engagement, motivation, and resilience in students. In S. L. Christenson, A. L. Reschly, & C. Wylie (Eds.), *Handbook of research on student engagement* (pp. 541–562). New York, NY: Springer.
Browne, G., Gafni, A., Roberts, J., Byrne, C. & Majumdar, G. (2004). Effective/efficient mental health programs for school-age children: A synthesis of reviews. *Social Science and Medicine, 58*, 1367–1384.
Cadima, J., Leal, T., & Burchinal, M. (2010). The quality of teacher-student interactions: associations with first graders' academic and behavioural outcomes. *Journal of School Psychology, 48*(6), 457–482.
Catalano, R. F., Hawkins, J. D., Berglund, M. L., Pollard, J. A., & Arthur, M. W. (2002). Prevention science and positive youth development: Competitive or cooperative frameworks? *Journal of Adolescent Health, 31*(6SUPPL.), 230–239.
Chandrashekhar, C. R. (2002). *Manualon students' counseling for college teachers*. Bangalore: Department of Collegiate Education, Government of Karnataka, and National Institute of Mental Health and Neurosciences, Bangalore.
Cohen, J. (2013). Creating positive school climate: A foundation for resilience. In S. Goldstein & R. B. Brooks (Eds.), *Handbook of resilience in children* (pp. 411–422). New York, NY: Springer.
Costello, E. J., Egger, H., & Angold, A. (2005). 10-year research update review: The epidemiology of child and adolescent psychiatric disorders: I. Methods and public health burden. *Journal of the American Academy of Child and Adolescent Psychiatry, 44*(10), 972–986.
Costello, E. J., Erkanli, A., & Angold, A. (2006). Is there an epidemic of child or adolescent depression? *Journal of Child Psychology and Psychiatry, 47*(12), 1263–1271.
Costello, E. J., Mustillo, S., Erkanli, A., Keeler, G., & Angold, A. (2003). Prevalence and development of psychiatric disorders in childhood and adolescence. *Archives of General Psychiatry, 60*, 837–844.
Doll, B. (2013). Enhancing resilience in classrooms. In S. Goldstein & R. B. Brooks (Eds.), *Handbook of resilience in children* (pp. 399–410). New York, NY: Springer.
Doll, B., & Cummings, J. A. (Eds.). (2008). *Transforming school mental health services*. Thousand Oaks, CA: Corwin Press.
Espelage, D. L., & Poteat, V. P. (2012). Counseling psychologists in schools. In N. Fouad & L. Subich (Eds.), *APA handbook of counselling psychology: Practice, interventions, and applications* (Vol. 2, pp. 541–566). Washington, DC: American Psychological Association.

Essau, C. A., Conradt, J., & Petermann, F. (2000). Frequency, comorbidity, and psychosocial impairment of depressive disorders in adolescents. *Journal of Adolescent Research, 15*(4), 470–481.

Essau, C. A., Lewinsohn, P. M., Seeley, J. R., & Sasagawa, S. (2010). Gender differences in the developmental course of depression. *Journal of Affective Disorders, 127,* 185–190.

Farrington, D. P., & Ttofi, M. M. (2009). School-based programmes to reduce bullying and victimization. *Campbell Systematic Reviews No. 6.* Oslo, Norway: Campbell Corporation.

Fazel, M., Hoagwood, K., Stephan, S., & Ford, T. (2014). Mental health interventions in schools in high-income countries. *The Lancet Psychiatry, 1*(5), 377–387.

Fekkes, M., Pijpers, F. I., & Verloove-Vanhorick, S. P. (2005). Bullying: Who does what, when and where? Involvement of children, teachers and parents in bullying behaviour. *Health Education Research, 20*(1), 81–91.

Fergusson, D. M., Horwood, L. J., Ridder, E. M., Beautrais, A. L. (2005). Subthreshold depression in adolescence and mental health outcomes in adulthood. *Archives of General Psychiatry, 62* (1), 66–72.

Fombonne, E. (2001). Is there an epidemic of autism? *Pediatrics, 107,* 411–413.

Gansle, K. A. (2005). The effectiveness of school-based anger interventions and programmes: A meta-analysis. *Journal of School Psychology, 43,* 321–341.

Gross, J. (Ed.). (2008). *Getting in early.* London: Smith Institute and the Centre for Social Justice.

Hanko, G. (2001). 'Difficult-to-teach' children: Consultative staff support as an aspect of inclusive education: Sharing expertise across national and cultural boundaries. In J. Visser, H. Daniels, T. Cole (Eds.), *Emotional and Behavioural Difficulties in Mainstream Schools* (pp. 47–62). Oxford: Elsevier.

Harden, A., Rees, R., Shepherd, J., Brunton, G., Oliver, S., & Oakley, A. (2001). *Young people and mental health: A systematic review of research on barriers and facilitators.* London: EPPI-Centre, Social Science Research Unit.

Harwood, V., & Allan, J. (2014). *Psychopathology at school: Theorizing mental disorders in education.* Abingdon, United Kingdom: Routledge.

Hen, M., & Sharabi, A. (2014). Teaching the teachers: Emotional intelligence training for teachers. *Teaching Education, 25,* 375–390. https://doi.org/10.1080/10476210.2014.908838.

Horowitz, L., & Garber, J. (2006). The prevention of depressive symptoms in children and adolescents: A meta-analytic review. *Journal of Consulting and Clinical Psychology, 74*(3), 401–415.

Jennings, P. A., Frank, J. L., Snowberg, K. E., Coccia, M. A., & Greenberg, M. T. (2013). Improving classroom learning environments by cultivating awareness and resilience in education (CARE): Results of a randomized controlled trial. *School Psychology Quartely, 28,* 374–390.

Jennings, P. A., & Greenberg, M. T. (2009). The pro-social classroom: Teacher social and emotional competence in relation to student and classroom outcomes. *Review of Educational Research, 79,* 491–525.

Kapur, M. (1997). *Mental health in Indian schools.* New Delhi: Sage.

Kapur, M., & Cariappa, I. (1979). Training in counselling for schoolteachers on emotional problems of school children. *International Journal of Advances in Counseling, 2,* 109–115.

Kauffman, J. M., & Landrum, T. J. (2013). *Cases in emotional and behavioural disorders of children and youth* (3rd ed.). Pearson: Boston.

Kim-Cohen, J., Caspi, A., E Moffitt, T., Harrington, H. L., Milne, B., & Poulton, R. (2003). Prior juvenile diagnoses in adults with mental disorder: Developmental follow-back of a prospective-longitudinal cohort. *Archives of general psychiatry, 60,* 709–717.

Kourkoutas, E. (2008). An ecosystemic psychodynamic intervention for children with mild psychosocial problems and academic difficulties: Prospects and limits of the evaluation process. In C. Canali, T. Vecchiato, & J. K. Whittaker (Eds.), *Assessing the "evidence-base" of intervention for vulnerable children and their families* (pp. 434–438). Padua, Italy: Zancan.

Kourkoutas, E. (2012). *Behavioural disorders in children: Ecosystemic psychodynamic interventions within family and school context.* New York, NY: Nova Science.

Lang, I. A., Marlow, R., Goodman, R., Meltzer, H., & Ford, T. (2013). Influence of problematic child-teacher relationships on future psychiatric disorder: Population survey with 3-year follow-up. *The British Journal of Psychiatry, 202,* 336–341.

Lewinsohn, P. M., Klein, D. N., & Seeley, J. R. (2000) Bipolar disorder during adolescence and young adulthood in a community sample. *Bipolar Disorders* 2(3.2), 281–293.

Loades, M. E., & Mastroyannopoulou, K. (2010). Teachers' recognition of children's mental health problems. *Child and Adolescent Mental Health, 15*(3), 150–156.

Manickam, L. S. S., Saravanan, S., Nithya, H. M., & Susheela, S. (2005). Counseling problem children: Evaluation of school mental health programme in rural Chennai, South India. *2GCTE Journal of Research and Extension Education, 1*(1), 17–32.

Manjula, M. (2016). Academic stress management: An intervention in pre-university college youth. *Journal of the Indian Academy of Applied Psychology, 42*(1), 105–13 (2016).

Manjula, M., Roopesh, B. N. Philip, M. (2015). *Stress management in youth: A preventive intervention.* Project report submitted to Indian Council of Social Science Research, New Delhi.

Meltzer, H., Gatward, R., Corbin, T., Goodman, R., & Ford, T. (2003). *The mental health of young people looked after by local authorities in England.* London: The Stationery Office.

Merikangas, K. R., He, J. P., Burstein, M., Swanson, S. A., Avenevoli, S., Cui, L., et al. (2010). Lifetime prevalence of mental disorders in US adolescents: Results from the National Comorbidity Survey Replication–Adolescent Supplement (NCS-A). *Journal of the American Academy of Child & Adolescent Psychiatry, 49*(10), 980–989.

Monsen, J., & Graham, B. (2002). Developing teacher-support groups to deal with challenging child behaviour: The staff sharing scheme. In P. Gray (Ed.), *Working with emotions: Responding to the challenge of difficult pupil behaviour in schools* (pp. 130–149). London, United Kingdom: Routledge.

Murthy, RS. (1993). Child Mental Health: Policies in India – Perspectives and Developments in the National Context in Child Mental Health – Proceedings of the Indo-US Symposium. In Kapur M., Kellam S., Tarter R.,Wilson R. (Eds.), *NIMHANS –ADAMHACollaboration 1993.*

Nagpal, J. (2011). Expressions 2009: Delhi experience. Symposia/workshops. *Indian Journal of Psychiatry, 53,* 10–26.

National Mental Health Programme for India. (1982). *Ministry of Health and Family Welfare, Government of India.* New Delhi: Directorate General of Health Services (DGHS).

National Policy for persons with disabilities. (2006). *Ministry of Health and Family Welfare, Government of India.* New Delhi: Directorate General of Health Services (DGHS).

Neven, R. S. (2010). *Core principles of assessment and therapeutic communication with children, parents and families: Towards the promotion of child and family wellbeing.* Routledge.

Patton, G. C., Coffey, C., Romaniuk, H., Mackinnon, A., Carlin, J. B., Degenhardt, L., et al. (2014). The prognosis of common mental disorders in adolescents: A 14-year prospective cohort study. *The Lancet, 383*(9926), 1404–1411.

Payton, J., Weissberg, R. P., Durlak, J. A., Dymnicki, A. B., Taylor, R. D., Schellinger, K. B., et al. (2008). *The positive impact of social and emotional learning for kindergarten to eighth-grade students: Findings from three scientific reviews.* Chicago, IL: Collaborative for Academic, Social, and Emotional Learning.

Ramkumar, G. S. (2015). Mental health provisions in schools of Kerala: A narrative overview of programmes and interventions. *Kerala Journal of Psychiatry, 28*(1), 82–93.

Reef, J., Diamantopoulou, S., van Meurs, I., Verhulst, F. C., van der Ende, J. (2011). Developmental trajectories of child to adolescent externalizing behavior and adult DSM-IV disorder: Results of a 24-year longitudinal study.*Social Psychiatry and Psychiatric Epidemiology, 46,*1233–1241.

Reddy, R., Rhodes, J. E., & Mulhall, P. (2003). The influence of teacher support on student adjustment in the middle school years: A latent growth curve study. *Developmental Psychopathology, 15*(1), 119–138.

Rendall, S., & Stuart, M. (2005). *Excluded from school: Systemic practice for mental health and education professionals.* Hove, United Kingdom: Routledge.

Rohner, R. P., & Khaleque, A. (2010). Testing central postulates of parental acceptance-rejection theory (PAR Theory): A meta-analysis of cross-cultural studies. *Journal of Family Theory and Review, 2*(1), 73–87.
Rothy, D. M., & Leavey, G. (2006). Mental health help-seeking and young people: A review. *Pastoral Care in Education, 24*(3), 4–13.
Sarva Shiksha Abhiyan (SAA). (2014). *19th Joint Review Mission,* State Report. Kerala.
Sawyer, M. G., Arney, F. M., Baghurst, P. A., Clark, J. J., Graetz, B. W., Kosky, R. J., et al. (2001). The mental health of young people in Australia: Key findings from the child and adolescent component of the national survey of mental health and well-being. *Australian & New Zealand Journal of Psychiatry, 35*(6), 806–814.
Sayal, K., Hornsey, H., Warren, S., MacDiarmid, F., & Taylor, E. (2006). Identification of children at risk of attention deficit/hyperactivity disorder: A school-based intervention. *Social Psychiatry and Psychiatric Epidemiology, 41*(10), 806–813.
Schmidt, N. R. (2010). Core principles of assessment and therapeutic communication with children, parents and families: Towards the promotion of child and family wellbeing. New York, NY: Routledge.
Schonert-Reichl, K. A., Kitil, M. J., LeRose, M., Sipl, M., Lina Sweiss, L., et al. (2016). Social & emotional learning and teacher education: What do we know and where do we go from here? *White Paper Prepared for HopeLab.* The University of British Columbia: Vancouver.
Simpson, R., & Mundschenk, N. A. (2012). Inclusion and students with emotional and behavioural disorders. In J. P. Bakken, F. E. Obiakor, & A. F. Rotatori (Eds.), *Behavioural disorders: Practice concerns and students with EBD. Advances in special education* (Vol. 23, pp. 1–22). Emerald Group Publishing Limited.
Singh, S., & Manjula, M. (2010). *Suicidal risk, childhood adversity and psychological functioning in college students.* Unpublished dissertation submitted to NIMHANS, Bengaluru.
Singhal, M., Manjula, M., & Vijay Sagar, K. J. (2015). Perceived stigma and satisfaction in adolescents: Results from a school-based depression prevention programme. *Andhra Pradesh Journal of Psychological Medicine, 16*(1), 54–61.
Soyingbe, A. A., Ogunyanwo, O. O., Onadipe, T. O., Adetoyi, H. E., & Adetayo, O. P. (2013). Roles of teachers in the promotion of mental health among secondary school students in Ijebu-Ode local Government area, Ogun State, Nigeria. *International Journal of Humanities and Social Science Invention, 2*(1), 29–34.
Srinath, S., Girimaji, S. C., Gururaj, G., Seshadri, S., Subbakrishna, D. K., Bhola, P., et al. (2005). Epidemiological study of child & adolescent psychiatric disorders in urban & rural areas of Bangalore, India. *Indian Journal of Medical Research, 122,* 67–79.
Tol, W. A., Barbui, C., Galappatti, A., Silove, D., Betancourt, T. S., Souza, R., et al. (2011). Mental health and psychosocial support in humanitarian settings: Linking practice and research. *The Lancet, 378*(9802), 1581–1591.
Waddell, C., McEwan, K., Peters, R., et al. (2007). Preventing mental disorders in children: A public health priority.*Canadian Journal of Public Health, 98,*174–178.
Weare, K., & Nind, M. (2011). Mental health promotion and problem prevention in schools: What does the evidence say?. *Health Promotion International, 26*(1), i29–i69.
Wells, J., Barlow, J., Stewart-Brown, S. (2003). A systematic review of universal approaches to mental health promotion in schools. *Health Education, 103*(4), 197–220.
Whear, R., Marlow, R., Boddy, K., Ukoumunne, O. C., Parker, C., Ford, T., et al. (2014). Psychiatric disorder or impairing psychology in children who have been excluded from school: A systematic review. *School Psychology International, 35*(5), 530–543.

Chapter 14
The Importance of Recreational Activities to Assess and Prevent Bullying

Ana Carina Stelko-Pereira, Jessica Elena Valle and Lucia C. A. Williams

Abstract This chapter reviews the literature on bullying, exploring important aspects of its definition, as well as its consequences, followed by a discussion on the importance of recreational activities to identify bullying involvement, and to intervene in the problem. Bullying negatively impacts emotional, social, and academic development, as it is associated with mental health problems, psychosomatic complaints, interpersonal difficulties, and poor academic performance. Recreational activities have an important role in child development, as toys and games allow children to acquire different skills associated with healthy pro-social relationships. Thus, recreation has an educational as well as a social function, in the sense that it is a source of learning, favouring socialization. Several studies report the association between lack of friendships and bullying, indicating that bullying victims have fewer friends, or no friends at all, and are less involved in multiplayer games. Furthermore, children who do not participate in extracurricular activities have more chances of being a bullying perpetrator. Therefore, investigations into targeted recreational activities may not only provide clues on bullying occurrence, but can also be a resource to attenuate or eliminate the problem. In this context, recreational activities may be an important strategy to reduce violence among students, due to the acquisition of social skills, peer appreciation, increase in well-being of participants, expression of positive feelings, and negative ones, which could deter aggressive behaviours. Thereby, the importance of recreational activities in the school context is highlighted as one of the main strategies to intervene in bullying prevention. Studies that present recreational strategies to prevent bullying will be

---

This chapter is part of a Brazilian research project, which received grant #458956/2014-7, by the first author from the Brazilian National Council for Scientific and Technological Development (CNPq).

A. C. Stelko-Pereira
Ceará State University (Universidade Estadual do Ceará, UECE), Fortaleza, Brazil

J. E. Valle · L. C. A. Williams (✉)
Federal University of São Carlos (Universidade Federal de São Carlos, UFSCar), São Carlos, Brazil
e-mail: luciacawilliams@gmail.com

S. Deb (ed.), *Positive Schooling and Child Development*,
https://doi.org/10.1007/978-981-13-0077-6_14

described, as well as the description of promising low-cost activities developed by the authors in Brazil, such as board games and classroom folders, along with the evidence that they encompass positive strategies to prevent bullying.

Keywords Bullying · Recreational activities · Games · Student School

Introduction

The importance of recreational activities for child development, such as playing with toys and games, is well established (Pellegrini 2009). This chapter explores the importance of recreational activities to identify bullying involvement and to intervene in the problem. However, before we argue about the role of recreational activities to prevent bullying, we contextualize the phenomenon with a brief review of literature on bullying.

Bullying: An Urgent Problem in Need of Prevention

Bullying refers to a situation where a student is intentionally, repeatedly, and over time, exposed to negative actions by peers (Olweus 1993). This phenomenon has particularities differentiating it from other kinds of violence, such as the restriction to occurrence among peers, its repetitiveness and persistence over time, the intentionality of aggressive behaviours, which do not result from arguments and point of view divergences, and the inequality of power among participants, leading the victim to a situation where he/she cannot prevent or defend him or herself (Olweus 1993, 2013). The inequality of power among bullying participants is not restricted to physical strength, but may also include differences in social status, popularity, and cognitive abilities, among others. Thus, customarily, students in vulnerable conditions are victims of bullying (Guerin and Hennessy 2002; Lamb et al. 2009; Vaillancourt et al. 2003).

Bullying participants may be characterized as bullies or perpetrators, those who practice the action; victims, those who suffer aggressions; victim-perpetrators or bully-victims, those who are assaulted by stronger perpetrators, and assault weaker peers; and witnesses, those who stand by and witness the violence but do not participate directly (Olweus 1993; Orpinas and Horne 2006). Additionally, the aggression may be shown in a direct way, such as punching, kicking, cursing, and giving depreciative nicknames, or in an indirect way, such as deliberate exclusion, spreading rumours, among other examples (Hamburger et al. 2011; Lamb et al. 2009).

Bullying is an international problem, occurring in countries with better socioeconomic conditions, as well in medium- or low-income countries. Craig et al. (2009) performed a study of bullying prevalence, gathering data from 40 countries, in which they found that 26% of participants had some kind of bullying involvement: 12.6% as victims; 10.7% as perpetrators; and 3.6% as victim-perpetrators. Nevertheless, Fleming and Jacobsen (2009) pointed out that countries with better socioeconomic conditions have shown bullying prevalence involvement varying from 5 to 57%, whilst in low- or medium-income countries this prevalence could vary from 12 to 100%. These authors conducted a survey in 19 middle-income countries (Upper middle-income, middle-income and lower middle-income) and low-income countries, identifying that, in general, 34.2% of participants suffered bullying, with the rates varying from 7.8 to 60.9% among countries which participated in the survey (Fleming and Jacobsen 2009).

According to the literature, bullying involvement may present consequences to participants, in the short or long term (Albuquerque et al. 2013; National Academies of Sciences, Engineering, and Medicine 2016). Victims are likely to have anxiety disorders, depression, suicidal thoughts, low academic achievement, and school evasion (Cornell et al. 2013; Due et al. 2005; Holt et al. 2015). In the long term, victims may be socially isolated, with attachment difficulties, and problems in the work environment (Wolke and Lereya 2015). Nevertheless, not only are victims impacted by this phenomenon, perpetrators may also get involved in substance abuse, criminal activities, gang membership, low academic achievement, and school failure (Farrington et al. 2011; Valdebenito et al. 2015). Bully-victims experience more negative impacts due to the role combination, presenting more depressive disorders and severe anxiety, as well as more chances of substance abuse. In addition, witnesses may feel guilty for not contributing to the interruption of the aggression, as well as fearing being the next victims (Albuquerque et al. 2013; National Academies of Sciences, Engineering, and Medicine 2016; Rigby 2003).

In the face of the high prevalence and the amplitude of the negative effects of bullying involvement, prevention and intervention efforts for the problem have been recurring. Studies have pointed out, however, the inefficiency of mere punitive actions—such as the compulsory transference of students to other schools, forcing the perpetrator to apologize to the victim—as well as the implementation of surveillance cameras and metal detectors in schools (National Academies of Sciences, Engineering, and Medicine 2016). On the other hand, social skills training, promotion of a positive school climate, the enhancement of teaching quality in classes, making the subject more relevant to students with more participation from them, increasing supervision during recess, and informative meetings with parents have been considered promising strategies (National Academies of Sciences, Engineering, and Medicine 2016).

Latest Evidence on Recreational Activities in Bullying Prevention

Playful activities are characterized by the practice of social interaction through games, toys, and recreation (Baliulevicius and Macário 2006). These activities described as leisure and fun (Bustamante 2004) are considered of major importance to human development due to the fact that their impact goes beyond leisure, as a way of promoting learning (Mauricio 2007; Moreira and Pereira 2008; Roloff 2010). Through playful elements, it is possible to convey contents and knowledge, combining them with recreational activities and games, so that one is able to learn how to play in an intuitive way (Kishimoto 1996; Roloff 2010).

Recreational activities promote motor, cognitive, psychological, and social development, enabling the student to acquire fine motor abilities and motor coordination. In addition, they stimulate curiosity, creativity, and imagination, providing concentration and attention, new concept development, shaping values and character, developing language and thought, acquiring knowledge and self-knowledge, promoting autonomy, self-esteem, and self-confidence, and developing peer relations (Baliulevicius and Macário 2006; Barros 2012; Bertoldo and Reschell 2000; Roloff 2010; Schwarz et al. 2006; Smith 2006). Through games and play, important social values may be learned, such as: the importance of communication; expression of positive and negative feelings; of respect, equality, solidarity, and teamwork (Barros 2012; Carvalho 2012; Roloff 2010). Therefore, playing is important for development and learning, as well as the establishment of good social interaction.

Nonetheless, the playful element is still little explored in the school context (Marcellino 2011; Roloff 2010), in spite of the fact that studies have already pointed out that extracurricular activities and/or leisure, encourage social skill development and social problem solving, providing a buffer to at-risk behaviours (Farb and Matjasko 2012; Riese et al. 2015).

Recreational strategies have been used, in the school context, as a way of identifying or assessing the presence of bullying, and also as a tool to prevent bullying, as seen below.

Recreational Activities as a Strategy to Assess Bullying

Self-report instruments are commonly employed to evaluate the prevalence of bullying (Hamburger et al. 2011), in which participants respond questions about whether or not they have experienced it as victims or have themselves engaged in bullying perpetrations. Despite their importance, these instruments present some disadvantages, as respondents may not be capable of an accurate evaluation of his/her involvement in bullying, in addition to the possibility of feeling insecure when describing the involvement, especially when they are perpetrators (Seixas 2005). In light of these difficulties, complementing this evaluation method is important.

One recreational method that may be used to identify bullying involvement is the *Prosocial Cyberball Game.* Riem et al. (2013), originally adapted the cyberball virtual game, in which players toss a ball, to study the effects of oxytocin on prosocial behaviour during a game with female adults. Subsequently, Vrijhof et al. (2016) investigated the application of the *Prosocial Cyberball Game* with 133 Dutch students from 9 to 17 years of age. The results showed that players compensated for the social exclusion of an unknown peer, by tossing the ball more often to that player in compensation conditions, compared to the fair play condition. On the other hand, players identified as bullying perpetrators tossed the ball significantly less to the excluded player. These data, beyond enabling the identification of complicit bystander, passive bystander, and active defender, also indicate the importance of investigating the role of bullying witnesses, as their behaviour may influence the occurrence of aggression.

Another interesting strategy to evaluate bullying using a recreational strategy, is *Mii-School,* developed by Spanish researchers (Carmona et al. 2010). It is a 3D virtual reality school simulator, where 17 school scenarios are shown containing dialogues among characters. Five of such situations in the interactive video game involve bullying, and the remaining ones investigate problematic behaviours, such as substance abuse. The evaluated student chooses a character (male or female) and proceeds to indicate which role he/she would adopt in situations involving the classroom and playground. The player may, for instance, run away or protest, among other actions. The attractiveness, comprehension, and easiness in answering these scenarios were well evaluated by 65 students, with an average age of 14.6 years. *Mii-School* also had its psychometric characteristics evaluated by Torres et al. (2012), showing an adequate level of internal consistency to the bullying dimension (0.7). The instrument comprehends two relative factors in terms of bullying: victimization and perpetration.

Another method involves school observations and asking questions about how interactions occur in students' playful moments, such as at recess. Craig et al. (2016) asked students whom they liked to talk to and sit near at recess. The authors noticed that the more rejected students in playful and less-structured moments were also the ones who were rejected during class activities, in addition to being identified as bullying victims by themselves, the classmates, and teachers. The authors highlight the importance of performing more contextual bullying assessments, especially taking into account children's interaction in recreational moments, such as recess, for example.

Recreational Activities to Prevent or Intervene in Bullying

Recreational activities are not only resources to assess bullying, as they may also be employed for the prevention of and intervention on this serious problem. For instance, Carvalho (2012) used recreational cooperative activities with 457 students from Grades 3–4, in two schools from Paraná State, in Southern Brazil.

These activities were carried on for 15 weeks and involved different constructs, such as rules, self-knowledge, and knowledge about peers, body awareness, equality notion, cooperativeness, teamwork, and recommended actions against bullying. Comparing pre- and post-intervention assessments, a decrease in bullying victimization was observed, with a prevalence decline of victims from 34 to 21%; an increase of non-victimized students, from 55.3 to 63.2%; an increase in calling for help on the part of bullying witness students, (prior 13.6% and post 18.4%), suggesting that recreational activities enhance the socialization and cooperation among students, enabling a reduction in bullying victimizations.

Additionally, Barros (2012) verified whether the use of games and recreation during school recess could prevent bullying with 393 9–10-year-old children from public schools in Paraná State, Brazil. For the duration of six weeks, recreational material—such as games, toys, including skipping ropes, playing with rubber bands, ring tossing, chess—were provided to students at recess. Pre- and post-intervention assessments showed significant positive results only in the number of students who tried to help bullying victims (from 4.5 to 9.2%). Although not significant, other results presented a positive modest trend: a decrease in bullying victimization percentages from 26.5 to 20.4%; an increase in non-victimized students from 57.5 to 66.8%; a decrease in bullying perpetration from 8.5 to 2.6%. Thus, we need further studies with more complex methodology (Randomized Controlled Trials—RTC, for example) to further explore the methodology used by Barros (2012) as helpful to develop healthy relationships in students.

Caballo et al. (2011) also investigated the effects of a play-based intervention with 193 students ranging from 9 to 14 years (average 11.2), from two private schools in Granada, Spain. The intervention consisted of a group application, during 14 weeks, of a programme called *Jugando y Aprendendo Habilidades Sociales* (*Playing and Learning Social Skills*) (JAHSO), based on a game aimed to develop social skills required for good coexistence and also to extinguish undesired behaviours, such as aggression. Prior to the game application, there were presentations about social skills, including concepts and components, such as expression of feelings, interpersonal problem solving, etc. The game, in turn, had activities about social skills, where daily interpersonal situations were recreated in a way that players would have to demonstrate the required skills and knowledge to deal with such situations. Results comparing pre to post-test assessment indicated a statistical significant decrease in relational victimization (prior $M = 48.26$ and post $M = 44.70$); in physical victimization (prior $M = 13.35$ and post $M = 11.48$); and in physical aggression (prior $M = 8.88$ and post $M = 7.42$), as well as in witnesses' support of perpetrators (prior $M = 13.55$ and post $M = 10.72$).

Furthermore, Bandura et al. (2017) investigated the association between participation in leisure activities and risk behaviours, including bullying involvement in a study with 10,279 students who were 11, 13, and 15 years old, from schools in the Czech Republic. Results showed that students who practiced some kind of artistic activity had less probability of being bullying perpetrators (OR = 0.62, 95% CI = 0.38–0.99, $p < 0.05$), and victim-perpetrators of bullying (OR = 0.22, 95%

CI = 0.09–0.59, $p < 0.01$), when compared to those who did not practice any kind of leisure activity. Nevertheless, no significant results to other kinds of leisure activities were found.

Bullying Prevention Through Arts and Sports

The practice of sports may also contribute to bullying prevention. Based on analysis of interview answers of 62,215 American parents of students from 6 to 17 years, Riese et al. (2015) identified the existence of a negative relation between taking part in extracurricular activities and bullying perpetration. Children who did not participate in extracurricular activities presented higher frequency in bullying perpetration (22%) when compared to students who participated in extracurricular activities. Those who engaged in a combination of sports and non-sportive extracurricular activities presented minor frequencies (11%) of bullying perpetration, compared to 17% for those who participated only in sportive activities and 16% to those who participated only in non-sportive extracurricular activities. Therefore, the combination of different modes of extracurricular activities predicted less bullying behaviours. The authors remark that engagement in extracurricular activities is associated with positive development due to the acquisition of important skills and increase of self-esteem, resulting from the exposure to several people and activities.

In a similar way, Curelaru et al. (2011) performed a study with 1,100 Romanian students who answered a questionnaire about whether they practiced sports, how much they enjoyed such practice, and their concepts on violence. The researchers noticed significant negative correlations, albeit weak, between the practice of sports and bullying ($r = -0.10$). In addition, those who affirmed enjoying and/or practicing sports in their free time were less favourable to bullying perpetration than those who did not enjoy nor practiced sports in their free time. According to the authors, sports are opportunities to release negative feelings, learning about fairness and respect for others, particularly when the goal of the activity is not only physical fitness, but also learning about principles associated with overcoming obstacles, cooperation, and fair play.

Merlim and Pereira (2013) investigated whether the practice of sports would prevent the occurrence of bullying, in a study with 1,818 students from three public schools in Portugal, from Grades 5–9, with average age of 12.8 years, ranging from 10 to 18 years. Results showed that the percentage of bullying victimization was smaller among students who practiced some kind of sport outside of school (24.2%), particularly group sports (22.7%), when compared to those who did not practice any sports (32.7%). These data suggest that taking part in extracurricular sports activities might buffer bullying because children who practice sports may feel more confident, in addition to presenting higher social skills, and thus are able to interact better with peers, handling victimization better.

Twemlow et al. (2008) highlighted the importance of sports for bullying prevention by defending that martial arts training could be a strategy to change aggressive behaviours and attitudes, since traditional martial arts focus on the psychological, spiritual, and non-aggressive aspects of the sport and is associated with a decrease in aggressiveness. With this goal, Twemlow et al. (2008) evaluated the Gentle Warrior Programme, an intervention based on traditional martial arts especially directed to decreasing aggressiveness in schools as part of creating a Peaceful School Learning Environment (CAPSLE), aimed at reducing school violence. To alter the attitudes towards violence, the Gentle Warrior Programme offers instructions to students, guided by a philosophy of peace and non-aggression, teaching self-control, respect, empathy, self-protection techniques, and problem solving.

Twemlow et al. (2008) recruited 254 students from Grades 3–5 of American public schools to participate in the Gentle Warrior Programme. The Programme was applied in three sessions of 45 minutes each, focusing on non-aggressive techniques, respect, self-control, relaxation, and also in self-protection techniques, such as blocking, escaping, defensive positioning, and balancing. Results showed that participation in the programme was significantly associated with changes towards aggression. This effect was moderated by the gender of participants, with a decrease in aggression in post-programme measures for boys only ($\beta = -0.31$, $t = -5.34$, $p < 0.001$). In addition, programme participation was also significantly associated with changes towards witnesses, which were also moderated by gender. Thus, there was an increase in the attitude of helping victims after the programme, but only for the boys ($\beta = 0.15$, $t = 2.28$, $p < 0.05$). Finally, results indicated the mediating effect of empathy in reducing aggressiveness ($t = -1.75$, $p = 0.08$), and in attitudes towards victims ($t = 2.06$, $p < 0.05$). Thus, changes towards aggression and attitudes of helping victims occurred due to a change in empathy.

Other activities associated with bullying prevention refer to the inclusion of music components in the school context. Ziv and Dolev (2013) conducted a pilot study, in Israel, to assess whether calming music background, through its effect on arousal and mood, could create a pleasant atmosphere and reduce bullying occurrence. In the first week prior to the intervention, 56 students, from two different Grade 6 classes, answered a questionnaire on bullying and a questionnaire on arousal, after recess for three consecutive days. In the second week, calming background music was played during recess for three consecutive days and children answered the same questionnaires again. In the third and last week, the calming background music was removed and participants answered the questionnaires. The results showed a significant decrease in bullying occurrence during the phase in which the calming background music was played. These preliminary data suggest that the soothing components of music may be combined with other intervention strategies to create a positive school climate and reduce bullying occurrence.

Del Arroyo et al. (2014) were also interested in the importance of musical resources to bullying prevention. The authors conducted a qualitative study in which the lyrics of 10 Spanish hip-hop songs addressing the theme were analyzed. The songs evaluated bullying involvement negatively, pointing the perpetrator as someone less satisfied with life, and the victim with feelings of inadequacy, depressive symptoms, and even suicidal ideation. The authors suggest that the hip-hop songs should be listened to, and dramatized at schools, along with graffiti drawing and break-dancing as bullying prevention strategies.

Haner et al. (2009) defend that an arts-based curriculum is particularly important in bullying prevention for its capacity in altering students' thoughts and feelings. The authors claim that arts are especially important because they inspire socially responsible behaviours, providing the needed model to help students face adversity. Haner et al. (2009) examined how a curriculum based on art activities would serve as a resource in bullying prevention analyzing the effects of an opera performance to 104 students, from five Grade 4–5 classes of three Canadian schools. The opera *Elijah's Kite* was chosen as it may provide socioemotional learning to students, by eliciting emotions that stem from music, the performing arts, and dance. *Elijah's Kite* also includes a choir of local students, maximizing the connection with the audience. Moreover, five students from each school were invited to participate in the opera, which had elements such as power differences, changes in social status, empathy, and tolerance. Post-intervention results showed a significant statistical difference in knowledge towards bullying by participants with an increase in the average from $M = 4.47$ to $M = 5.10$. In addition, a significant statistical difference in bullying victimization was observed (a decrease from $M = 0.84$ to $M = 0.67$). These data suggest that opera, although it does not comprise an autonomous programme, may be a promising resource in multidimensional programmes in bullying prevention.

Joronen et al. (2011), in turn, propose that dramatic theatre and role-playing are important resources to prevent bullying by giving non-violent models, in addition to the promotion of social skills, empathy, expression of feelings, self-knowledge, and empowerment. These authors evaluated the effects of a drama programme on victimization and perpetration of bullying. 134 students from eight classes from Grades 4–5 in two schools with similar demographics, in Finland, took part in the programme by answering self-report questionnaires on the bullying experience. One school served as a comparison group and the other received the intervention, which consisted of classroom dramatizations guided by the teachers, involving topics on friendship, bullying, and tolerance. In addition, homework to be performed with parents was assigned, in which students, for instance, had to interview the parents about bullying occurrences. In addition, parenting meetings were held in the school, so that parents could learn to use drama to enhance parent–children relations. Results from Jorenen et al.'s (2011) study indicated a statistically significant decrease in bullying victimization, with a decline of 20.7% (prior 58.8% and post intervention 38.1%). The authors remarked that using applied drama and theatre methods in the classroom may improve children's relationships at school.

Bullying Prevention Through Information and Communication Technology (ICT)

Not only artistic and sports activities, but recreational resources of Information and Communication Technology (ICT) may also be helpful in bullying prevention. The researchers from Portugal, Raminhos et al. (2016), highlighted that the use of interactive technologies, such as videogames, may result in productive bullying prevention, if made to teach and alter behaviours. Raminhos et al. (2016) developed the game called *Stop Bully* for computers and tablets, aiming to promote empathy, resulting from attitude changes when learning about bullying. The target audience involved 10–12 year olds, identified as victims and bystanders of bullying. In the beginning of the game, the player chose between the role of victim or bystander, among different available characters for each profile. The player, then, had to choose which level he/she wanted to play, and according to the levels recreate a situation or a narrative involving the school. The player is confronted with challenges and bullying situations, where he/she has to make decisions in which the consequences are reflected in the scores obtained. The player only moves forward in the game when he/she reaches the minimum score. The game was assessed by volunteer players and valid evidence was obtained concerning the characters, different levels, and impact of the game, indicating that this tool has potential to intervene in schools in bullying prevention.

Along the same line, Sapouna et al. (2010) assessed the effectiveness of a game called *Fear Not!* (Fun with Empathic Agents, to achieve Novel Outcomes in Teaching) in reducing bullying victimization by teaching problem-solving skills, and encouraging students to think and evaluate a range of answers in dealing with victimization. 1,129 students from 7 to 11 years of 27 schools, from England and Germany, participated in the study. The game was composed of 3D animations, containing a school and students. The game's episodes presented bullying situations, where the player observed, and then interacted, with the virtual victim suggesting a way of dealing with the occurrence and preventing future ones; the consequences of this suggestion were subsequently presented to the player. The game was played by students for 30 minutes, on three consecutive weeks in a non-randomized control trial design.

Sub-sample analysis from Sapouna et al.'s study (2010) found a significant effect on escaping victimization only for UK children (adjusted RR, 1.90; CI, 1.23–2.57). UK children in the intervention group experienced decreased victimization rates at the first follow-up compared with controls, even after adjusting for baseline victimization, gender, and age (adjusted RR 0.60; 95% CI, 0.36–0.93). The authors concluded that the virtual learning intervention designed to help children experience effective strategies for dealing with bullying had a short-term effect on escaping victimization for prior identified victims, and a short-term overall prevention effect for UK children, which are encouraging results for this new technology, although further investigation is recommended.

Olenik-Shemesh et al. (2014) also evaluated a game involving a virtual reality in three dimensions to promote knowledge and alter behaviours related to bullying and cyberbullying, called Anti Bullying Village for Kids and Teens (ABV4KIDS), where each player has a character who moves around several environments of the village (such as a Parliament, movie theatre, and so on). The village was built throughout the period of two years with the participation of adolescents from several countries, guided by experts. To assess the impact of the ABV4KIDS intervention, 60 Israeli students answered five questionnaires in two moments, 34 were from the Control Group (who did not play the game) and 26 from the Experimental Group (who played the game). Prior to the intervention, the groups were similar in knowledge on bullying and cyber bullying, and face-to-face victimization. The results of intervention were somewhat inconclusive, perhaps due to the small sample (although, this is not indicated by the authors). Olenik-Shemesh et al. (2014) did mention that the participants enjoyed the game.

Another bullying preventive programme that also uses virtual strategies is KiVa (Salmivalli et al. 2010), elaborated in Finland. This programme consists of 10 face-to-face school activities of 90 minutes each, through virtual (videogame), and printable educational worksheets to parents, based on the importance of the bystanders' role in decreasing bullying. There is also a differentiated approach to the teacher to handle bullying disclosures, which consists of talking to the victim separately, then to the perpetrator, and in another moment to the students who may support the victim. The activities occur in a virtual school, and the game has three levels: (1) The first level is called "I know", in which bullying is presented, the face-to-face taught concepts are revised, and questions are made in order to verify learning; (2) The second level, called "I can", includes conflict situations where the player should indicate how he/she would respond and there is the option of accessing other characters' thoughts, as well as verifying the consequences of the elected actions; (3) The third level, called "I do", involves the player describing how he/she had been using the virtual and face-to-face learnt strategies in daily situations.

The KiVa programme was assessed in a large sample of 8,237 children from grades 4–6 (10–12 years) involving 78 schools, 39 as controls (Kärnä et al. 2011) with many positive results, including decreases in self-reported bullying and self-reported victimization. The programme was also tested in in Italy with 2,042 students in a RTC study with positive results, particularly to Grade 4 students (Nocentini and Menesini 2016), and is presently been tested in Chile also in a RTC study (Gaete et al. 2017).

In general, there are not many bullying prevention programmes using recreational activities with ICT with solid methodology. Nocentini et al. (2015) conducted a systematic review of studies assessing bullying ICT-mediated interventions using PsychInfo, Scopus, and Pubmed's database. The authors concluded that ICT tools are under-used in bullying prevention, a somewhat surprising fact as most children enjoy them, and there is an urgent need to test them with rigorous methodology. Coincidentally, the same authors were responsible for testing the KiVa programme with large enough samples and RCTs in several countries, which is desirable.

Our Experience with Recreational Anti-bullying Tools

In addition to virtual games, more traditional games such as card games, board games, and flyers with word-search activities, among others, may be employed with less cost than virtual games, a needed alternative in developing countries. Such games may maximize learnt information and skills as they allow for face-to-face interaction. In our country, Brazil, development, and use of recreational activities to prevent bullying are still scarce. Thus, as members of the Brazilian *Laboratory for Violence Analysis & Prevention* (LAPREV—www.ufscar.br/laprev), the authors made efforts to develop and assess recreational materials for bullying intervention.

For instance, Stelko-Pereira and Williams (2013) elaborated an anti-bullying folder to be printed on a dual sided paper sheet, containing four games. (The Portuguese folder is available on LAPREV's website). The games tell the story of six bullies (three boys and three girls), with different ethnic features: (1) The first game consists of a maze where the player should relate the name of the character to his/her verbalizations through the correct pathway; (2) The second game is a crossword puzzle, in which the student fills out the blank spaces with the name of the characters; (3) The third refers to a word-search, and the player searches and identifies bullying consequences; (4) The last activity involves drawings and a story with the character's verbalizations that students may colour.

Stelko-Pereira and Williams (2013) assessed the social acceptance of the folder with 70 students, from Grades 6–9 in a mid-size city of São Paulo State, Brazil. The folder activity and correction of the material lasted about 40 minutes, and the results indicated that the majority of participants (85%) reported having enjoyed the material, which was considered attractive, easy to understand, and that it promoted the intended discussions. However, the effectiveness in reducing bullying still remains to be assessed. We conducted an assessment of a school violence prevention programme in Brazil (Stelko-Pereira and Williams 2016), but the programme targeted independent variables mainly teacher behaviours, well-being, and their assessment of how much bullying occurred and, thus, the folder was not analyzed as a component.

Stelko-Pereira et al. (submitted) assessed the attractiveness of three additional games: (1) *Say No to Bullying* presents questions related to social skills and bullying through a recreational card game; (2) *Super Student: An anti-bullying Activist,* a children's board game with dice and themes related to school bullying, including its consequences and the expression of feelings; and (3) *The Conciliators,* a board game that simulates a Courthouse where players have the opportunity to analyze bullying episodes and propose solutions through social problem solving. Consumer satisfaction was assessed in a Grade 5 class of 30 students aged 10–12 in a public school of Fortaleza, in Northeast Brazil. Each game was used by students on a different day and was evaluated as attractive and relevant by the majority of the class. More than 80% of the students affirmed that they had learnt new information with the games, more than 70% indicated that they would know what to suggest to a peer who suffers bullying, and more than 70% indicated that the games were easy to comprehend, and that they felt motivated to play. As in the folder previously described, these last games remain to be assessed in terms of their anti-bullying efficiency.

Issues and Concerns, Recommendations and Conclusion

One may argue that serious subjects, such as bullying, must be only approached by formal methods, such as reading materials and lectures. We tried to show in this chapter that recreation might be used as a strategy to learn about this detrimental and common problem.

Dr. Stuart Brown is a psychiatrist who founded the National Institute for Play, in California, who does pioneering work showing the importance of playfulness to human development. Dr. Brown first became interested in the topic of play by analyzing the life of murderers and noticing one commonality: the lack of play in childhood. He cites data showing that children who play more become more intelligent and clever adults and he affirms that playing (in which he includes humour, games, roughhousing, and fantasy) should also be present in adult routines (Brown 2008). The same author also describes a concern that is shared by the authors of this chapter, referring to the fact that society increasingly values intellectuality and formal scholarly content, disregarding the importance of play, which according to several studies presented here, is fundamental to the promotion of healthy interpersonal relations and, consequently, to the prevention, identification, and confrontation of a relevant social problem, like bullying.

Similarly, Keil (2011), an entrepreneur based in Bulgaria, reinforces that the opposite of play is not work, but depression, and that when the human potential of play is devaluated, the future of a nation is at risk, as playing enables us to learn how to soften thoughts, evaluate strategies, solve problems, and feel motivated. Indeed, learning to interact with other human beings should not be done through aversive strategies, violence, or punishment, but through positive strategies, such as play or recreation, for example.

Thus, there are several creative possibilities of recreational strategies from different parts of the world, which were presented in this chapter, aimed at preventing bullying, from traditional board and card games to virtual games, from listening to music, to singing, acting, and engaging in different types of dramatization, among others. These strategies have been well accepted by the target audience and present promising effects. Nevertheless, we need, in general, more research about their effects in terms of anti-bullying efficacy and impact.

We do not want to give the impression, in this chapter, that recreational activities per se are sufficient to curb and prevent bullying. The literature shows that what works in bullying prevention is a combination of many variables: programmes that are long-term, systemic and that intervene in all school components, including students, parents, and educators. In addition, one should not forget the importance of mental health professionals in helping children who are victimized by bullying, children who are bullying perpetrators, and a combination of the two, in addition to helping their parents. But we strongly believe that recreational activities are beneficial and, thus, should be part of the bullying intervention package.

References

Albuquerque, P. P., Williams, L. C. A., & D'Affonseca, S. M. (2013). Efeitos tardios do bullying e Transtorno de Estresse Pós-Traumático: Uma revisão crítica [Long term effects of bullying and post traumatic stress disorder: A literature review]. *Psicologia: Teoria e Pesquisa, 29*(1), 91–98. https://doi.org/10.1590/s0102-37722013000100011.

Baliulevicius, N. L. P., & Macário, N. M. (2006). Jogos cooperativos e valores humanos: Perspectiva de transformação pelo lúdico [Cooperative games and human values: Transformation perspectives through playing]. *Revista Fitness & Performance Journal, 5*(1), 48–54.

Bandura, P., Sigmundova, D., Sigmund, E., Geckova, A. M., van Dijk, J. P., & Reijneveld, S. A. (2017). Participation in organized leisure-time activities and risk behavior in Czech adolescents. *International Journal of Public Health, 62,* 387–396. https://doi.org/10.1007/s00038-016-0930-9.

Barros, P. C. (2012). *Jogos e brincadeiras na escola: Prevenção do bullying entre crianças no recreio. [Playing at school: Bullying prevention in children during recess.]* Doctoral Dissertation. Universidade do Minho, Portugal.

Bertoldo, J. V., & Reschell, M. A. (2000). Jogar e brincar: Representando papéis, a criança constrói seu próprio conhecimento [Children construct their own knowledge through role-playing]. *Revista do Professor, 16*(61).

Brown, S. (2008). *Play is more than fun: Its vital.* Retrieved from https://www.ted.com/talks/stuart_brown_says_play_is_more_than_fun_it_s_vital?language=pt-br.

Bustamante, G. O. (2004). Por uma vivência escolar lúdica [For a playful school experience]. In G. M. Schwartz (Ed.). *Dinâmica lúdica: Novos olhares [Playful dynamics: New perspectives]* (pp. 55–68). Barueri, SP: Ed. Manole.

Caballo, V. E., Calderero, M., Carrillo, G. B., Salazar, I. C., & Irurtia, M. J. (2011). Acoso escolar y ansiedad social en niños (II): Una propuesta de intervención en formato lúdico [Bullying and social anxiety in children (II): Proposal of a new recreational intervention programme]. *Behavioral Psychology, 19*(3), 611–626.

Carmona, J. A., Espínola, M., Cangas, A. J., & Iribarne, L. (2010). Mii-School: New 3D technologies applied in education to detect drug abuses and bullying in adolescents. *Tech-Education, 73,* 65–72. https://doi.org/10.1007/978-3-642-13166-0_10.

Carvalho, J. E. (2012). *Os benefícios das atividades lúdicas para a prevenção do bullying no contexto escolar [The benefits of recreational activities for bullying prevention in the school context]*. Doctoral Dissertation. Universidade do Minho, Portugal.

Cornell, D., Gregory, A., Huang, F., & Fan, X. (2013). Perceived prevalence of teasing and bullying predicts High School dropout rates. *Journal of Educational Psychology, 105*(1), 138–149. https://doi.org/10.1037/a0030416.

Craig, J. T., Samantha J., Gregus, S. J., Elledge, L. C., Pastrana, F. A., & Cavell, T. A. (2016). Preliminary investigation of the relation between lunchroom peer acceptance and peer victimization. *Journal of Applied Developmental Psychology, 43,* 101–111. https://doi.org/10.1016/j.appdev.2016.01.005.

Craig, W., Harel-Fisch, Y., Fogel-Grinvald, H., Dostaler, S., Hetland, J., Simons-Morton, B., et al. (2009). A cross-national profile of bullying and victimization among adolescents in 40 countries. *International Journal of Public Health, 54,* 216–224. https://doi.org/10.1007/s00038-009-5413-9.

Curelaru, M., Abalasei, B., & Cristea, M. (2011). Psychosocial correlates of the need for physical education and sports in high school. *Journal of Social Sciences, 7*(4), 521–528.
Del Arroyo, G. M., Relinque, C. S., Ruiz, D. M., & Ochoa, G. M. (2014). La música hip-hop como recurso preventivo del acoso escolar: Análisis de 10 canciones de hip-hop en español sobre bullying [Hip-hop as a preventive resource for bullying: Analysis of 10 Spanish hip-hop songs about bullying]. *Qualitative Research in Education, 3*(1), 1–30. https://doi.org/10.4471/qre2014.34.
Due, P., Holstein, B. E., Lynch, J., Diderichsen, F., Gabhain, S. N., Scheidt, P., et al. (2005). Bullying and symptoms among school-aged children: International comparative cross sectional study in 28 countries. *European Journal of Public Health, 15*(2), 128–132. https://doi.org/10.1093/eurpub/cki105.
Farb, A. F., & Matjasko, J. L. (2012). Recent advances in research on school-based extracurricular activities and adolescent development. *Development Review, 32,* 1–48. https://doi.org/10.1016/j.dr.2011.10.001.
Farrington, D. P., Loeber, R., Stallings, R., & Ttofi, M. M. (2011). Bullying perpetration and victimization as predictors of delinquency and depression in the Pittsburgh Youth Study. *Journal of Aggression, Conflict and Peace Research, 3,* 74–81. https://doi.org/10.1108/17596591111132882.
Fleming, L. C., & Jacobsen, K. H. (2009). Bullying among middle-school students in low and middle income countries. *Health Promotion International, 25*(1), 73–84. https://doi.org/10.1093/heapro/dap046.
Gaete, J., Valenzuela, D., Rojas-Barahona, C., Valenzuela, E., Araya, R., & Salmivalli, C. (2017). The KiVa antibullying programme in primary schools in Chile, with and without the digital game component: Study protocol for a randomized controlled trial. *Trials, 18*(75), 1–9. https://doi.org/10.1186/s13063-017-1810-1.
Guerin, S., & Hennessy, E. (2002). Pupils' definitions of bullying. *European Journal of Psychology of Education, 17,* 249–262. https://doi.org/10.1007/BF03173535.
Hamburger, M. E., Basile, K. C., & Vivolo, A. M. (2011). *Measuring bullying victimization, perpetration and bystander experiences: A compendium of assessment tolls.* Atlanta, G.A.: Centers for Disease Control and Prevention, National Center for Injury Prevention and Control.
Haner, D., Pepler, D., Cummings, J., & Rubin-Vaughan, A. (2009). The roles of arts-based curricula in bullying prevention: Elijah's Kite—A children's opera. *Canadian Journal of School Psychology, 25*(1), 55–69. https://doi.org/10.1177/0829573509349031.
Holt, M. K., Vivolo-Kantor, A. M., Polanin, J. R., Holland, K. M., DeGue, S., Matjasko, J. L., et al. (2015). Bullying and suicidal ideation and behaviors: A meta-analysis. *Pediatrics, 135*(2), 496–509. https://doi.org/10.1542/peds.2014-1864.
Joronen, K., Konu, A., Rankin, H. S., & Astedt-Kurki, P. (2011). An evaluation of a drama programme to enhance social relationships and anti-bullying at elementary school: A controlled study. *Health Promotion International, 27*(1), 5–14. https://doi.org/10.1093/heapro/dar012.
Kärnä, A., Voeten, M., Little, T., Poskiparta, E., Kaljonen, A., & Salmivalli, C. (2011). A large-scale evaluation of the KiVa anti-bullying programme: Grades 4–6. *Child Development, 82,* 311–330. https://doi.org/10.1111/j.1467-8624.2010.01557.x.
Keil, S. (2011). *A manifesto for play, for Bulgaria and Beyond.* Retrieved from www.ted.com/talks/steve_keil_a_manifesto_for_play_for_bulgaria_and_beyond.
Kishimoto, M. T. (1996). *Jogo, brinquedo, brincadeira e a educação [Games, toys and play in education].* São Paulo: Cortez.
Lamb, J., Pepler, D. J., & Craig, W. (2009). Approach to bullying and victimization. *Canadian Family Physician, 55*(4), 356–360.
Marcellino, N. C. (2011). *Pedagogia da Animação [Animation Pedagogy].* Campinas, SP: Papiros.
Mauricio, J. T. (2007). *Aprender brincando: O lúdico na aprendizagem* [*Learning by playing: The playful in learning*]. Retrieved from http://www.profala.com/arteducesp140.htm.
Melim, F. M. O., & Pereira, B. O. (2013). Prática desportiva, um meio de prevenção do bullying n aescola? [Sports as means of bullying preventing at school?]. *Movimento, 19*(2), 55–77.

Moreira, S., & Pereira, B. (2008). *As atividades lúdico-desportivas nas práticas de lazer em crianças do 1º ciclo* [*Recreational and sports activities in children's leisure at the Primary School*]. Master's thesis. Portugal: Universidade do Minho.

National Academies of Sciences, Engineering, and Medicine. (2016). *Preventing bullying through science, policy, and practice*. The Washington, D.C.: National Academies Press.

Nocentini, A., & Menesini, E. (2016). KiVa anti-bullying programme in Italy: Evidence of effectiveness in a randomized control trial. *Prevention Science, 17,* 1012–1023. https://doi.org/10.1007/s11121-016-0690-z.

Nocentini, A., Zambuto, V., & Menesini, E. (2015). Anti-bullying programmes and information and communication technologies (ICTs): A systematic review. *Aggression and Violent Behavior, 23,* 52–60. https://doi.org/org/10.1016/j.avb.2015.05.012.

Olenik Shemesh, D., Heiman, T., & Rabin, E. (2014). Virtual anti-bullying village project for coping with bullying and cyberbullying within virtual learning environment: Evaluation research. *International Journal of cyber Society and Education, 7*(2), 97–124. https://doi.org/10.7903/ijcse.1147.

Olweus, D. (1993). *Bullying at school: What we know and what we can do*. Oxford, U.K.: Blackwell.

Olweus, D. (2013). School bullying: Development and some important challenges. *Annual Review of Clinical Psychology, 9,* 751–780. https://doi.org/10.1146/annurev-clinpsy-050212-185516.

Orpinas, P., & Horne, A. M. (2006). Bullies and victims: A challenge for schools. In J. R. Lutzker (Ed.), *Preventing violence: Research and evidence-based intervention strategies* (pp. 147–165). Washington: American Psychological Association.

Pellegrini, A. (2009). *The role of play in human development*. New York: Oxford University Press.

Raminhos, C., Cláudio, A. P., Carmo, M. B., Gaspar, A., Carvalhosa, S., & Candeias, M. J. (2016). A serious game-based solution to prevent bullying. *International Journal of Pervasive Computing and Communications, 12*(2), 194–215. https://doi.org/10.1108/IJPCC-04-2016-0022.

Riem, M. M. E., Bakermans-Kranenburg, M. J., Huffmeijer, R., & Ijzendoorn, M. H. (2013). Does intranasal oxytocin promote prosocial behavior to an excluded fellow player? A randomized controlled trial with Cyberball. *Psychoneuroendocrinology, 38,* 1418–1425. https://doi.org/10.1016/j.psyneuen.2012.12.023.

Riese, A., Gjelsvik, A., & Ranney, M. L. (2015). Extracurricular activities and bullying perpetration: Results from a nationally representative sample. *Journal of School Health, 85*(8), 544–552. https://doi.org/10.1111/josh.12282.

Rigby, K. (2003). Consequences of bullying in schools. *The Canadian Journal of Psychiatry, 48*(9), 583–590.

Roloff, E. M. (2010). *A importância do lúdico em sala de aula* [*The importance of recreation in the classroom*]. Paper presented at the X Anais da Semana de Letras, Porto Alegre, Brasil. Retrieved from http://ebooks.pucrs.br/edipucrs/anais/Xsemanadeletras/comunicacoes/Eleana-Margarete-Roloff.pdf .

Salmivalli, C., Kärnä, A., & Poskiparta, E. (2010). Development, evaluation, and diffusion of a national anti-bullying programme, KiVa. In B. Doll, W. Pfohl, & J. Yoon (Eds.), *Handbook of youth prevention science*. New York, N.Y.: Routledge.

Sapouna, M., Wolke, D., Vannini, N., Watson, S., Woods, S., Scheinder, W., et al. (2010). Virtual learning intervention to reduce bullying victimization in primary school: A controlled trial. *Journal of Child Psychology and Psychiatry, 51*(1), 104–112. https://doi.org/10.1111/j.1469-7610.2009.02137.x.

Schwarz, L., Erbs, C., Weber, F., & Silva, M. R. (2006). *Princípios de uma reflexão do lúdico e a infância [The beginings of a reflection on playing and childhood]*. Paper presented at the Anais da XVIII Encontro Nacional de Recreação e Lazer, Curitiba, Brasil.

Seixas, S. R. (2005). Violência escolar: Metodologias de identificação dos alunos agressores e/ou vítimas [School Violence: Methodologies to identify student bullies and/or victims.]. *Análise Psicológica, 23*(2), 97–110.

Smith, P. K. (2006). O brincar e os usos do brincar [Playing and its uses]. In J. R. Moyles (Ed.), *A excelência do brincar [The excellence of playing]* (pp. 25–38). Porto Alegre: Artmed.

Stelko-Pereira A. C., Martins Júnior, A. T., Moraes, B. C., Alves, D. L. G., de Bezerra, L. L. A. L., & da Silva, S. R. (submitted). *Avaliação de jogos de prevenção ao bullying por estudantes do ensino fundamental* [*Evaluation of bullying prevention games by primary students*]. Manuscript submitted for publication.

Stelko-Pereira, A. C., & Williams, L. C. A. (2013). "Psiu, repara aí!": Avaliação de fôlder para prevenção de violência escolar ["Hey there, look at this!": Folder assessment to prevent school violence]. *Psico-USF, 18*(2), 329–332.

Stelko-Pereira, A. C., & Williams, L. C. A. (2016). Evaluation of a Brazilian school violence prevention project (Violência Nota Zero). *Pensamiento Psicólogico, 14*(1), 63–76. https://doi.org/10.11144/javerianacali.ppsi14-1.ebsv.

Tewmlow, S. W., Biggs, B. K., Nelson, T. D., Venberg, E. M., Fonagy, P., & Twemlow, S. T. (2008). Effects of participation in a martial arts-based antibullying programme in elementary schools. *Psychology in the Schools, 45*(10), 947–959. https://doi.org/10.1002/pits.20344.

Torres, J. A. C., Cangas, A. J., García, G. R., Langer, A. I., & Zárate, R. (2012). Early detection of drug use and bullying in secondary school children by using a three-dimensional simulation programme. *Cyberpsychology, Behavior and Social Networking, 15*(1), 43–49. https://doi.org/10.1089/cyber.2010.0589.

Vaillancourt, T., Hymel, S., & McDougall, P. (2003). Bullying is power: Implications for school-based intervention strategies. *Journal of Applied School Psychology, 19,* 157–176. https://doi.org/10.1300/J008v19n02_10.

Valdebenito, S., Ttofi, M., & Eisner, M. (2015). Prevalence rates of drug use among school bullies and victims: A systematic review and meta-analysis of cross-sectional studies. *Aggression and Violent Behavior, 23*(1), 137–146. https://doi.org/10.1016/j.avb.2015.05.004.

Vrijhof, C. I., Bulk, B. G., Overgaauw, S., Lelieveld, G., Engels, R. C. M. E., & IJzendoorn, M. (2016). The prosocial cyberball game: Compensating for social exclusion and its associations with empathic concern and bullying in adolescents. *Journal of Adolescence, 52,* 27–36. https://doi.org/10.1016/j.adolescence.2016.07.005.

Wolke, D., & Lereya, S. T. (2015). Long-term effects of bullying. *Archives of Disease in Childhood, 100*(9), 879–885. https://doi.org/10.1136/archdischild-2014-306667.

Ziv, N., & Dolev, N. (2013). The effect of background music on bullying: A pilot study. *Children & Schools, 35*(2), 83–90. https://doi.org/10.1093/cs/cdt006.

Chapter 15
All Work and No Play: The Importance of Extracurricular Activities in the Development of Children

Bangalore N. Roopesh

Abstract Academics play a significant role in shaping one's life. It has a direct influence on one's future career, health, and standard of living. Recognizing this, a majority of the parents send their children to school. Considering the importance of academics, they lay enormous emphasis on marks and grades, ignoring extracurricular activities. Extracurricular activities being non-academic, the widespread tendency is to regard them as not important. Therefore, until recently, encouragement and participation in organized or structured extracurricular activity has largely been voluntary and restricted to a few schools and/or children belonging to upper social strata. Though almost all schools have at least one period in a week devoted to physical education/training, on many occasions, due to the lack of resources, children are left on their own to play or do whatever they want. Sometimes, if the syllabus is not completed, even this one period is taken up for academics. Not knowing the value of extracurricular activities, several schools use extracurricular activities period as a privilege, which is taken away every time a child shows undesirable behaviour. Though extracurricular activities have several indirect and direct benefits in academics as well as in non-academics, not many are aware of it. Research over several decades has shown that participating in one or more structured extracurricular activities has physical, emotional, psychological, academic, and social benefits. These benefits range from improvement in general health, emotional regulation, study skills, subject grade points, and aptitude test scores to increase in self-esteem. In addition, it also teaches respect for social values, customs, rules, and individual differences. On the other hand, participation in structured extracurricular activities has been shown to reduce negative and delinquent behaviours. Given the extent of benefits, it becomes imperative to advocate incorporating extracurricular activities into the regular schedule of all schools throughout the country.

Keywords School · Students · Extracurricular activities · India Development

B. N. Roopesh (✉)
Department of Clinical Psychology, NIMHANS, Bengaluru, India
e-mail: bn.roopesh@gmail.com

S. Deb (ed.), *Positive Schooling and Child Development*,
https://doi.org/10.1007/978-981-13-0077-6_15

Introduction

Several centuries ago, humans used to spend much of their time in the wild by walking, running, or climbing in search of food or working in the fields growing food. Until a few decades ago, almost all people were involved in some form of physical work as part of their livelihood, such as agriculture, carpentry, weaving, and grinding. Further, the daily work required them to travel significant distances on foot. The leisure hours were usually spent in interacting with neighbours in the community, either chatting, sharing information, participating in local governance, or watching stage shows. Children usually learned the family occupation and household work during some part of the day and, at other times, they were left free to play and interact among peers. These activities usually took care of the physical, psychological, emotional, and social needs of the children.

With the industrial and technological advancement, there was more reliance on equipment, machines, and automobiles. This automatically reduced the emphasis on physical and prolonged labour, and increased the focus on intellectual work. This greatly reduced the barriers of learning one particular skill or choosing a particular profession due to physical or social restrictions.

Earlier, people had to significantly spend several years to learn and master a particular skill as a vocation. However, industrial and technological progress has created different jobs that require different skill sets. This has led to a situation where all children can learn basic education up to a level and then decide which specialization to take up, depending upon the prospects of being gainfully employed. Given the near-certainty of procuring employment with appropriate education, the stress on academics has increased manifold. People have realized the importance of academics, as, in many instances, it has a direct influence on a person's standard of living and their future. In the majority of countries, academic education has been considered as the only way to change the socio-economic status of the family. This can be understood in terms of Maslow's hierarchy of motivation, where, when the food and safety needs aren't met the focus is more on obtaining these goals rather than other higher order needs. Only when the basic needs, such as hunger and safety, are taken care of, do person think about other activities. In an economy where academics are given utmost priority, and where it is difficult to make a career out of extracurricular activities, there is little encouragement to take up or pursue such activities.

Nowadays there is a race to score maximum marks or GPA in the exams. Aiming for the maximum marks or GPA in itself not problematic, but the stress or the pressure that is imposed on the child or adolescent is enormous. The race to get into a few premier institutions or universities is such that some schools train or coach children towards this goal from Grade 1 onwards. Given this environment, everything from intelligence, to the worth of the child, is judged by what marks or grade the child obtains in the exams.

It is a known fact that children vary in their capabilities with respect to intelligence, temperament, academics, and the ability to handle stress. Not all children will be able to score high marks. If the focus is mainly on grades, then those children who are not able to get higher grades might start perceiving themselves as failures or might develop low self-esteem or self-worth. This, in turn, might lead some children to end up having anxiety and depression (Kumaraswamy 2013; Jayanti et al. 2015; Martinez and Fabiano 1992). On the other hand, for a child to have good health and a holistic development, focus should not merely be on academics.

Development of a person requires both nature and nurture. It is aptly said that nature is expressed through nurture. This emphasizes the importance of nurture in the development of the person. Development is more than mere growth and involves different domains, such as physical, language, cognitive, emotional, and social. For each of these domains to develop age-appropriately and in coherence with other domains, adequate 'nurture' is required. Development, both physical and mental, usually follows a pattern, and some domains, such as language, have critical periods which are sensitive to the extent of stimulation received for adequate development (Berk 2008; Hurford 1991). Along the same lines, the period from birth to late adolescence can be considered an important period, where a child will go through tremendous changes before becoming an adult (Berk 2008). The changes involve physical growth and pubertal changes, neuronal growth and brain maturation, temperament changes leading to personality pattern, from being dependent on care-takers to being independent, from being ego-centric to fighting for a societal cause (Santrock 2011). All these changes require adequate inputs and exposure, without which development might not be complete or it may not be coherent.

Academics alone do not provide necessary ingredients for a person to have a holistic development. On the other hand, not all children can do well in academics, due to various reasons, such as subnormal level of intellectual ability and specific learning disabilities (Rumberger 1987, 1995). In these situations, extracurricular activities provide additional support or they become the sole avenue for the growth and development of the child.

Extracurricular Activities

The term 'extracurricular activities' usually refers to activities that fall outside the scope of the regular academic institutional curriculum, or course. It ranges from completely or partially organized activities connected with school, to activities that are not connected with school. If performed on a regular basis, unstructured activities such as painting, playing a musical instrument, or other similar activities can also be considered extracurricular activities (Burr 2012). Extracurricular activities usually do not offer any direct academic credit; however, it can provide additional value to the person's academic achievement, especially when applying for higher education or employment.

Some of the following criteria are important to be considered as an extracurricular activity:

- The activity where a child or adolescent is required to spend sufficient amount of time to practice a skill set to develop a talent.
- An activity that is usually acknowledged and/or practiced by other people. Playing football is easily considered as an extracurricular activity, compared to, say, collecting different footballs.
- An activity that has some importance and/or contributes value to the common good. For example, moderating a blog on teenage problems would be such an activity, in contrast to just surfing the internet.

Types of Extracurricular Activities

The common perception of extracurricular activities is usually restricted to activities related to sports, music, and performing arts. There is no consensus on how to classify extracurricular activities. Feldman and Matjasko (2005) described extracurricular activities in terms of sports, clubs, organizations, and student-managed work programmes. Guest and Schneider (2003) classified them as sports versus non-sports. Eccles et al. (2003) and Fredricks and Eccles (2005) categorized them as team sports activities involving school, performing arts, and academic clubs. However, there are a wide variety of activities that can come under the umbrella term of extracurricular activities. Most extracurricular activities are usually carried out as part of a team or group or clubs. These activities can be grouped into activities related to

- Sports and athletics (such as, football, hockey, basketball, and cricket)
- Music (such as, singing, playing instruments, choir groups)
- Performing arts (such as, drama, puppetry, and dancing)
- Academics (such as, Maths club, Science club and Computer club)
- Art (such as, photography, painting and sculpting)
- Outdoor/adventure (such as, mountaineering, hiking and biking)
- Health and fitness (such as, Yoga, martial arts and Tai chi)
- Language (such as, English club, French club and Chinese club)
- Community/social (such as, Environmental, animal rights and gender equality clubs)
- Volunteering (such as, Red Cross and tutoring underprivileged children)
- Technology (such as, Blogging and movie making club)
- Media (such as, University radio station, college newspaper and creating videos for YouTube channel)
- Political (such as, Youth United Nations and Youth Parliament)
- Religious (such as, Church, *Madrasa*, and Temple)
- Other organized groups (Such as, Scouts, Guides and Chess)

Though extracurricular activities range from sports and performing arts to literary clubs, activities like popular sports and performing arts often endure for a long time in a person's life, even after the completion of school or college. Other activities, such as environmental club or English club, usually last for shorter duration, or only for as long as the person is associated with that particular school or college.

There are different theories (Astin 1999; Chickering 1969) about how extracurricular activities help in the overall development of a child or an adolescent. Chickering's psychosocial development theory (Chickering 1969) proposes seven vectors known as tasks, which students have to go through to develop identity. They are: developing intellectual, manual skills and interpersonal competence; ability to manage emotions; moving through autonomy towards independence; developing mature interpersonal relationships; establishing identity; developing purpose; and developing integrity. Astin's Involvement Theory (Astin 1999) describes the child's involvement in terms of the quality and quantity of the physical, as well as psychological, energy that s/he invests in school/college experience. The involvement usually consists of immersion in academics, involvement in extracurricular activities, and interaction with school staff. The greater the student's involvement in school, the greater will be the learning and personal development. His theory stresses the significance of holistic experience and believes that success is the sum total of experiences which can occur inside and outside of the school.

Adolescents generally spend about 80% of their waking hours outside the school (Zaff et al. 2003). Extracurricular activities facilitate students to excel in different aspects which the school environment does not provide. Due to the non-academic nature, there is a general tendency to regard extracurricular activities as unimportant, and until a few years back, participation in extracurricular activities has been more a matter of choice, and restricted mainly to a few elite schools. On the other hand, modern households generally do not provide much training in initiative and responsibility. Given this, the importance of participating in extracurricular activities becomes even more significant.

Though the most important functions of extracurricular activities appear to be physical and psychological, it is actually social in outlook. More than a century ago, John Dewey said that "education is a process of living and not a preparation for future living" (Dewey 1897), and that schools should facilitate this by providing activities and opportunities.

Benefits of Extracurricular Activities

On the whole, adolescents' involvement in extracurricular activities has been consistently and positively associated with better physical and mental health, higher academic grades, improved Information Communication Technology (ICT) skills, increased independent study skills, lower school dropout rates, lower academic burnout, higher academic aspirations and achievement, better peer relationships, increase in discipline, reducing delinquent behaviour, less alcohol and drug abuse, higher life satisfaction, improved self-image, increased self-esteem and promote cross-ethnic relationship in a multi-ethnic environments (Babenko and Mosewich 2017; Caruso and Gill 1992; Crosnoe 2002; Eccles et al. 2003; Feldman and Matjasko 2005; Fox and Corbin 1989; Hoffmann and Xu 2002; Janssen and LeBlanc 2010; Johnson and Taliaferro 2011; Knifsend and Juvonen 2017; Mahoney 2000; Mahoney and Cairns 1997; Mahoney et al. 2003; Mahoney et al. 2006; Marsh and Kleitman 2003; Sharp et al. 2003). Substantiating the benefits of extracurricular activities, Bucknavage and Worrell (2005) found that 93% of the youth who are academically bright also participated in extracurricular activities.

The positive effects and the benefits of the participation in extracurricular activities are not universal and permanent. Even though all extracurricular activities have desirable effects, not all result in similar benefits. Blogging might increase writing skills, facilitate greater social visibility, and increase self-esteem, but may not accrue the additional benefits of physical fitness, and team involvement, which are result of playing football. Similarly, participating in an extracurricular activity for a short duration cannot guarantee the same benefits for the long term. Research indicates that the benefits of participating in extracurricular activities (especially those that involve physical activity) in academics are short-term and the benefits accrue only if one participates regularly in an activity (Taras 2005; Bird et al. 2013). On the other hand, there are common benefits irrespective of the type of extracurricular activity. This is especially true with regard to self-esteem. Pol and Roopesh (2016), in this regard, found that children who are regularly involved in organized sports activities, and children who are regularly involved with organized music and instruments, did not differ with respect to self-concept, self-esteem, and psychological well-being. However, both groups had significantly higher self-concept, self-esteem, and psychological well-being compared to children who were not involved with any regular extracurricular activities.

There are several mechanisms and processes suggested about how adolescents benefit from participation in extracurricular activities. It can be through being part of a group and having a sense of belonging, engaging in pro-social activities, observing and imitating positive role models, or having an opportunity to spend time in a safe place (Boratav 2005; Eccles and Barber 1999; Mahoney et al. 2006). Other mechanisms proposed are academic-related benefits that may happen due to learning how to structure time and focus on extracurricular activities (Chin and Harrington 2007). As participating in extracurricular activities increases their confidence level, behavioural adjustment and social-emotional competencies, students may try harder and persist with the task, thereby overcoming the difficulty in academics (Aronson 2002; Durlak et al. 2011).

In terms of the mechanism, Chin and Harrington (2007) considered the possible advantages of studying music, such as learning to focus, development of fine motor skills, and improvement in social skills. This highlights the importance of direct effects on the brain, with respect to cognitive functions such as attention and concentration, as well as visuospatial motor skills. It is a widely accepted fact that almost all of our behaviour can be traced to brain functions (Coon and Mitterer 2016). This can be applied as well to the beneficial effects of participation in extracurricular activities. The brain of children and adolescents is a developing brain, and it reaches maturity only in the early twenties (Klingberg and Betteridge 2012). Given this, there can be a direct benefit of extracurricular activity on the brain with respect to various neuropsychological functions. For example, learning to play a musical instrument that has strings has been shown to increase neural connections in the areas of the brain involved in musical perception and finger movements (Kolb and Whishaw 2008). Further, playing an instrument requires one to repeatedly practice and remember multiple tunes and sequences, which can all directly stimulate the brain areas that are responsible for working memory and sequential learning. Working memory and sequential processing are an important component in any type of learning, especially academics. As mentioned above, research in this regard has shown that children who are good in music also perform well in academics (Cabanac et al. 2013). Apart from the direct benefits with respect to cognitive functions, a few researchers argue that participation in extracurricular activities confers benefits, of group participation and healthy peer relationships, on those adolescents who face hardships in their lives due to economic or social conditions (Boratav 2005; Guttman 1994).

With respect to negative behaviours, there are several explanations as to how extracurricular activities can reduce negative or violent behaviours and promote positive personality development. Extracurricular activities enable adolescents to learn social and intellectual skills that are required to handle different situations and diverse environments. Further, through peer interaction, group activities can encourage adolescents to participate in and contribute to their community, which, as a result, might help in creating a sense of belongingness to the community and, in the process, also enhance self-esteem (Eccles et al. 2003). The whole process of being part of and contributing to the society might act against negative behaviours by channelling the energy of the adolescent in a positive direction. Substantiating this, it has been observed that adolescents who participate in extracurricular activities have been shown to reduce risky behaviours such as alcohol and substance abuse (Blum et al. 2003: Darling 2005; Eccles et al. 2003). Another way in which being involved in extracurricular activities reduces deviant behaviours might be, that children who have behaviour problems seldom receive encouraging and positive reinforcement from people around them. Research has also shown that children with deviant behaviours usually have inconsistent disciplining in their life (Halgunseth et al. 2013), and have deficits in social skills (Merrell and Gimpel 1998; van der Stouwe et al. 2016), which make it difficult for them to have and indulge in behaviours that are positively reinforced. Participation in any regular extracurricular activity usually involves written or unwritten rules and regulations, which everybody needs to follow. This provides consistency for adolescents. Further, as mentioned above, regular participation encourages togetherness among the participants, which increases bonding and 'we-feeling'. In addition, participation can entail praise and positive reinforcements. This consistency, togetherness, 'we-feeling', praise, and reinforcements, can provide a new interaction pattern to an adolescent and can have significant positive effects in reducing negative behaviours.

Studies have also shown that participation in extracurricular activities has far reaching benefits; from benefits in academics and reducing risky behaviours. It provides children and adolescents with an opportunity to learn moral and ethical values, social as well as life skills, and improve interpersonal communication (Fozzard 1967; Sybouts and Krepel 1984). Extracurricular activities further provide situations and challenges that inculcate persistence, teach emotional regulation, and help to learn time management and problem solving skills (Denson et al. 2015; Larson et al. 2006). On the other hand, participation in extracurricular activities increases friendship, teamwork, and social support; it has been shown to decrease negative emotions, such as boredom and loneliness (Shernoff and Vandell 2007). Smoll and Smith (2002) in their study, opined that involvement in athletics can increase perseverance, build character, and inculcate respect for rules. Similarly, Burton et al. (2000), discussed that participation in arts-related activities may enhance creativity, imagination, fluency, as well as critical and divergent thinking. Apart from enabling adolescents to cope with life challenges, participating in extracurricular activities helps in providing new goals and helps to discover new meaning in life (Nesan 2009).

Studies also point out the differential effects of participation in different types of extracurricular activity. Eccles and Barber (1999) found that participation in Church and volunteering has a direct association with academic achievement, and inverse association with engagement in risky behaviour. This indicates that participating in religious groups and activity helps in academics and decreases undesirable behaviour. They further found that participation in the performance arts is positively correlated with academic achievement. However, participation in athletics is positively correlated with academic achievement and also, surprisingly, to alcohol use. Guest and Schneider (2003) found that participation in both athletic as well as non-athletic activities (music and drama clubs or student government) was positively shown to be associated with academic achievement and educational expectations. Similarly, Denny (2007) showed that higher musical involvement in young adolescents had significant positive association with higher educational and occupational expectations.

Choice of Extracurricular Activity

The choice of a particular extracurricular activity is determined by many factors. Rosenberg (1972) believes that a student is usually influenced by several factors while choosing an extracurricular activity, which Rosenberg claims is based on the perceived involvement, which can be either inclusive or exclusive. According to him, the 'inclusive activity' is usually the one that tries to attract more members. Success is measured by the degree to which the activity attracts maximum members. Inclusive activity generally tends to be social in nature and may have planned or unplanned gatherings. The objective is primarily social, and the members usually belong to the same friendship groups. On the contrary, 'exclusive activity' has relatively less members; the membership is open to people who have a specific skill set or who wish to attain it. Here, there is less social involvement. No one activity can be entirely inclusive or exclusive, for it can vary from individual to individual, school to school, and year to year (Rosenberg 1972).

There are several factors that determine what activity an adolescent is involved in. These range from cultural, geographical, and family values, to socioeconomic status, feasibility, talents, and interests of the student, to the gender. Child-rearing practices with more focus on one's own culture might make a person believe that traditional dance forms are better than more contemporary dance forms. Similarly, geographical location also influences the choice within an activity; people from south India might opt for Bharatanatyam (a South Indian dance form) rather than Kathak (a North Indian dance form). Similarly, people with a familial aversion against dancing on stage might prohibit their children from practicing dance, but there may not be any such restrictions for learning singing.

Apart from the above factors, the physical condition, talents and interest of the student matters in the choice of extracurricular activities. A physically weak student usually tends to avoid outdoor contact sports and might choose non-contact indoor sports, or activities related to academics or performing arts. Similarly, feasibility also determines what activity one gets to choose. If a desired activity is not possible to participate in, due to financial, distance, or time-related issues, then the student will not be able to participate in that particular activity. Therefore, she or he can choose another activity that is feasible based on cost, distance, or time.

Adolescents' participation in activities varies across different countries. With respect to extracurricular activities, there are more studies carried out in the US compared to other countries, and, within these studies, athletics is the most commonly studied activity (Bucknavage and Worrell 2005) and the most frequently reported on adolescents (Feldman and Matjasko 2005; Worrell and Bucknavage 2004). Larson and Verma (1999) found that adolescents in Europe spend more time in activities related to music, whereas adolescents in US spend more time playing sports. It is also observed that, compared to high-income economies or communities, overall there is significantly less participation by lower-income economies (Mahoney et al. 2004). Similarly, studies also highlight that minority populations are under-served with respect to extracurricular activities, compared to majority populations (Linville and Huebner 2005).

Gender and Extracurricular Activities

In terms of gender, studies have found that girls across nations generally participate in more diverse extracurricular activities than boys, and boys participate more in athletics than girls. Further, boys are known to participate in more team sports and unorganized activities compared to girls, and the participation of girls is observed to be significantly more for individual sports, socializing, academic activities (speech & debate clubs), activities such as music and drama, and organized group activities compared to boys (Buser and Humm 1980; Eccles and Barber 1999; Eccles et al. 2003; Feldman and Matjasko 2005; Larson and Verma 1999; Mahoney et al. 2005; Posner and Vandell 1999). Hill and Clevan (2005) further highlight that girls usually participate in non-contact sports such as volleyball, swimming, dance, aerobics and gymnastics, whereas boys participate more in contact sports such as football, soccer, and hockey.

Further, it is often the interaction of gender and socio-political factors that determines participation in a particular activity. For example, boys participate more in leisure time activities compared to girls in non-industrial countries, whereas in industrialized countries, these differences in terms of available time to participate in extracurricular activities did not emerge (Larson and Verma 1999).

Things were not the same earlier for girls. There were significant negative biases and stereotypes with respect to the participation of girls in sports and athletics (Sherrow 1996). In recent years, the participation of girls in recreational, competitive (boxing and wrestling) and extreme sports (inline skating, skateboarding and snowboarding) has increased (Zimmerman and Reavill 1998). Despite increasing participation of girls in sports, gender stereotypes still prevail. Boys are encouraged from childhood to participate in competitive and aggressive team sports, whereas girls are taught to be content with individual, aesthetically pleasing, sports and activities, such as gymnastics and figure skating (Schmalz and Kerstetter 2006). In this regard, McClung and Blinde (2002) studied how women athletes identify with gender issues. They explored women athletes' experiences and perceptions with respect to sports. The authors observed that the women athletes made three distinct identifications that: (a) "their status in sports is secondary compared to men"; (b) their perception that women's sport "doesn't really matter"; and (c) society's perception of women athletes, who were generally stereotyped as being "masculine", "tomboy", or "lesbian" (McClung and Blinde 2002). This can be easily observed in how much attention and remuneration sports played by women garners. For example, there is constant debate on the lower payment received by female professional tennis players, and the significantly lower media attention given to women's cricket, hockey, or football. Given this, there is an urgent necessity to increase female participation in sports and athletics.

Factors Affecting Extracurricular Participation

Factors affecting participation in extracurricular activity can be broadly divided into 'within school' and 'out of school' factors. Within school, factors such as inadequate and limited facilities and equipment (such as playground, sports room, and sports equipment), lack of well-trained and motivated human resources (such as coaches and instructors), financial limitations, socioeconomic status of the school, poor planning on the part of school management, overemphasis on curricular activities, excessive workload on teachers, crowded classrooms and large number of students in school, can adversely affect student participation (Jenkinson and Benson 2010).

Out of school factors that hinder participation in extracurricular activities are parents' education, socioeconomic status and occupation of the parents, physical and mental health of the parents as well as the student, poor peer support, inadequate encouragement and guidance for extracurricular activities, overemphasis on curriculum, lack of motivation, negative parental attitude about physical activity, and restricted socio-politico-cultural atmosphere, such as places having civil war (Jenkinson and Benson 2010). With respect to parents' education and physical and mental health, it was observed that the mother's education level and her health status is seen to be more relevant for a child's participation in extracurricular activities, compared to father's education level and health (Hansen et al. 2003; Feldman and Matjasko 2005; Peters and Mullis 1997).

Conclusion

Given the pervasive importance of extracurricular activities in overall growth and development of children and adolescents, it is imperative for various stakeholders to act in favour of promoting extracurricular activities as a regular part of the course in school and colleges. Not all children are able to engage in all types of activities. Given this, there should be ample opportunity for students to choose from different types of activities that cater to their physical condition, ability, and interests. These should be effectively implemented in every school, and at all levels. For the same, every government should enact policies and provide financial and other resources to facilitate active participation in different activities. Additionally, there should be recruitment of trained human resources, such as coaches and trainers, from both genders in every school. Apart from these, teachers should be trained so that they can encourage and supervise students in a particular activity. In this regard, clubs can be started in every school that cater to different types of extracurricular activities, such as sports club, martial arts club, skating club, music club, dance club, piano club, language club, debate club, and so on. Schools should accommodate time for these activities as part of regular school timings. Further, schools should provide adequate and appropriate equipment for these activities. Every year, grade, school, zonal, state, and national level programmes, and competitions, should be held to increase motivation and healthy competition. In addition, trainers and teachers should receive continuing education every few years to update their knowledge and skill set related to the particular activity that they are supervising. To increase the adherence, every school can be asked to prepare a report to be submitted to the education department and these reports need to be evaluated and feedback given about the performance and what extra needs to be done. A system to rate schools based on their performance in encouraging, facilitating, and developing extracurricular activities in students can be started.

Apart from the school, parents should also be informed to facilitate and encourage their children's participation in extracurricular activities. Parents should avoid blindly enforcing their own interests and beliefs on their children's activities. Rather, they should know their child's abilities and interests, and adjust accordingly. A child might show interest in a particular activity in the beginning, but later might lose interest or change it to some other activity. Parents should evaluate these instances and take an unbiased decision keeping the best interest of the child.

On the other hand, there are some parents who enrol their children in multiple extracurricular activities leading to activity overload. If children are in multiple activities, it might lead to undue stress and they might not get enough time to live their childhood. Children need extracurricular activities, but at the same time, they also need free time for themselves to play whatever they like and love. These can be anything from an informal game of marbles, playing on a swing, reading a story book, knitting a friendship band, playing hopscotch, playing hide-and-seek, to just being lost in their own make-believe world. This helps them to realize their own interests, talents, and creativity, rather than those imposed by parents and society.

References

Aronson, J. (2002). Stereotype threat: Contending and coping with unusual expectations. In J. Aronson (Ed.), *Improving academic achievement: Impact of psychological factors on education* (pp. 279–301). San Diego: Academic Press.

Astin, A. W. (1999). Student involvement: A developmental theory for higher education. *Journal of College Student Development, 40,* 518–529.

Babenko, O., & Mosewich, A. (2017). In sport and now in medical school: Examining students' well-being and motivations for learning. *International Journal of Medical Education, 8,* 336–342.

Berk, L. E. (2008). *Child development* (8th ed.). India: Prentice Hall.

Bird, K. S., Tripney, J., & Newman, M. (2013). The educational impacts of young people's participation in organized sport: A systematic review. *Journal of Children's Services, 8,* 264–275.

Blum, R. W., Halcon, L., Beuhring, T., Pate, E., Campell-Forrester, S., & Venema, A. (2003). Adolescent health in the Caribbean: Risk and protective factors. *American Journal of Public Health, 93,* 456–460.

Boratav, H. B. (2005). Negotiating youth: Growing up in inner-city Istanbul. *Journal of Youth Studies, 8,* 203–220.

Bucknavage, L. B., & Worrell, F. C. (2005). Academically talented students' participation in extracurricular activities. *Journal of Secondary Gifted Education, 16,* 74–86.

Burr, B. L. (2012). *Do extracurricular activities help adolescents develop academic self-efficacy? Evidence for how and why.* M.Sc. dissertation submitted to the Brigham Young University, paper 3268.

Burton, J. M., Horowitz, R., & Abeles, H. (2000). Learning in and through arts: The question of transfer. *Studies in Art Education, 41,* 228–257.

Buser, R. L., & Humm. W. L. (1980). Special report on co-curricular offerings and participation. Springfield, 111: Illinois State Board of Education.

Cabanac, A., Perlovsky, L., Bonniot-Cabanac, M. C., & Cabanac, M. (2013). Music and academic performance. *Behavior and Brain Research, 256,* 257–260.

Caruso, C. M., & Gill, D. L. (1992). Strengthening physical self-perceptions through exercise. *Journal of Sports Medicine, 32,* 426–447.

Chickering, A. W. (1969). *Education and identity*. San Francisco: Jossey-Bass.

Chin, C. S., & Harrington, D. M. (2007). Supporting the development of musical talent. *Gifted Child Today, 30,* 40–47.

Coon, D., & Mitterer, J. O. (2016). *Introduction to psychology: Gateways to mind and behaviour*. New Delhi: CENGAGE Learning Custom Publishing.

Crosnoe, R. (2002). Academic and health-related trajectories in adolescence: The intersection of gender and athletics. *Journal of Health and Social Behavior, 43,* 317–335.

Darling, N. (2005). Participation in extracurricular activities and adolescent adjustment: Cross-sectional and longitudinal findings. *Journal of Youth and Adolescence, 34,* 493–505.

Denny, E. (2007). To what extent does participation in extracurricular music affect the future aspirations of 11-12-year-olds? A small-scale investigation. *British Journal of Music Education, 24,* 99–115.

Denson, C. D., Stallworth, C. A., Hailey, C., & Householder, D. L. (2015). Benefits of informal learning environments: A focused examination of STEM-based program environments. *Journal of STEM Education, 16,* 11–15.

Dewey, J. (1897). My pedagogic creed. *The School Journal, 54,* 77–80.

Durlak, J. A., Weissberg, R. P., Dymnicki, A. B., Taylor, R. D., & Schellinger, K. B. (2011). The impact of enhancing students' social and emotional learning: A meta-analysis of school-based universal interventions. *Child Development, 82,* 405–432.

Eccles, J. S., & Barber, B. L. (1999). Student council, volunteering, basketball, or marching band: What kind of extracurricular involvement matters? *Journal of Adolescent Research, 14,* 10–43.

Eccles, J. S., Barber, B. L., Stone, M., & Hunt, J. (2003). Extracurricular activities and adolescent development. *Journal of Social Issues, 59,* 865–890.

Feldman, A. F., & Matjasko, J. L. (2005). The role of school-based extracurricular activities in adolescent development: A comprehensive review and future directions. *Review of Educational Research, 75,* 159–210.

Fox, K. R., & Corbin, C. B. (1989). The physical self-perception profile: Development and preliminary validation. *Journal of Sport and Exercise Psychology, 11,* 408–430.

Fozzard, P. R. (1967). *Out-of-class activities and civic education*. Strasbourg: Council of Europe.

Fredricks, J. A., & Eccles, J. S. (2005). Developmental benefits of extracurricular involvement: Do peer characteristics mediate the link between activities and youth outcomes? *Journal of Youth and Adolescence, 34,* 507–520.

Guest, A., & Schneider, B. (2003). Adolescents' extracurricular participation in context: The mediating effects of schools, communities, and identity. *Sociology of Education, 76,* 89–109.

Guttman, C. (1994). *On the right track: Servol's early childhood and adolescent development programming in Trinidad and Tobago*. Paris: United Nations.

Halgunseth, L. C., Perkins, D. R., Lippold, M. A., & Nix, R. L. (2013). Delinquent-oriented attitudes mediate the relation between parental inconsistent discipline and early adolescent behaviour. *Journal of Family Psychology, 27,* 293–302.

Hansen, M. D., Larson, W. R., & Dworkin, B. J. (2003). What adolescents learn in organized youth activities: A survey of self-reported developmental experiences. *Journal of Research on Adolescents, 13,* 25–55.

Hill, G., & Cleven, B. (2005). A comparison of 9th grade male and female physical education activities preferences and support for coeducational groupings. *The Physical Educator, 62,* 187–197.

Hoffmann, J. P., & Xu, J. (2002). School activities, community service, and delinquency. *Crime and Delinquency, 48,* 568–591.

Hurford, J. R. (1991). The evolution of the critical period for language acquisition. *Cognition, 10,* 159–201.

Janssen, I., & LeBlanc, A. (2010). Systematic review of the health benefits of physical activity and fitness in school-aged children and youth. *International Journal of Behavioral Nutrition and Physical Activity, 7,* 40.

Jayanti, P., Thirunavukarasu, M., & Rajkumar, R. (2015). Academic stress and depression among adolescents: A cross-sectional study. *Indian Pediatrics, 52,* 217–219.

Jenkinson, K. A., & Benson, A. C. (2010). Barriers to providing physical education and physical activity in Victorian state secondary schools. *Australian Journal of Teacher Education, 35,* 1–18.

Johnson, K., & Taliaferro, L. (2011). Relationships between physical activity and depressive symptoms among middle and older adolescents: a review of the research literature. *Journal for Specialists in Pediatric Nursing, 1,* 235–251.

Klingberg, T., & Betteridge, N. (2012). *The learning brain: Memory and brain development in children*. USA: Oxford University Press.

Knifsend, C. A., & Juvonen, J. (2017). Extracurricular activities in multiethnic middle schools: Ideal context for positive intergroup attitudes? *Journal of Research on Adolescence, 27,* 407–422.

Kolb, B., & Whishaw, I. Q. (2008). *Fundamentals of human neuropsychology*. USA: Worth Publishers.

Kumaraswamy, N. (2013). Academic stress, anxiety and depression among college students: A brief review. *International Review of Social Sciences and Humanities, 5,* 135–143.

Larson, R. W., Hansen, D. M., & Moneta, G. (2006). Differing profiles of development experiences across types of organized youth activities. *Developmental Psychology, 42,* 849–863.

Larson, R. W., & Verma, S. (1999). How children and adolescents spend time across the world: Work, play, and developmental opportunities. *Psychological Bulletin, 125,* 701–736.

Linville, D. C., & Huebner, A. J. (2005). The analysis of extracurricular activities and their relationship to youth violence. *Journal of Youth and Adolescence, 34,* 483–492.

Mahoney, J. L. (2000). School extracurricular activity participation as a moderator in the development of antisocial patterns. *Child Development, 71,* 502–516.

Mahoney, J. L., & Cairns, R. B. (1997). Do extracurricular activities protect against early school dropout? *Developmental Psychology, 33,* 241–253.

Mahoney, J. L., Cairns, B. D., & Farmer, T. W. (2003). Promoting interpersonal competence and educational success through extra-curricular activity participation. *Journal of Educational Psychology, 95,* 409–418.

Mahoney, J. L., Eccles, J. S., & Larson, R. W. (2004). Processes of adjustment in organized out-of-school activities: Opportunities and risks. *New Directions for Youth Development, 101,* 115–144.

Mahoney, J. L., Harris, A. L., & Eccles, J. S. (2006). Organized activity participation, positive youth development, and the over-scheduling hypothesis. *Society for Research in Child Development Social Policy Report, 20,* 1–30.

Mahoney, J. L., Larson, R. W., Eccles, J. S., & Lord, H. (2005). Organized activities as developmental contexts for children and adolescents. *Organized activities as contexts of development: Extracurricular activities, after-school and community programs*, 3–22.

Marsh, H. W., & Kleitman, S. (2003). School athletic participation: Mostly gain with little pain. *Journal of Sport and Exercise Psychology, 25,* 205–228.

Martinez, A. M., & Fabiano, P. (1992). *Stanford students' health needs assessment 1990, Student Health Center*. Cowell: Stanford University Report of Stanford CA.

McClung, L., & Blinde, E. (2002). Sensitivity to gender issues: Accounts of women intercollegiate athletes. *International Sports Journal*, 117–133.

Merrell, K. W., & Gimpel, G. A. (1998). *Social skills of children and adolescents: Conceptualization, assessment, treatment*. New York: Psychology Press.

Nesan, D. (2009). *Co-curricular activities in schools*. International Debate Education Association (www.idebate.org/debatabase/).

Peters, H. E., & Mullis, N. C. (1997). The role of family income and sources of income in adolescent achievement. In B.-G. Duncan (Ed.), *Consequences of growing up poor*. New York: Russell Sage Foundation.

Pol, S., & Roopesh, B. N. (2016). *Extracurricular activities, self-esteem, self-concept and psychological well-being in adolescents*. Unpublished M.Phil. in Clinical Psychology dissertation submitted to National Institute of Mental Health and Neuro Sciences, Bengaluru.

Posner, J. K., & Vandell, D. L. (1999). After-school activities and the development of low-income urban children: A longitudinal study. *Developmental Psychology, 35,* 868–879.

Rosenberg, M. (1972). *Society and the adolescent self-image*. Princeton: Princeton University Press.

Rumberger, R. W. (1987). High school dropouts: A review of issues and evidence. *Review of Educational Research, 57,* 101–121.

Rumberger, R. W. (1995). Dropping out of middle school: A multilevel analysis of students and schools. *American Educational Research Journal, 32,* 583–625.

Santrock, J. W. (2011). *Adolescence* (12th ed.). India: McGraw Hill Education India Pvt. Ltd.

Schmalz, D., & Kerstetter, D. (2006). Girlie girls and manly men: Children's stigma consciousness of gender in sports and physical activities. *Journal of Leisure Research, 38,* 536–557.

Sharp, C., Blackmore, J., Kendall, L., Greene, K., Keys, W., Macauley, A., et al. (2003). *Playing for success: An evaluation of the fourth year*. Nottingham: Department for Education and Skills.

Shernoff, D. J., & Vandell, D. L. (2007). Engagement in after-school program activities: Quality of experience from the perspective of participants. *Journal of Youth and Adolescence, 36,* 891–903.

Sherrow, V. (1996). *Violence and the media: The question of cause and effect*. Millbrook Press.

Smoll, F. L., & Smith, R. E. (Eds.). (2002). *Children and youth in sport: A biopsychosocial perspective*. Kendall Hunt Publishing Company.

Sybouts, W., & Krepel, W. J. (1984). *Student activities in the secondary schools*. Westport: Greenwood.

Taras, H. (2005). Physical activity and student performance at school. *Journal of School Health, 75*(6), 214–218.

van der Stouwe, T., Asscher, J. J., van der Hoeve, M., Laan, P. H., & Stams, G. J. J. M. (2016). Social skills training for juvenile delinquents: Post-treatment changes. *Journal of Experimental Criminology, 12,* 515–536.

Worrell, F. C., & Bucknavage, L. B. (2004). Participation in extracurricular activities by students attending assisted and prestige schools in Trinidad. *Caribbean Curriculum, 11,* 129–147.

Zaff, J. F., Moore, K. A., Pappillo, A. R., & Williams, S. (2003). Implication of extracurricular activity participation during adolescence on positive outcomes. *Journal of Adolescent Research, 18,* 599–630.

Zimmerman, J., & Reavill, G. (1998). *Raising our athletic daughters: How sports can build self-esteem and save girls' lives*. New York: Doubleday.

Chapter 16
Quest for a Therapeutic Anodyne for the Degenerating Teacher—Student Relationship in New India

S. Visaka Devi

Abstract The Teacher-Student relationship in India was a much revered one in ancient times. Today, one can notice a drastic change that has crept into this relationship. Crucial factors have effected this change. The chapter aims to discuss major crises on a research orientation to bring about positive amendments to keep India secure from the onslaught of social anomalies. School plays a vital role in moulding the personality of a child and this, in turn, is calibrated with individual Teacher–Student relationships, with merits as well as deficiencies, though the latter has a large impact on the child's psyche. In contemporary India, the factors that debauch Teacher-Student relationships are as follows: (a) Teacher-training and education programmes merely develop on the remains of an outmoded teacher-training system that hardly delves into the psychic and social problems of the new Indian Teacher-Student relationship; (b) The teaching profession is dominated by women who multitask, with no social support system as in the West. Here, women manage both the domestic and professional fronts in the perpetuation of a patriarchal system. Expectations of women's contributions to the conduct of a family are the same as before; this leads to students being at the receiving end of the frustrations of the teacher; (c) Teaching as a profession is often a mere lucrative choice, rather than one of passion; (d) Periodical, professional counselling for teachers and students, that orients and refreshes them to face challenges, animosities, hostilities, and exploitations is yet another grave gap; (e) Failure of teachers to recognize, appreciate and encourage talents; (f) Failure to identify and address behavioural issues in students while considering each individual student's familial background; (g) Inflation in student intake that fractures inter-personal relationships; (h) students with attention deficit; (i) Rise of prejudice, unscrupulousness, and impatience among teachers; (j) Teacher awards and legalized 'teacher-gift' systems in schools (often in private institutions) endanger the personality-moulding of students, which is part of teaching, and encourage a score-oriented teaching system; (k) commercialization of the education system sanctions the growth of innumerable private schools run by untrained, unskilled,

S. V. Devi (✉)
Department of English, Pondicherry University, Puducherry 605014, India
e-mail: visakasajan17@gmail.com

S. Deb (ed.), *Positive Schooling and Child Development*,
https://doi.org/10.1007/978-981-13-0077-6_16

profit-oriented businessmen with clandestine political backing; and (l) philistinism and degeneration of moral values caused by easy Internet accessibility in India. The article intends to analyze each of these, punctuated with suggestions that would attempt to contribute a social panacea.

Keywords Therapy · Students · Schools · Teachers · Relationship
New India

Introduction

"Is there a change in the interpersonal teacher–student bond today, compared to what it was many years ago?" This question may have multiple answers, each from a different perspective: psychological, social, personal, and individual. Quite undeniably, the origins of this change are rooted in the various social changes that have occurred over the last three decades, which in turn, directly or indirectly, have affected the teacher–student bond as well. The changes, to enumerate a few, were those that swept over India on a massive scale, such as: the increase in Multinational trade, connectivity through the World Wide Web, economic progress that was coupled with the sudden insatiable surge for higher education. To a large extent, all of these left an indelible and reprehensible impact on both the young and the young adult Indian. However, the changes that occurred in the youth in terms of values, attitude, and the related 'social changes' both have their roots in the changes in the atmosphere of upbringing, in both the domestic and the social front. Consciously or unconsciously, changes have diffused into all possible Indian social spheres, though its negatives are conveniently pushed under the carpet. The reason for this wilful ignorance is due to the contemporary Indian psyche that focuses more on ruthless economic progress that overlooks all ethics of conduct which are in fact more vital for social well-being.

The transition, one has to keep in mind, perhaps began with the shift from the intrinsic, philosophic, 'Gurukul-ism', to an extrinsic, information and economy-oriented 'Google-ism', which introduced a number of inexplicable, tradition-defiant, and serendipitous changes that often devalued many a traditional norm across the nation, which in turn affected the teacher–student relationship too. According to Mathur,[1] the basic change happened with money having become the driving force in Education. The relationship between the teacher and student, which was once treated with awe, was diluted and what ultimately emerged was the business attitude of 'I-pay-and-you-get-paid' among students. This attitude gradually increased much more in the recent times, especially with the advent of Google that gave students greater access to information that shaped them into self-made Intellectual Gurus which gave them a new conviction that they could function minus any monitoring by parents or teachers.

[1]www.campusdiaries.com/stories/the-changing-dynamics-of-teacher-student.

Thus the following discussion would take into consideration the roots of what actually changed the teacher–student bond, the dual responsibility on the part of both teachers and students, the social agents that were responsible for it, the pros and cons of such changes, and the necessary amendments that might possibly draw its rampage to a halt.

To identify specific reasons for the change, we need to locate specific issues that upset the social system: First, there was an abandonment of teaching of value systems in institutions; second, the employability of women/mother paradoxically resulted in removal of familial support systems, as a remorseless patriarchal attitude failed to acknowledge the woman's monetary contribution to the family, and expected her to toil alone at both the work and home fronts, leading to an adverse impact especially on women who were teachers.[2]

Abandonment of Teaching of Value Systems

A vacuum seems to inhabit the teacher–student bond in the Indian school system today. Obviously, this has been the outcome of the absence of values/moral education which, whether one enjoyed teaching or learning it in the past, was an integral part of the curriculum. Today, that has been crippled in multifarious ways, as cordiality, understanding, tolerance, sharing, caring, attitude, behaviour, and flexibility are all meagre remnants that hold no significance at all. As a result, both teacher and student nurse a mutual malice that has invaded their psyche in the form of ego. It is important to recall, that the same subject, called value instruction, was once taught and learnt without any bias or prejudice, though often in the form of moral or religious instruction. Today, the scene differs drastically as all value instructions are intricately combined with religious values, that too with such fanatical spirit that, unlike olden times, any moral aspect shared in classrooms would be trapped in religious polemic. As a result, the education system in India has removed value education from the curriculum, possibly owing to the fanatic religious connotations attached to it. Thus, such instructions, which otherwise could have inspired both the teaching and learning process, were curbed and ultimately silenced. This change then, invaded the young as they were more easily adept, sensitive and change-prone and preferred total independence from anything that reigned over them.

Employment of Women/Mothers

While the value change and its impact were visible in the attitudinal and relationship aspects of teachers and students, it is also vital to note, that the change also affected women and mothers. For, with economic progress, many women became

---

[2]www.thehindu.com/opinion/open-page/working-vs…moms/article5740972.ece.

working women. Most women were also ready for change as well, as they were, for too long, bound by the stringency of Indian traditions. Thereby, the urge to take up lucrative jobs, with total economic independence, became stronger in them.

Working parents which included mothers were/are engrossed with creating a world of 'dream-come-true' for their most often 'single' child or, at the most, two. As a result, total freedom and a huge stress unconsciously weighed heavily upon both the young, as well as parents, in three major forms: (a) the young or adolescents, on the one hand, who cautiously manoeuvred through the onslaught of change positively; on the other, (b) a disproportionate number of uncared-for young and adolescents at home who were lost either due to stressed/over-demanding parents or who were lost in the world of the Internet; and (c) uncaring/callous/self-absorbed parents also grew in number, lost to their children as they too were engrossed with either work or with the follies of modernity or other socially detrimental, unethical practices. Both parents and the young/young adults suffered a mutual, irretrievable loss and uncertainty owing to the aforementioned factors.

As a result, the moulding of the personality of young students which usually developed at home and evolved further at school, lost its foothold in the face of the unprecedented changes that affected the new, change-craving-Indian.

New Economic Freedom and Lax Ethical Codes

Besides this, the fine parenting of yesteryears deteriorated further, in the nuclear family system. This worsened the social attitude and there were more unprecedented changes in the ethics, values, interests, and focus even among contemporary parents, who now had gained independence from the binding ties and demands of the joint-family system. Their attention was now occupied with other things: economic freedom (often ruthless); absence of absolute commitment to their families; insatiable aspirations for higher positions (often in the name of elevating family status and sometimes even at the cost of familial bonding); worst of all, there were other unethical engagements that took away their attention completely from their families and their commitments to them. Some parents even chose extreme freedom either by way of extra-marital affairs or alcoholism, or other forms of indulgence that gave them absolute freedom to make unlimited choices at the cost of an organized, legal family system (Such aspects are not going to be analyzed in depth as they are case-specific).

Failed Teacher Education Agenda and Deprivation of Psychological Understanding to Students

Consequently, the economic freedom of parents, their high or low status, their positive professional commitments, or negative familial conduct, all of these affected the young. The impact was huge both on the early and the late adolescents, who usually consider themselves absolutely mature yet are unable to make any sensible decision. Thus, whatever emanated from a student's home atmosphere either strengthened or enfeebled them. This made them either confident or insecure especially when facing an adverse situation in school or criticism from their peer group or teachers. When they became incapable of coping with either their peers or with academic pressure or some other form of exploitation which they normally would prefer to share with others, they began seeking support or attention. At such junctures, they largely depended on their teachers. But the teaching community, by then wrapped-up in its own self-indulgent engagements, which ought to have offered them understanding, utterly failed them. Most often the crumbling of the teacher–student relationship began in such contexts, closely followed by related rupture in the social system too, for the roots of what ought to be a stable social systems had already caught the disease.

If the young are subjected to afflictive, disturbing, or partially disturbing conditions at home, at school they tend to suffer varied levels of stress that are manifested in myriad ways. They, then, turn out to be either hyperactive or hypersensitive or attention-seeking or turn out to be bullies exhibiting deplorable behaviour, which are hardly noticed by teachers, or if noticed, are considered severely punishable offences. These students are branded 'badly-behaved, dull-heads' and given many more such belittling attributes. Such derisive remarks push them further into the abyss of vulnerability, provoking them to be more adamant and outrageous in their behaviour.

On the other side are those students from peaceful and happy homes, who tend to be confident, smart, and highly independent. There are chances that in such instances, teachers who are traumatized, over-stressed at home or at work, who tend to be irritable, impatient, and, at times, even envious of such students. Such students are constantly assaulted by adverse, sarcastic remarks by thoughtless teachers, who mutilate the vital potential of their tender minds. What ultimately resonates in their young minds are the echoes of ineffaceable verbal abuses that affect their entire personality.

While the early part of this discussion speaks about the changed Indian set-up and the need for value education which has been overlooked, the following focuses on the need for periodical guidance through counselling for teacher educators, trainees, and trained teachers. This provides scope for updating and finding solutions for current issues and specific cases that would help bring about a changed attitude and adept problem-solving resolutions mostly among teachers and additionally in students too.

Who Needs to Be More Responsible?

Before discussing the questions raised, reports on the erratic whimsicalities of teachers have to be assessed and the following reports offer sufficient vindication of the issues in question. Hardly any school in India or teacher training institution takes practical cues from the above instances for these have become obsolete, nor do they offer periodical counselling (as part of a modernized system). Mere psychological counselling for day-to-day issues themselves can lead to a person being branded insane or a nervous wreck. Similarly, simple basic needs of the young to be heard, and solutions, answers, or guidance to their problems, which need to be provided, are unabashedly ignored. Even patience on the part of a teacher to listen to the personal woes of a student, be it a truth or a lie, to give him the benefit of the doubt even, is missing. Neither a troubled student nor a student who has poor IQ, or behavioural issues or some kind of learning difficulties has any space in the Indian classrooms in an otherwise generous nation that has reservations for many other social and religious segments. Unlike many other professional fields, practical application of the theories in class rooms is merely an abstract notion and remains simply in the realm of textual theory. They are meant for academic appraisals or a degree while application of theories into practice, in class room realities, while tackling a certain situation related to a stressed student, for instance, is a utopian dream in India. Even behavioural case-specific training is hardly given to the teacher-trainee; much of the focus is on teaching principles. Behavioural psychology, though part of the teacher training programme, posits only textual and not reality-based instances. Forums and hands-on workshops that would generate more substantial evidence-based experience are missing in the teacher-training programmes. As a result, what is offered by teacher-educators to the trainees lags behind in periodical updating, and practical counselling on the newer much more challenging issues of the contemporary times are unknown to the trainers and trainees.

Finding Measures to Overcome Lapses in Teachers and Teacher Education Programmes

The questions that have been raised so far are about the inability to cope with the large-scale chaotic social changes, which have shaken the Indian socio-economic set-up, the transitions that have overtaken even the most responsible parent population, the outmoded teacher education and practice system, a mismatched teacher-training system that fails to accommodate or consider relevant, contextual changes. All of these have uprooted the possibility of a sound utility-orientation. What, then, persist are varied forms of social menaces that are pernicious to a healthy social system. For, it is the school atmosphere that conditions the psychological strength of the young. In normal circumstances, an institution acts as a complementary system that further trains and enhances what a child learns at home. It is in the context of an educational atmosphere that the teachers' influences have a bearing on the young and serve to install impeccability in their minds. But, indifference, impatience, petulance, sarcasm and excess criticism on the part of a teacher, can also deform positive personality developments in the young. For, in the case of such situations, a student is caught unawares, that too in adolescence, as well as in the midst of drastic social changes. He, thereby, loses his grip over the contingencies that soon over-take his sensibilities too. It is important to revamp the teacher education programme, to encompass a larger psychological orientation, for, as rightly put "… the role of a teacher, as a mentor to channelize, filter and adapt […] information to a child's level of understanding cannot be undermined, let alone be ruled out. Of course, the change in perspective with … education as commodity, teacher as a service provider and parent as client has led to a loss of respect among the students. …respect, which was integral to the classroom atmosphere, has simply flown out of the window".[3]

Assessment of Possibilities: Pros and Cons

Is the situation correctable? Can the entire teaching population of a nation known for its plurality of sorts be brought under the ambit of a revamped teacher education system? A country like Finland took six years to re-train its teaching–learning system. In contradiction to the past scenario, in India, teachers of the present times seem to have popularized the art of exploitation of students in myriad ways that have further soured the bonding. Ramandeep Kaur's comprehensive views about the deteriorating standards of relationship between teachers and students highlight certain crucial facts about the height of exploitation of students by teachers. He quotes the gory incident of a teacher and Principal of Thakur Vidhya Mandir who hired his ex-students for Rs. 50,000/- to kill his wife; the ruthless incident of a student in Chennai who killed himself after being thrashed and stripped by his teacher; the tragic plight of a student who lost his vision after a teacher threw a duster at him; all these add to the instances of petulance and erratic behaviour among teachers (Kaur 2013). The most appalling truth of all is Kaur's observation on the open, free access to the Internet to both teachers and students who can access erotic and obscene sites at their will. Such exposure not only devalues behavioural ethics but also dismisses discipline absolutely from the lives of the young, no matter what arguments one can present in its favour. The mixture of reasons for exploitation of the young have various entry points that could be enumerated as: the timidity of the student; the self-vested interest of the teacher; the indifference of parents; or also their fear of further maltreatment of their loved ones by the concerned teacher.[4]

Certain tragic reports are worth discussing. Raj Chengappa reports in India Today, of a young boy, Sudhanshu, a Grade XI student, who hanged himself on the day of his results. They found a suicide note on his bed in which he wrote: "Bye

[3]http://timesofindia.indiatimes.com/city/nagpur/Modern-student-teacher-relationship-is-of-understanding-each-other/articleshow/22304311.

[4]http://www.mapsofindia.com/my-india/education/changing-teacher-student-relationship.

everybody. I'm committing suicide. Nobody else is involved. I have decided to end my life because the pressure has started to get to me and I cannot take it any longer. I love my family and I hope they will understand. I love my brother Siddharth and I would like to wish him all the best for the future… I hate the Eco teacher but I'm not doing this because of her".[5] Though the point about the 'Eco' teacher is subtle, it is a matter that cannot be brushed aside as slight and dismissible. There are thousands of Sudhanshus in India whose psychological strengths, confidence levels, and abilities have been brutally assaulted, mutilated, and demeaned by many a thoughtless 'teacher owing to her/his irrationality, ego and vanity. This could be out of sheer lack of understanding, tolerance, patience, tact and attitude on the part of a teacher who is poorly trained who works merely on the basis of immature assumptions that she's always right and refuses to make a balanced psychological assessment of the appeals or even demands of students. As Poonam Batra points out, the core aim of the teacher as an agent whose role is to bring about a social transformation, with the right focus on the practitioner's skills, is no more on the agenda. Instead, what is given primary importance is the idea that teacher education programmes provide easy job opportunities and serve to universalize education. The same report also points out how schools are ill-equipped to handle such issues and that many of the Indian education systems encourage merely an exam-orientation.

Reverse Instances

However, one has to accept the truth that often the present day set-up is that there is also a reverse possibility of occurrences, of teachers taken to task for questioning or chiding or reprimanding a student even for a grievous fault. For instance, the vague promise of rectifying measures in the case of aggressive students, get ruled out as well with the undue intervention of over-protective or influential parents who do not want their young to be questioned or corrected even in the instance of a mistake that needs to be controlled or checked, or at times when the young often seem to have imbibed erroneous behavioural aspects from home.[6]

The repercussion of such thoughtless interventions on the part of parents is a curb on the freedom of teachers and other authorities to implement disciplinary measures or codes of conduct even in seriously reprehensible contexts. Though such extreme cases are rare, one such incident in the recent times is worth recalling. It is of a recent video clipping that went viral on social media of two boys—Vishal and Vikky—of a *Kendriya Vidyalaya* in Bihar in North India, sons of a local gangster beating up another boy inside a classroom, threatening to thrash him up

[5]http://indiatoday.intoday.in/story/growing-number-of-students-commits-suicide-over-exams/1/194023.html.

[6]www.mapsofindia.com/my-india/education/changing-teacher-student-relationship.

again if they were implicated.[7] These incidents though sparse, reflect the haphazard lifestyle and upbringing of the young. They are neither monitored nor cared for by parents and teachers; they are unfortunately at the mercy of the reckless contingencies of modern life, to grow to adulthood on their own. What kind of adults would these young become, is a formidable question that remain better unasked and unanswered; for if the same trend continues the future of the young would be nerve-chilling.

Matters of Social Abhorrence

A recent issue of *The Hindu* reported the possibility of greater rise in young suicides (which already has multiplied in comparison with the past) in the coming years in India, which evokes a sense of social remorse when one considers the profundity of the issue. It is a fact that all society has to be held responsible for such repugnant moulding in educational institutions, by either over indulgent or indifferent parenting. Given all these facts about the young, the moulding yet of the young, is undeniably a social responsibility and a major part of it needs to be holistically nurtured by teachers with whom the young spend a major part of their lives. "More programmes for prevention are needed, programmes that strengthen the rights of adolescents and young people, that respond to their daily needs and hopes, and that help to protect them from harm and prevent them from inflicting harm on others" (Bhabha 2014, p.132).

A Diagnosis of Reasons

However, the reason behind this is that the condition in India today is that schools are either result-oriented or score oriented. The job of the teacher is blithely reduced to being robotic in attitude, as one who needs to merely ensure completion of syllabi and maintain the hundred percent result which adds to the reputation of the school. The question whether a student has understood the subject or whether he learnt it mechanically to score well, is something that the system ignores, just as it ignores the psychological issues of students. Such academic onslaughts cause heavy damage to the psyche of a student. The reason for this is because, schools today have turned into appendices of MNC's that are profit- and fame-oriented. Strategic, practical, well-planned, and organized measures to mould the personality of the young play no part in the curricula. Schemes that promote excessive, unimpassioned commitments that elicit work among school teachers through awards, medals, honours and gifts are trendier today. It is rare to find teachers who are

[7]http://indiatoday.intoday.in/story/bihar-school-student-thrashed-gangster-sons/1/786824.html.

genuinely committed and passionate about being teachers in the true sense of the word and the few that are there are lost in the debris of calamitous politics, of economic power, of reckless hankering after repute and thus remain muted.

Causes and Set-Backs in Teacher-Education and Emphasis on Revamping Course Work

The haste with which syllabi are completed, the mechanical, systematic routine that is practiced by teachers, the lack of a binding, intellectual and emotional rapport with students, have become additional factors that immolate the remains of a teacher–student bond that once existed, until the advent of the web that wrapped us all in its nefarious conceit. However, yet another unpardonable oversight is the random cattle-herding of school teachers through undergraduate teacher-training programmes. The major drawback here is that the teacher training and education programmes merely survive on the reminiscences of an outmoded teacher training system that hardly delve into the psychic and social mishaps of the young or the new Indian teacher–student relationship. It also fails to give updated directives to teachers who are also parents and human beings with emotional set-backs. As a result, as Liu observes of the American and Chinese school set-up, it needs to be understood that, in India too, the teacher–student relationship rests solely on the comfort and confidence that the teacher builds for her students; she needs to be the hub that should strive to build such a strong bond between her and her student (Liu, 1997, p. 157). Unfortunately, this is absolutely lost in new India. Pomeroy observes that the bonding fails and the discredited young have no grasp over how they should behave (Pomeroy, 1999, p. 470). This incompetency on the part of teachers emanates from the failed graduate programme in the discipline of teacher education. For the programme in India still relies on the outmoded syllabi of colonial times, especially in terms of practical applications and in rising up to contextual variations. In other words, much of the programme remains unaltered and deprived of a revamping that would suit the needs of the times. The syllabi, therefore, do not add relevant tips and strategies to tackle the modern young. Poonam Batra points out that the evolution of teacher-education in India mimicked models of the 'monitorial and pupil teacher systems' prevalent in twentieth century Britain and is now considered appropriate for a large mass of teachers. This approach to the education of Indian school teachers has remained unchanged for half a century […] (Batra, 2009, p. 129).

This failure to educate the new teacher to cope with the belligerency of the new phenomenal young is the crux of the whole issue that undermines the teacher–student bond in India. The teacher education programmes need to revamp their syllabi according to the current social conditions which bear multifarious challenges of the times or the syllabi would continue to remain a mismatch to the contemporary young whose characteristics are an absolute contrast to the traditional school kids of yesteryear. Reports between the years 2000 and 2017 in India are a clear vindication of the reckless imbalances that have set into this bonding. As Poonam Batra (2009) states, first of all, there is no connection between the structure of the curriculum and the social milieu of school kids. Secondly, there is mere mechanical rendering of the syllabi rather than encouraging teaching and understanding with passion; besides, she clearly points out that there is no way a 'student-teacher' can analyze her own biases and beliefs, and suggests that the teacher education system should develop its own advanced, enriched attitudes, dispositions, habits and interests; She states that, "The odd mix of a technical-rationalist approach embedded in a matrix of folk pedagogies shape the practice of training teachers and therefore the practice of teaching children in much of the country" (p. 9).[8] The above observations clearly ratify the arguments presented so far. For there is indeed a glaring mismatch in the syllabi which was created for the teacher-trainee of the yesteryears and its incongruous persistence to prevail even in the face of today's chaotic social matrix.

Identifying Challenges for Women as Teachers

Women as mothers and as teachers are a complex and a dual issue. On the one hand, as Vidya Subramaniam points out, there could be specific reasons why a woman chooses to work or remain at home. Her contributions at the home front and official front, either way, are enormous and unaccountable.[9] Nowhere does she receive the support that is due to her. On the other hand, the oppressive trend against women that so lulled the Indian social set-up 60 years back, even now roosts in the same nest and continues to remain unchanged even until 2017. While some women enjoy job opportunities and entrepreneurship and are dexterous at managing both duties well, there are many, especially those who belong to the lower middleclass, who scuffle with duties at home and the workplace. The services of most women are neither acknowledged nor accepted as crucial. There is constant criticism whether women work at home or outside. The sense of appreciation is denied to her. Lack of acknowledgement, especially by peer groups and more especially by superior male authorities, deprives women of psychological self-esteem leading them to sheer frustration. This happens at the home front too where the women as mothers, wives, and daughters-in-law are severely criticized for their inability to cope with individual demands that differ with each person and with each family type. However, whether a woman works in an MNCs or serves as a teacher her plight is the same when it comes to rating her as an employee. While women who officiate top positions in MNCs and IT sectors may have to wait for a span of time for their assignments to be assessed, women who serve as teachers

[8]www.teindia.nic.in/Files/jrm/PPTs/TE Vision and Curricular Thrusts PB.ppt.

[9]www.thehindu.com/opinion/open-page/the-working-mother…/article2354405.ece.

tend to receive criticism on a daily or weekly basis. This almost instantaneous criticism also enfeebles their spirits to try harder or to gain time to expedite their rectification process, be it in terms of upgrading knowledge or attitude. While this is the case with most teachers that are sensitive, teachers who have a high self-esteem suffer ego-issues or related complexes and penalize students in turn to vent their emotions. Ibarra, Ely and Kolb, (2013) in the Harvard Business Review in the context of women in leadership roles, point to the 'Identity shift' that women undergo and the expectation of acknowledgment which is the fundamental motive to any training centre which actually focuses on the larger purpose of a profession. But they also point out that quite often women "have no power to determine their own success". Setbacks are considered as their own faults.[10] The point that needs to be considered here, is that, in what way do teacher education training programmes which train the prime, most pivotal profession that grooms the rest of the world, pay attention to such issues? Do these programmes offer practical training or suggestions to overcome such stringent conditions where teachers are found guilty of misdemeanour or are found to be at fault in handling student-related challenges, or even when their hard work is subjected to severe criticism, and is cast to the onslaught of professional rivalry? Is it safe for future trainees to brush off the teacher's faults and set-backs as her own individual fault? The answer is 'no', as teaching is a unique profession that cannot be taken for granted and set aside for another time. For the obvious reason that, it is those in the teaching profession that create the rest of the world around us and the people therein.

Mandates for the Contemporary Teacher and Teacher-Education Programmes

This thereby forms the very crux of the whole discussion meant to describe the various factors above that affect the teacher–student relationship. For, even though the young are considered as capable of fine potentials, still, their behaviour cannot be taken for granted nor can it be considered uniform or static among the whole lot of them that belong to the same age group. Each individual is from a different and specific social background and the teacher, in special, has to be well-equipped, with different operatives to face challenging contexts. In short, the teacher's job is comparable to that of a Defence personnel who needs to rise to the hour, to the need of the time and is required to be on the alert with the required abilities 'to be' and perform changes in the lives of their wards. Teaching is not merely the provision of knowledge and awareness but it is also creating consciousness of what it is to be a human being, and the values of being well-mannered, and most important of all, to be a good human too. This overall moulding is the most catalytic duty of a teacher, which in turn would very naturally render a fine society and a finer social system.

[10]https://hbr.org/2013/09/women-rising-the-unseen-barriers.

This is best described by Vakil (2016), a policy maker with Tata Trusts, who describes this as "behaviour management".[11] Puhan et al. (2013) draw our attention to the ethics in teacher education. They maintain that there is a gap between the prescriptive methods of Teacher Education and practical applications. This lack of proper coordination thus fails to cater to a holistic application of the principles. The following questions they raise add greater relevance to the point made here: "What training implications stem from the conceptions of teachers regarding ethics and the way it is learned? Which ethical concepts emerge? Is it possible for a deontological code of the teaching profession and training to be articulated in the ethical regulation of the profession? What is the position of teachers in terms of ethical training? To what extent are they satisfied with the training received?"[12]

The most vital arguments the critics bring forth through their study is that of 'self-disclosure', on the part of teachers. Self-disclosure is seen as a mode that offers a directive to students. For, when teachers share their own frustrations discreetly and carefully with students, considering the varying levels of students' psychological abilities and disabilities, those themselves become a sample pattern of emotional regulations for them. These sample patterns then would enable students to channelize their own spirits positively in such similar frustrating situations. Similarly, unlike at homes, the teacher should prudently shun chastising students in the presence of others in school which could leave an inerasable impression in their minds. According to Ramanathan and Parvathy (2012) who remark that "Administering punishment to a student in school is not the same as chastising a child in a family setting. A school is a public space and cannot afford the privacy and containment of shame that a home may. Punishment by a teacher is invariably meted out in the presence of the peer group and even when administered in private, the knowledge of such an act cannot be kept secret, assailing the self-esteem of the errant student".[13]

However, the most important of all is the unrelatedness of theory in Teacher education to class room realities. Yet another crucial suggestion is to bring about flexibility of relevance while handling different student types and the need for persevering with value-oriented education.[14] The best remedial measures in teacher education programme would be to encourage periodical discussions through live interactions between teacher-educators and trainees, between students and teachers; periodical counselling for teacher-educators for updating latest issues, professional discussions between teachers of various categories with a balanced moderator; sharing live, unbiasedly narrated instances from classrooms with counsellors, educators, and colleagues in order to arrive at a resolution applicable to most related contexts, besides value oriented lectures for all categories of teachers, educators,

---

[11]www.hindustantimes.com/…/teaching-teachers…India…/story-Cj9z5ihSwW04YTMKx.

[12]http://pubs.sciepub.com/education/2/12A/1/.

[13]http://www.thehindu.com/opinion/open-page/no-place-for-fear-in-classroom/article2932688.ece.

[14]http://pubs.sciepub.com/education/2/12A/1/.

students and parents, which would at least partially remove the gory instances that are on the increase of late.

Vidhya Srinivasan, in her article "Great students make great teachers", points out to certain relevant points such as, professionalism in the skills and appearance of a teacher, accessibility, love and care, innovative teaching strategies and collaborative team work as essentials of a good teacher.[15] There needs to be mutuality in these aspects and the methods have to develop into positive magnetism between teachers and students. Such aspects on a research footing should be made an integral part of teacher-education. At the outset, though, these may seem simple and easily applicable, with varying degrees of attitude on the part of a teacher and student; a hands-on training alone in exacting contexts would help enrich such experience. A teacher who nurtures ego in her mind would never be able to crawl out of her own traumas and prejudices nor provide care, support, and attachment to students; especially to students that are difficult to manage.

To a great extent, the most difficult students often are the most vulnerable and malleable compared to the 'adhesive' types who outgrow true attachment in the long run. However, simple, direct, spontaneous appreciation could bring around even the most weak or the most difficult student. While this is the case on the one hand, on the other, a blatant truth in the modern context about teachers is their inability to appreciate achievements of their wards. Instead, what surfaces often in classrooms is their ego against the little skills, achievements and pranks of their own students. Either ways it results in curt criticism or sarcasm on the part of the teacher and the student is crudely demoralized.

Mandates for Dual Behavior Variants

Often in such contexts the blame is on students though, "However it is not always easy to be warm and supportive…" as Jennnings and Greenberg put and they further observe, that teachers "… regularly face situations that provoke anger, contempt, disgust, sadness, and frustration, to develop and maintain healthy relationship with their students teachers must find appropriate ways to express (or inhibit) their feelings in classroom setting…Although teachers recognize the importance of regulating their emotions and think they are keeping their feelings hidden from their students, often they are less successful than they imagine" (Jennings and Greenberg 2009 p. 500). The critics further observe that it is more in such contexts that a teacher has to muster up much patience as a reserve to elicit more positive outcomes and responses from her challenging and defiant students. The teacher is a responsible agent and she has to keep in mind that the behavioural differences amounting to misdemeanour could be owing to socially generated

---

[15]http://www.thehindu.com/features/education/great-students-make-great-teachers/article7619381.ece.

differences that have influenced her attitude against that of the concerned student. This may be a fact hard to comprehend but has been proven by Jantine L. Spilt, of University of Amsterdam and her research fellows.[16] In the Indian context, these socially generated difference could be basically economic background, exposure, ethnic background, religion, caste, etiquette, manners, and even countenance in certain cases.

There is a grave necessity for teachers to give students maximum understanding at the adolescent stage; for the victimization of the young that pervades different corners of education are myriad, unfathomable, and often clandestine too. These are inflicted upon them, often without provocation, especially in the contemporary scenario. Various forms of victimization which could be physical, psychological, or emotional are meted out to them and the confused adolescent succumbs to the impact. From being bullied by their peers to being exploited for various purposes, the young, in majority, suffer in silence. This alters their entire outlook towards life. The experiences could be: bullying, derogatory references, beating, harsh familial altercations, deliberate rejection, comparisons with fellow class mates, sexual assaults and abuse, deliberate betrayals, austere, aggressive home atmosphere, academic stress, childhood trauma, discriminations of sorts (a common social matrix in India), deprivation of normal legitimate rights, poverty and its related complexes; all of these are common among the young. An important area of future investigation … (should be) the extent to which young people perceive that adults in their schools practice the behaviors that undermine their sense of worth as a person (for example, ridicule, public embarrassment, violation of privacy, social comparison) and the extent to which these practices undermine their social and emotional well-being (Bhabha, 2014). This could create attention deficit with little understanding from the teachers' side. The adolescent is hardly equipped to face the onslaught and would rather dampen up his emotions. He is so traumatized, that he resorts to venting the frustration through some manifestation or the other which would vary with each individual. A consistent pattern of this may or may not be decipherable to the average teacher. Besides, but for a handful of them, the rest of them gulp down the humiliation and tend to psychologically suffer the consequences, and surrender to the circumstances. These instances undoubtedly have a horrific bearing on their lives and on their personality in the long run. Hartjen and Priyadarsini (2012) comment that, "victimized young people register a variety of psychological and emotional problems that often have a long term impact and sometimes require therapy" (Hartjen and Priyadarsini, 2012, p. 345). This may lead to psychological adjustment problems, low academic performance, aggression, attention-seeking, low self- esteem, fear psychosis, impulsive and boorish reactions and many more (Jennings and Greenberg, 2009, pp. 346–347).

[16]https://www.ncbi.nlm.nih.gov/pmc/articles/PMC3399930/.

Inflation Versus Emotional Issues

Yet another frustrating factor that may aggravate a synchronized inter-personal relationship between the teacher and the student is the over-crowded classroom, which makes this a remote possibility. In such cases, the grim reality for the teacher is the difficulty of uneven distribution of attention and in the decision-making of what or who actually deserves priority. Situations may arise where the priority could be the weaker ones, or the slow learners, or the troublesome ones; or the demand could be to provide more elaborations on some topic or the other under discussion. However, if the number is too large, that is, if the strength of the class exceeds a maximum of 30, then even the most conscientious teacher would find it hard to cope with the varying demands thus leading to stress and irritability. As a result, the teacher thereby would naturally prefer to focus merely on the syllabus and inevitably ignore the behaviour of her students. Such cramming of classes is a common condition in India, even in institutions of Higher Education where the inflation is hardly addressed with disproportionate number of teaching community. Of course, there are prescriptions made by Educational bodies for maintaining certain meaningful norms but effective practice of these norms is arduous to most administrators who hold top positions. In fact, even school principals, in their statements to reporters, have openly confessed such issues. But the large-intake trend, with inadequate planning of Human resource and supportive Infrastructure are big issues in India. This continues even today, in spite of the fact that students too, have confessed academic failure owing to the large mass in class in which they are left to fend for themselves.[17] While such large intake is mimicked by most institutions, considering the passivity and Governmental disregard in bringing about practical and effective transitions in teacher-education programmes to cope with the inflation in student numbers, the issues obviously will largely remain unaddressed for the next couple of decades. In this context, though dilution of quality education is indeed unpardonable, the most loathsome issue is the psychological malevolence this condition leaves upon the teacher too. While an over-crowded class room distorts priorities, Koomen and Spilt add that there is also possible failure among teachers in sustaining a professional and emotional balance. This is owing to the inadequacy in the teacher education programmes that should in fact enable teachers, to maintain a 'distant-emotional-bonding' with her students. In a crammed class room of nearly sixty students, though, such individual bonding could be impossible. Nevertheless, what needs to be noticed here is the impossibility of maintaining 'professional and emotional balance', a vital requirement in teachers. For, if the teacher is of the sensitive, internalizing type, with regard to her relationships with students, it may prove difficult for her to maintain the said balance.[18] While a few smart teachers who practice distant emotional bonding, succeed in maintaining

[17]http://indianexpress.com/article/chandigarh/lack-of-teachers-huge-number-of-students-behind-poor-class-xii-results-govt-schools-4681939???/.

[18]springer.com/article/https://doi.org/10.1007/s10648-011-9170-y.

objectivity all through with their students, the other internalizing type often succumb to emotionality and excessive reactions to the slightest variation in her students' attitude. This widens the scope for conflicts and disparities in the bonding between them. Therefore, this is yet another grave factor that the teacher-educators and related programmes need to equip their trainees with. For, "These programmes need to be informed by reality in the field and the testimonies of [these] young men and women. They must build from empathy with the anxieties of adolescents regarding the commitments and responsibilities they undertake…" (Bhabha, 2014, p. 303).

Flaws and Recommendations

In yet another context, Bolia and Aggarwal (2016), in an article in *The Indian Express*, comment on the ineffectiveness of formal education in India. "India does not have enough teachers, who can even understand, let alone practice, the methods being recommended by the various frameworks". The statement is appropriate in the context of the teacher education framework which is incongruous; an irrelevant appendix that flaunts the education system of the colonial times. In other words, "India's formal education system behaves like an industry of the colonial era. It neither recognizes the current needs of students nor provides the desired infrastructure." They also add that "India needs extensive experiments in education.… A similar rethinking is needed for pedagogy and teacher-training, laws and regulations, and emotional and integral development…. In this process, policymakers should be facilitators, not implementers. They should improve the capacity of the failing public infrastructure, provide authority to the capable institutes, and allow flexibility.[19]

Conclusion and Way Forward

To conclude, our society has been battered by various questionable and iniquitous transitions. These transitions have been rapid and have rendered many of our systems obsolete. The basic requirement to alleviate this insane invasion would be a well-planned execution of practical and effective resolutions that focus chiefly on the young population of India. Educational institutions could serve as the hub of such a make-over and teachers alone can co-ordinate a change as that. Unfortunately, ever since the privatization of educational institutions, a tawdry incentive-culture has seeped into school premises. Though government does set norms for establishing schools, often private schools are sanctioned with

[19]http://indianexpress.com/article/opinion/columns/what-teachers-must-learn/.

deliberate oversight of many rules. A BBC news report states that private schools are profit based and observes that "Private, for-profit schools are a reality—and they perform both well and badly".[20] While there are controversial opinions on the non-profit and profit-oriented private schools in India, the glaring fact is that private schools are a haven compared to the many dysfunctional government schools in India. If government schools functioned as much as the private ones and if either of these could work with finely trained teachers and if teacher-training could enhance that possibility, what more could India ask for? It is still not too late as there are options that could well steer us away from the risk of marooning our educational institutions. And that could be brought about only as Dev Lahiri points out by "… a serious revamping of curriculum to move away from the current content and test and teacher-driven model to one that enhances curiosity, creativity, and sharpens the ability to apply that knowledge to the real world". [21]

We will have to invest heavily in teacher-training. Teaching should be an 'aspirational' career and those making the choice must be professionally trained and handsomely remunerated. Perhaps there is some merit in the idea of creating an 'elite corps' like the IAS with several top-class training academies all over the country. The private sector must be encouraged, but closely monitored. Today's investors unfortunately view a school only through the 'profit-prism'.[22] In order to transform this dream into a reality there definitely needs to be a revamping of the teacher-education programmes with more focus on hands-on experience and deliberations of day-to-day issues reported from schools during their hands-on training period.

The reformations introduced in the programme should take into consideration, the following factors: choice of teaching as a profession for passion's sake; revamping teacher-education programmes with regard to the needs of hour, with constant debates and deliberations between educational authorities, parents, teachers and students; annual updating of changes in campus, student psyche, and social systems to bring about contextual changes in Teacher education programmes and educators syllabi; trainees' exposure and regular reports on challenging situations; trainees' submission of peculiar, periodical case-studies for generating (hands-on) information, to Education authorities; reintroduction of positive orientation of relevant behavioural ethics; psychological counselling and orientations to teachers and students; sizing down numbers of students in classes; syllabi that evoke curiosity to knowledge rather than marks-oriented examinations; invoking students to pursue interest-based activities; well-trained teaching community that would rise up to nurture, care, and train; objectivity, emotional and intellectual balance in trainees; strict revamped laws that eliminate profit-oriented awards and incentives for teachers that are purely enslavement-operatives; uniform norms that

[20]http://www.bbc.com/news/business-20641059.

[21]http://indianexpress.com/article/opinion/columns/school-education-job-market-delink-indian-system-professions-column-2892085/.

[22]See Footnote 20.

abolish profit, and mechanical marks-oriented private schools; instantaneous elimination of laborious tasks; promotions and over-time incentives to teachers in private schools; behaviour-regulating personality development programmes in schools for both teachers and students; meditation and yoga to overcome stress; frequent cultural, craft, and talent oriented activities; assignment-free vacations for all; encouraging innovations in teachers and students; gradation of schools by students graduating in the final year of the +2. These and more such innovations alone could possibly overcome the monotonous colonization of students, teachers, and the teacher-education system.

References

Bhabha, J. (Ed.). (2014). *Human rights and adolescence*. University of Pennsylvania Press.

Hartjen, C. A., & Priyadarsini, S. (2012). *The global victimization of children: Problems and solutions*. Springer Science & Business Media.

Hughes, J. N. (2011). Longitudinal effects of teacher and student perceptions of teacher-student relationship qualities on academic adjustment. *The Elementary School Journal, 112*(1), 38–60.

Hughes, J. N. (2012). Teacher–student relationships and school adjustment: Progress and remaining challenges. *Attachment and Human Development, 14*(3), 319–327. https://doi.org/10.1080/14616734.2012.672288.

Jennings, P. A., & Greenberg, M. T. (2009). The pro-social classroom: Teacher social and emotional competence in relation to student and classroom outcomes. *Review of Educational Research, 79*(1), 491–525. https://doi.org/10.3102/0034654308325693.

Liu, J.-Q. (1997). The emotional bond between teachers and students: Multi-year relationships. *Phi Delta Kappan, 79*(2), 156.

McClowry, S. G., Rodriguez, E. T., Tamis-LeMonda, C. S., Spellmann, M. E., Carlson, A., & Snow, D. L. (2013). Teacher/student interactions and classroom behavior: The role of student temperament and gender. *Journal of Research in Childhood Education, 27*(3), 283–301.

Pomeroy, E. (1999). The teacher-student relationship in secondary school: Insights from excluded students. *British Journal of Sociology of Education, 20*(4), 465–482.

Spilt, J. L., Koomen, H. M., & Thijs, J. T. (2011). Teacher wellbeing: The importance of teacher–student relationships. *Educational Psychology Review, 23*(4), 457–477.

E-sources

Batra, P. (2011). http://teindia.nic.in/Files/jrm/PPTs/TE_Vision_and_Curricular_Thrusts_PB.ppt.

Batra, P. (2009). *Teacher empowerment: The education entitlement-social transformation traverse*. http://www.teindia.nic.in/e9-tm/Files/Poonam-Batra-Teacher-Empowerment-CED-6-2.pdf.

Batra, P. (October 1, 2005). http://www.teindia.nic.in/e9-tm/Files/NCF_documents/Poonam-Batra-Voice-Agency-Teachers-EPW_October-1-7.pdf.

Batra, P. (October 1, 2009).*Teacher education and class room practice in India*. http://episteme4.hbcse.tifr.res.in/review-volume/9-batra.

Bolia, N., & Aggarwal, S. (2016, February 1). *What Teachers Must Learn: India's education system is totally out of step with times*. The Indian Express. http://indianexpress.com/article/opinion/columns/what-teachers-must-learn/.

Britland, M. (2013, October 28). *Do teachers need to be qualified? Don't ask such silly questions*. The Guardian.

Chengappa, R. (2005, March 28). *Killer exams: How to revamp the system*. India Today. http://indiatoday.intoday.in/story/growing-number-of-students-commits-suicide-over-exams/1/194023.html.

Dix, P. (2010, February 9). *How to manage behavior in the class room*. The Guardian. https://www.theguardian.com/society/joepublic/2010/feb/09/pupil-behaviour-management-tips.

Fried, R. L. (2001). *The passionate teacher: A practical guide. Harvard Educational Review, 72* (4), 304. http://hepg.org/her-home/issues/harvard-educational-review-volume-72-issue-4/herbooknote/the-passionate-teacher_50. Boston: Beacon Press.

Gablinske, P. B. (2014). A *case study of student and teacher relationships and the effect on student learning*. University of Rhode Island. http://digitalcommons.uri.edu/cgi/viewcontent.cgi?article=1284&context=oa_diss.

Goodman, S. (2015, February 25). *The importance of teaching through relationships*. Edutopia, George Lucas Educational Foundation. https://www.edutopia.org/blog/importance-teaching-through-relationships-stacey-goodman.

Herminia, R. J., Deborah, E., & Kolb, M. (2013, September). *Women rising: The unseen barriers. Harvard business review*. https://hbr.org/2013/09/women-rising-the-unseen-barriers.

Kaur, R. D. (2013, June 24). *Changing teacher-student relationship*. Maps of India Site. http://www.mapsofindia.com/my-india/education/changing-teacher-student-relationship.

Lahiri, D. (2016, July 4). *School for the future: Education needs to be delinked from ideology and the job market*. The Indian Express. http://indianexpress.com/article/opinion/columns/school-education-job-market-delink-indian-system-professions-column-2892085/.

Lahiri, D. (2017, April 7). *Failing the student*. The Indian Express, http://indianexpress.com/article/opinion/columns/failing-the-student-board-examinations-scholls-universities-knowledge-children-student-4602662/.

Puhan, R. R., Malla, L. & Behera, S. K. (2013, June 24). Current ethical issues in Teacher Education: A critical Analysis on pre-service and in-service emerging teachers. *American Journal of Educational Research, 2*(12A), 1–7. https://doi.org/10.12691/education-2-12A-1. http://pubs.sciepub.com/education/2/12A/1/.

Ramanathan, H., & Parvathy, P. B. (2012, March 4). *No place for fear in the classroom*. The Hindu. www.thehindu.com/opinion/open-page/no-place…classroom/article2932688.ece.

Ramasundaram, A. (2011, August 14). *The working mother, a winner all the way*. The Hindu. www.thehindu.com/opinion/open-page/the-working-mother…/article2354405.ece.

Seharawat, Y., & Kumar Singh, R. (2016, October 14). *Student thrashed in Bihar school opens up: Gangster's sons threatened to kill me*. India Today. http://indiatoday.intoday.in/story/bihar-school-student-thrashed-gangstersons/1/786824.html.

Sharmal, S. (2013, September). *Modern-student relationship is about understanding each other*. Times of India. http://timesofindia.indiatimes.com/city/nagpur/Modern-student-teacher-relationship-is-of-understanding-each-other/articleshow/22304311.

Spilt, J., Hughes, J. N., Wu, J.-Y., & Kwak, O.-M. (2012, April). Dynamics of teacher-student relationships: Stability and change across elementary school and the influence on children's academic success. *Child Development, 83*(4), 1180–1195. doi:https://doi.org/10.1111/j.1467-8624.2012.01761. https://www.ncbi.nlm.nih.gov/pmc/articles/PMC3399930/.

Srinivasan, V. (2016, March 28). *Great students make great teachers*. The Hindu. www.thehindu.cosm/features/education/great-students…teachers/article7619381.ece.

Subramanian, V. (2014, March 2). *Working vs. stay-at-home moms*. The Hindu. www.thehindu.com/opinion/open…/working-vs.-stayathome-moms/article5740972.ec.

Tamang, V. (2017, May 31). *Lack of teachers, huge number of students behind poor class XII results: Govt schools*. The Indian Express. http://indianexpress.com/article/chandigarh/lack-of-teachers-huge-number-of-students-behind-poor-class-xii-results-govt-schools-4681939/.

Vakil, S. (2016, September 15). *Teaching teachers, the great challenge for India's education system*. The Hindustan Times. www.hindustantimes.com/…/teaching-teachers…india…/story-Cj9z5ihSwW04YTMKx.

Yasmeen, S., Nehru, A., Joshi, D., & Raghupathi, H. (2017, June). *License-permit-quota-raj-crushing-indias-private-schools*. http://www.educationworld.in/magazine/more/4870-licence-permit-quota-raj-crushing-indias-private-schools.

(January 15, 1976). *Indian women: Yesterday, today and tomorrow*. http://indiatoday.intoday.in/story/indian-women-yesterday-today-and-tomorrow/1/436978.html.

(March 2, 2017). *8 teachers in Rajasthan, rape student make video*. The Hindu. http://www.thehindu.com/news/national/8-teachers-in-rajasthan-rape-student-make-video/article17664574.ece.

Confederation of Indian Industry. (2013). *Towards-professional-preparation-teacher educators-Intel-CII*. http://www.teindia.nic.in/js/Towards-Professional-Preparation-TeacherEducators-Intel-CII.pdf.

Public Agenda. (May, 2004). *Teaching interrupted: Do discipline policies in today's public schools foster the common good*? https://www.publicagenda.org/files/teaching_interrupted.pdf.

National Association for the Education of Young Children. (2009, January). *The Mentor-Student Relationship—From Observer to Teacher*. Young Children. https://www.naeyc.org/files/yc/file/On%20Our%20Minds%20NAEYC.pdf. http://www.ncert.nic.in/html/pdf/schoolcurriculum/framework05/School%20and%20Classroom%20environment.pdf.

(2012, December 11). *Can Private Schools Teach the World*? BBC News. http://www.bbc.com/news/business-20641059.

Chapter 17
School Principals as Leaders: Major Research Trends and Future Directions

Bishakha Majumdar

Abstract Leadership in schools has been of interest to educational psychologists and policymakers for decades, owing to the significant impact it has on school outcomes such as school performance, school environment, satisfaction and commitment of the teachers, and psychological well-being of the students. The major trends that have appeared in school leadership research have evolved from essentially individual-centric explorations to more holistic and empowerment-oriented approaches, as indicated by the emergent themes of transformational leadership, distributive leadership, and shared leadership. Further, while earlier studies have focused on the nature and outcomes of effective school leadership, recent research has revealed that the effectiveness of a leadership style depends on the national culture and the consequent cultural values of the other members of the faculty and the students. This has led to school leadership being seen, unlike before, as a highly contextual competence. Finally, studies have also revealed situations that might ameliorate the impact of negative leadership, such as social support and school culture. This chapter traces the evolution of research in the field of school leadership to compute the major themes that emerged over the years, along with the important antecedents and outcome variables that have been explored. Of significant importance are their implications for management practices: for instance, exploring school leadership as a trainable attribute, or creating a school environment that enhances the impact of positive leadership practices. The chapter also explores the latest developments in the field, with special focus on the Indian educational scenario, and identifies future areas for research in this field.

Keywords Leadership · School · Principal · Teachers · Review

B. Majumdar (✉)
Organizational Behavior and Human Resource,
FORE School of Management, New Delhi, India
e-mail: f11bishakham@iimidr.ac.in

S. Deb (ed.), *Positive Schooling and Child Development*,
https://doi.org/10.1007/978-981-13-0077-6_17

Introduction

> You can have great teachers, but if you don't have a good principal, you won't have a good school.
>
> —Eli Broad, Founder, KB Home and SunAmerica (azquotes, n.d.)

Perhaps one of the most potent influences on a person's life in the early years, apart from the immediate circle of family and caregivers, is the school. Children spend, on an average, 10–15 years of their life in schools (Klein 2014), where they pick up basic knowledge about natural and human sciences, language and mathematics skills, and life skills. The school and its staff—the teachers, the principal, and the administrative personnel—exercise a considerable impact on how the society at large is functioning at any given moment. With increasingly frequent waves of technological advancements and demographic changes, the world today is dynamic and complex. To survive, be relevant, and train future personnel for such an environment, schools too need to be dynamic in adapting to the changing times, being responsive to the environment, resilient to shocks, and proactive rather than reactive in approach.

Leadership studies have found relevance in almost every professional context, and there has been a substantial amount of research devoted to the area of leadership in schools. The task of the school principal as a leader is especially complex, for s/he has to devote his/her skills to inspire and guide and maintain a delicate balance between two sets of people at any given time: the students and the teachers, who, by the virtue of age and maturity, differ astronomically in terms of their life goals, skills, and preferred leadership styles. The leadership in schools, headed by the principal, plays a major role in how schools deliver on core responsibilities, attract and retain personnel, and inspire generations of students to be valued members of society (Anderson 2017). According to Hall et al., "In our schools, districts, and education systems, we must have school leaders and effective leaders to achieve the results that our society requests and requires" (2016, 2).

In the following sections, we explore the development of the concept of school principal leadership, the theoretical bases, and the practice orientations, and the antecedents and consequences of effective leadership.

The Role of the School Principal

Since the beginning of organized schooling, schools traditionally have had a pyramidal structure across the world, headed by the Principal or the Head Master/Head Mistress, followed by the teachers, and then the non-teaching staff. The Principal is traditionally one who has been an educator himself or herself, or at least has had prolonged experience as an administrator in the education field. In the religious settings, the school principal additionally needs to hold a high position in the religious hierarchy, as in case of priests or nuns in Christian missionary schools, *maharaj*s or *sanyasini*s in Hindu religious schools, or *maulavi*s in Islamic *madrasa*s, to name a few.

Leithwood et al. opined that "School leadership is second only to classroom teaching as an influence on pupil learning" (2008, 27). However, there has been considerable discussion on the activities that the Principal should undertake in order to exercise this influence. One important distinction in this context is that between school leadership and school management. While school management is concerned with maintenance of operations of the school, school leadership also consists concerns with of developing individuals, shaping attitudes and behaviours, and improving school performance (Bush and Glover 2004; Dimmock 1999).

Further Hallinger et al. (1983) stated that a school principal has three major activities: setting the mission of the institution, overseeing the educational activities, and creating a positive environment for learning. On similar lines, Truong et al. (2017) stated that school leadership practices include organizational development, building the culture, and goal setting. Pont et al. (2008) state that the Principal has two major tasks in any educational institution:

1. Developing the organizational environment in a positive direction (Hoy et al. 1998).
2. Developing teaching styles and methods through detailed feedback (Freedman 2003; Fullan 1995).

Broadly speaking, the principal's task includes setting targets for the students (Knapp et al. 2010), developing a climate suitable for education (Goldring et al. 2009), developing leadership skills in teachers (Yukl 2009), improving teaching and professional learning (Louis and Miles 1990), and managing resources, processes, and data. The tasks of a leader in a school involve building systems that enhance capacities and build collaborations (Ng and Chan 2014) to achieve teaching goals.

In sum, according to Pont et al. (2008), the four important tasks of the school leader are as follows:

1. To support teachers develop professionally (OECD 2005), by improving the curriculum, evaluating teaching practices, promoting a collaborative work culture, and investing in professional development;
2. To define the goals of learning and to assess the students' performance, by setting school goals in adherence with national and international standards, using data to measure progress, and making needed interventions so that students achieve their potential;
3. To use resources strategically and align all activities in the school to achieve the goal of excellence in teaching and learning;
4. To interact with the community beyond the school such as other schools, policy makers, universities, communities, and social agencies, to create value through mutual assistance.

The task of the principal to link the school with the surrounding environment (Hargreaves et al. 2008) is highly crucial, although it is often neglected. Vogel et al. (2014) state that the task of a principal is to motivate and develop not only the teachers but also the students, their parents, and other staff. Such linkages should also extend to the community, law enforcement agencies, and sports clubs (Fullan 2013).

Fullan (2013) also suggested that the principal has a crucial role as a change agent, in preparing the school for changing situations and challenges. Principals get the school ready to meet the challenges of the future and the demands of the changing environment (Stoll et al. 2002). Mei Kin et al. (2017) demonstrated that the change leadership competences of principals have a positive effect on the change beliefs of teachers and their subsequent positive attitude towards change. In other words, principals who are effective change managers inspire teachers to be open to change and to work to make changes successful.

An important consideration in this context has been the extent to which principals maintain a balance between academic and non-academic leadership activities in the institution. Principals reportedly spend only up to 20% of their time in improving instructional methods (Dipaola and Hoy 2013) and only up to 7% of their time observing teachers in classrooms (Krajewski 2012). Bolman and Deal (2017) reported that principals with more formal education, and lady principals, prefer the role of instructional leaders, involved chiefly in academic pursuits, whereas principals with relatively lower education tend to engage more as general managers. However, as per Jones (2012), most successful elementary school principals reportedly devoted most of their time to academic pursuits.

School Leadership Styles: Major Types

School leadership varies from corporate leadership in its focus on academic enrichment, rather than profitability. Hence, the traditional theories of leadership have been re-conceptualized in the context of school leadership. School leadership styles vary in terms of the end goals that the principal is out to achieve, the amount of participation that is encouraged from the staff, and extent to which external agencies play a role in school management. The following sections categorize some of the major school leadership styles.

Instructional Leadership

This paradigm came into place during the 1980s' effective schools movement (Lezotte 2001). It holds that principals influence the school outcomes by positively affecting the instructional climate (Pan et al. 2015). A positive instructional climate is characterized by an inspiring curriculum, and an emphasis on academics, and caring and collegiality among the teachers, students, parents, and the community

(Witcher 1993). Based on the Far West Laboratory model, Hallinger (1989) reported that, as leaders, principals provide a clear mission to the school, which translates into an instructional focus for the teachers. This, in turn contributes, to student performance. Instructional leadership has been regarded as essential for school growth and initiatives (Lunenberg and Lunenberg 2013).

Colon (1994) used the Iceberg Model to explain instructional leadership. He stated that the principal's observable behaviour is a function of his/her vision, attitude, and knowledge, which, in turn, moulds the learner's behaviour. According to Krug (1992), instructional leadership is characterized by five specific behaviours:

1. *Framing the mission of the school and clearly communicating it to the stakeholders.* Blumberg and Greenfield (1986) stated that instructional leaders are characterized by clear, motivating goals, self-confidence and openness to others, tolerance for ambiguity, willingness to stretch the boundaries, analytical attitude, and control over the job role (Whitaker 1997)
2. *Providing resources that help teachers to carry out classes effectively.* This includes providing technical support (resources, training), emotional support (for health and welfare), and incentives (for professional growth) for teachers (Smith and Andrews 1989). Supervising teaching and providing 'prospective rather than retrospective' guidance
3. *Monitoring performance of students to ensure effective measurement and evaluation.* Principals contribute to instructional implement by being committed to and involved in curricular improvement, monitoring the performance of students and the teacher (Gersten and Carnine 1981)
4. *Promoting an exciting, supportive, and purposeful school environment.* Instructional leaders hold themselves, rather than the staff, responsible for the school climate. According to Niece (1993), instructional leaders tend to be people-oriented, interact regularly with subordinates, remain visible and accessible in the school, maintain network with other principals at the local, state, and the national levels, and have mentors for guidance in their professional activities.

Two more important activities of an instructional leader are co-ordination and troubleshooting through which the principal minimizes paperwork and record-keeping by the teachers as well as classroom interruptions (Duke 1982). This is done by discouraging absenteeism by students, reinforcing rules regularly and discarding redundant rules periodically, distributing resources fairly among the classes, visiting classrooms regularly, training the staff in conflict resolution and problem solving, and generating additional sources of revenue.

Shared/Distributed Leadership

The 'instructional leadership' paradigm views the principal as the primary provider of educational expertise, who sets the educational standards for the institution, and supervises the functioning of the teachers and the students. However, instructional leadership has been criticized to be paternalistic, which tends to elicit docility and passivity from followers (Marks and Printy 2003; Sheppard 1996). The hierarchical conceptualization of instructional leadership came into conflict with the participative management paradigms that became popular during the late 1980s (Marks and Louis 1997), leading to the rise of the paradigm of 'shared leadership'. Shared leadership in the educational context is an extension of instructional leadership that proposes decentralization of the school's leadership and management wherever decentralization is feasible. In this, the principals and the teachers collaborate on the development of the school rules and regulations, curriculum, teaching methods and assessment (Marks and Printy 2003). Thus, the principal is the "leader of instructional leaders" (Glickman 1989, 6), and the responsibilities for the development and maintenance of the school is shared by the principal and the teachers alike.

In 'shared instructional leadership', the principal bestows upon the teachers resources and support to execute and develop school functions. Therefore, the teachers assume responsibility for their own growth and development and solve school problems through collaborative enquiry (Reitzug 1997). Thus, the relationship is reciprocal as the personal resources of the individuals involved are utilized through coordinated actions (Marks and Printy 2003; Ogawa and Bossert 1995).

Shared leadership has been found to have several advantages over traditional instructional leadership. Research shows that principals rarely have the capacity to provide leadership for all the activities in a school (Ryabova 2010; Waldron and McLeskey 2010). This makes shared or distributed leadership critical for school development (Hoppey and McLeskey 2013; Spillane 2006). Owing to their close association with students, teachers possess valuable information about the students, which is useful in curricular development and devising standard teaching styles (Hallinger 1992). Greenlee (2007) reports that teachers' frustration often stem from their lack of understanding of the activities of the school beyond the classroom. Participation in leadership activities enhances the teachers' legitimacy (Little 1988), and improves the teacher's work experience as well as students' performance (Darling-Hammond and Goodwin 1993; Waldron and McLeskey 2010). Malloy and Leithwood (2017) demonstrated that shared or distributed leadership styles lead to planned alignment that, in turn, has a significant and positive relationship to academic optimism. Further, according to (Blase and Kirby 2000), educational reforms had a higher chance of success when teachers were involved than when teachers were not participating in the management, as the former are willing to take risks and try innovative teaching methods (Blase and Blase 1999).

Transformational Leadership

The concept of transformational leadership was popularized by Bass (1990) and further developed by Bass and Avolio (1993) in their 4 I's model. According to this theory, the task of the leader is to transform followers into leaders through idealized influence, inspirational motivation, intellectual stimulation, and individualized consideration (Avolio et al. 1999).

In the educational context, transformational leadership involves providing innovations for the organization, and empowering teachers to develop their decision making skills and emerge as partners in leadership (Conley and Goldman 1994; Leithwood 1994). Thus, it increases the participants' commitment to a cause by making them reach their fullest potential (Bass and Avolio 1993). Lai et al. (2014) demonstrated that transformational leadership by the school principals has a significant effect on continuance commitment and affective commitment of the teachers. Other advantages of transformational leadership include increase in commitment to change (Yu et al. 2002) and higher organizational commitment (Lai et al. 2014).

Leithwood and Jantzi (2005) described transformational leadership in schools as centring on three major areas:

1. *Mission Centred*: developing the school's vision, goals, and priorities
2. *Performance Centred*: providing intellectual stimulation, high performance motivation, and support to the teachers
3. *Culture Centred*: building a productive and collaborative school culture

Integrated Leadership

One major issue with transformational leadership is that it does not imply instructional leadership (Hallinger and Leithwood 1998). Hence the concept of 'integrated leadership' was proposed by Marks and Printy (2003), contending that the earlier models of leadership fail in promoting improvement and sustainability for the leader and the institution at the same time (Donaldson 2001). Instructional leadership is effective to the extent that teachers are committed to the purpose and vision of the principal. Transformational leadership, by sharing leadership responsibilities with the teachers, helps develop the teachers' commitment to causes, and builds their willingness to innovate and lead (Sheppard 1996). Integrated leadership, that fuses transformational and shared instructional leadership, helps in reducing the pressure on the principals in carrying the leadership responsibilities and, at the same time, does not deprive the school of the direction coming from the principal.

Learning Centred Leadership

In learning centred leadership, the focus is on developing in the teachers an attitude to learn and develop, which ultimately results in improved teacher and student performance. It is taken to be inclusive of instructional leadership, transformational leadership, collaborative leadership, and distributed leadership (Liu et al. 2016). It focuses on not only obtaining training for the teachers through workshops and training programmes (outside-in approach) (Cosner 2009), but also systematizing and reusing the professional knowledge available within the organization (Heck and Hallinger 2010).

Diverse Leadership

This concept was proposed by Bolman and Deal (1991), who proposed that leadership in schools is essentially conducted through four frames:

1. *Structure-oriented leadership*: In this, the focus is on the individual staff members' roles, associated tasks and the goals of the organization
2. *Human resources leadership*: Here, the leader focuses on satisfying individual staff members' needs and on the development of healthy interpersonal relations
3. *Politically-oriented leadership*: This focuses on the use of power by the leader and the approaches adopted to negotiate work situations
4. *Symbol-oriented leadership*: This involves creating an organizational image and history, through stories, values, rituals, and shared meanings (Sergiovanni 2008).

Holistic Leadership

The concept of holistic leadership was proposed by Brauckmann and Pashiardis (2011) and Pashiardis (2014), as a model to capture all the behaviours of school leaders that affect the performance of the students either directly or indirectly. It states that effective school leadership has five different elements:

1. *Instructional:* This involves creating teaching and instructional processes with clearly set goals. The target is to improve learning patterns and affect overall school achievement positively (Carrier 2011).
2. *Participative*: In this, the focus is on sharing responsibility and promoting participative management, through democratization of the decision-making process. This helps in developing followers as leaders and reducing the pressure on the principal (Mulford and Silins 2011).

3. *Structuring*: In this, the focus is on the designing of activities in the school in order to create clearly defined roles and responsibilities, and ensuring continuation and stability in the execution of duties. This includes implementation of policies and regulations and maintenance of order.
4. *Entrepreneurial:* In this, the principal focuses on the new opportunities for the schools and the changes that need to be brought about in the way the school is functioning, to keep up with the changing times (Zaidatol et al. 2014).
5. *Personnel development*: In this, the focus is on the professional development of staff and building their expertise, through training, role sharing, and guidance.

In a study on a Malaysian sample, Musa and Noor (2017) reported that principals tended to engage mostly in the instructional style and the structuring style, followed by personnel development and participation. Entrepreneurial style was the least reported among the principals.

Schools vary widely in their contexts, climates, and compositions, and hence the leadership style needed for an urban international school often differs significantly from that required in a small rural school. Further, school leadership styles change to adapt to cultural difference, leading to many new conceptualizations of school leadership. In addition to the major trends, the field of school principal leadership is seeing the rise of many emerging trends (Avolio et al. 2009). For instance, the Team-oriented approach to school leadership, which is similar to that of shared instructional leadership, is well-adopted in collectivist cultures like Japan, where teamwork is highly valued (Balazs 2007; Chen et al. 2017). Another such concept is that of compound leadership, in which school leadership is seen as the compounding of two essentially opposite actions: adoption and delegation (Uhl-Bien et al. 2007). In adoption, the school leader, or the principal, acts as a facilitator, who facilitates the teachers to adjust to the demands of the proposed teaching plans and encourages flow of information (Weberg 2012). In contrast, in case of delegation, the leader empowers the subordinate with the authority to work, design, and develop.

Outcomes of Principal Leadership

Numerous studies show that the principal is the most important factor in deciding the effectiveness of a school (see, for example, Robinson et al. 2007). According to Keefe et al., two things are needed for a productive school: "(1) a positive school learning climate and (2) a principal who supports the establishment and maintenance of this climate" (1985, 70–71). Edmonds (1982) identified leadership in the school as one of the five correlates of an effective school.

School principals, when effective as leaders, create a vision for their teachers and create goals amenable to collective efficacy (Anderson 2017). Principals who show a high regard for their employees build the self-esteem of their teachers, which in turn leads to greater acceptance and camaraderie between the teachers and the students (Beck and Hillmar 1987; Purkey and Smith 1983). Whitakar (1997) reported that principals who encourage creativity and innovation in teaching methods make staff members feel acknowledged for their efforts. Also, principals who are positively involved with teaching skills of the teachers make staff perceive the institutional climate as purposeful and positive. In a study conducted in Italy, Paletta et al. (2017) demonstrated that effective school leadership led to high job satisfaction and self-efficacy among the teachers.

Principals are key in developing the school culture (Peterson 2010) and in deciding whether the school will have a toxic culture (characterized by demoralization, negativism, and fragmentation) or a positive culture (characterized by morale, commitment, sense of purpose, and collegiality) (Deal and Peterson 2016). Pandey (1989), in his study on an Indian sample, revealed that the school climate has a positive impact on the teacher's morale, while Natarajan (2001) showed that an open climate enhances job satisfaction for the teachers. Beycioglu and Kondakçı, (2017) suggested that a bottoms-up approach to leadership that focuses on democratic management, authenticity, and sustainability help in creating a successful school system.

Principals also contribute to building enabling school structures that enhance faculty effectiveness and parental trust in schools (Tarter and Hoy 2004). Effective principals have also been found to contribute to social and community development, beyond the school walls (Sanders and Harvey 2002).

Effective leadership, particularly the tasks such as strategic resource management, defining goals, measuring success, and collaborating with external partners, is positively correlated with students' performance (Marzano et al. 2005; Robinson et al. 2007). Mitchell and Tarter (2016) reported that the principal's professional orientation towards leadership has a positive influence on academic optimism in school as well as professionalism among teachers, which, in turn influenced the achievement levels in schools (Biswas 2009; Cerit 2010). However, great emphasis on students' progress and performance is usually viewed negatively by the teachers who view the climate as non-conducive to risk-taking (Krug 1992). Similarly, while school autonomy is positively correlated to student's performance (OECD 2006), school autonomy has also been found to lead to role overload, and fatigue. Hence, adequate support is necessary for routine work while forcing instructional leadership (Pont et al. 2008).

Leithwood et al. (2008) state that effective leadership enhances the motivation and commitment of the teachers, as well as their capacities. At the same time, it has a positive effect on the working conditions. All these lead to improvement of school practices that in turn enhances school outcomes (Leithwood and Jantzi 2005).

Interventions to Develop Effective Leadership in Schools

There have been different opinions on what makes good school leaders. Some scholars recommend recruitment of talented leaders who have not previously been part of the school system, while others recommend recruitment of good teachers, who are already familiar with the school system (Darling-Hammond et al. 2002). It is also important that the leader has familiarity with the school settings and cultural contexts, because the knowledge, skills, and attitudes needed to lead a small village school are quite different from those needed to lead a large urban school (Leithwood et al. 2004). Studies show that it is difficult to attract and retain good people for school leadership (Knapp et al. 2003). Further, those who join are often not prepared for the demands of the job (Levine 2005; Young 2002). Again, unplanned succession of principals negatively affects the school's progress (Fink and Brayman 2006; Macmillan 2000). Having Inefficient leaders leads to greater attrition rates among teachers (Fiore 2004).

With the growing understanding of the importance of the leadership skills of principals for school improvement, and the reported shortage in the number of able candidates for the principal's position (Clayton 2014; Vogel et al. 2014), several interventions have been suggested to develop leadership skills in this population, to replace and supplement the traditional 'one shot workshops' (Davis et al. 2005; Peterson 2002). It is increasingly being recognized that earlier principles of school management may not suit twenty-first century educational institutions, and that there is a need to ensure a steady pipeline of future leaders to combat attrition and retirement in leadership posts (Pont et al. 2008). The National Commission for the Advancement of Educational Leadership Preparation (NCAELP) of USA recommends both preparatory and in-service programmes to enhance leadership skills of principals at different stages of their careers (Young 2002). The end goal is to create a set of shared values, beliefs, and knowledge about effective administrative practice (Knapp et al. 2003), and make the principals position-ready (Anderson 2017). According to Harvey and Holland (2011), the process of ensuring good leadership for schools includes the following: setting clear job descriptions for principals; providing good training for aspirants of the post; hiring selectively; providing on-the-job support; and evaluating principals regularly.

According to Davis et al. (2005), school principal development programmes have the following features:

Knowledge

Leadership programmes focus on imparting knowledge about theories of learning and teaching, change management, and organizational development. These also focus on theories of leadership, such as ethical and instructional leadership, overview of the values, contexts, and social systems in which a school functions, and related concerns such as diversity, equity, and holistic development.

Skills

School leadership programmes focus on skills such as collaborative decision-making, use of technology for school improvement (Knapp et al. 2003; Davis et al. 2005), critical thinking, reflection, managerial competence, and distributed leadership.

Methods

Leadership development programmes for school principals use a variety of instructional methods to facilitate adult earning and application of learnt information. Hence, the focus tends to be high on experiential learning and simulations. Methods employed include:

1. Field-based internships (Daresh 2001; Murphy 2006), where candidates deal with day-to-day problems of an administrator under the guidance of a mentor. Mentors are usually administrators of schools, or principals themselves, who impart knowledge through coaching, modelling, probing to assist self-reflection, counselling, and feedback (Daresh 2001; Lave 1991). Direct exposure to leadership tasks helps candidates develop the skills needed to excel on the task (Ng and Chan 2014).
2. Problem-based Learning (PBL), where theoretical knowledge is used to solve simulations complex problems from real life, and receive feedback through assessments (Hallinger et al. 2017).
3. Cohort groups, where the candidates for future leadership, as well as experienced leaders, are grouped into cohorts, where learning takes place through collaboration, mutual assistance, group learning, teamwork, and emotional and social support to solve actual work problems. Cohort groups have been found useful in developing skills among principals as well as developing networks that assist in further professional development. Further, they facilitate adult learning through collaboration with peers and feedback (AITSL 2015; Jensen et al. 2015).

In the USA, most schools have assistant principals, whose roles provide them with on-the-job exposure to the demands of the principals' work and prepare them to face the challenges (Militello et al. 2015). The quality of the training for leadership has been found to determine the quality of subsequent leadership (see Anderson 2017). Eckman (2017) explored the co-principal leadership model in a US school and found it beneficial for providing leadership stability and succession planning, and develop shared decision making. However, research also shows that most school leadership programmes are unable to prepare the leaders for the actual demands on the job (Lynch 2012).

School Leadership Research in India

India has one of the world's highest percentages of school dropouts, although, in recent times, it has made considerable progress in increasing school enrolment (Kingdon 2007). Despite the large body of research in this field, school leadership remains a topic that remains to be explored adequately, not only in India, but also across Asia (Truong et al. 2017). Several scholars have expressed the need for more extensive research in cross-cultural contexts to establish how principal leadership is a function of the national character (Mertkan et al. 2016; Walker and Hallinger 2015). It has been found that national culture plays a major role in determining the leadership style of school principals. Harris et al. (2017) demonstrated that school principals in South East Asia display instructional leadership.

Truong et al. (2017) reports that leadership in Vietnamese schools is strongly impacted by considerations of power, distance, and collectivism, as well as Confucian values (Hofstede 1991), while Japanese culture adheres to a team approach to leadership (Chen et al. 2017; Ishikawa 2012). Teachers in Singapore and Hong Kong were not open to participative management due to a strong sense of hierarchy and the need to have harmony, unlike teachers in Australia (Dimmock and Walker 2005).

Indian culture has a unique professional identity for the teachers. The traditional view is that of the teacher as *Guru*, which is very different from the western ideals of the professional concerned with selling academic services and performing bureaucratic functions (Kale 1970). Research done in the Indian setting on school leadership has shown both similarities and differences with the international trends (Sharma 2001). Khetarpal and Srivastava (2000) stated that the principals' behaviour, work practices, and interpersonal relations influence the schools' performance in the Indian context. In a study in an Indian sample, Arani and Abbasi (2004) revealed that professional growth and personal happiness lead to high engagement for teachers at work, as does a sense of control and interpersonal cooperation. Specifically, they proposed that a bureaucratic impersonal attitude of the principal, as well as micro-management of the staff, can have a detrimental effect on the morale of the teacher. Further, the impact of the principal's behaviour on the teachers' morale was seen to be much greater in case of the Indian sample than in case of an Iranian sample, suggesting the importance of the principal's role in Indian schools. Bhatnagar and Das (2014) report that Indian teachers look up to the school principal for resources and training, attitude modification of teachers, and inclusion programmes for children with special needs.

Directions for Future Research

Leadership by school principals is a topic that has considerable academic as well as practice-related significance. Effective school leadership, which is contextual and contemporary, helps in developing the institutions that form the base of a nation. The differences in the national culture and educational values in India and in the Western world necessitate that best practices of the western education system are re-explored for their effectiveness before adoption in the Indian system. Further, India being a vast country with wide geographical, sociological, and demographic variations, leadership practices need to be locally customized, rather than taking a 'one-size-fits-all' approach.

Another interesting topic might be the role of demographics in leadership by school principals. While the majority of school teachers in most countries are women, the representation of women in school leadership positions is below the average. Further, most women principals are found at the primary school level, rather than at the secondary school level (Pont et al. 2008). This finding is interesting, particularly in the light of the fact that, in many Asian countries including India, teachers do not regard male and female principals differently (Sharma et al. 2012). Further research is needed to know the impact of gender on school principals' leadership styles and effectiveness.

Principals are ineffective when tensions exist between school board and the principal, which can happen when: the board is either non-participative or overbearing; there is lack of clarity about the role of the board; and there is lack of skills in board members (Pont et al. 2008; Wylie 2007). Research is needed in the Indian context to explore the role of the school board in school effectiveness, and on the optimal level of participation by the school board in the school decision making.

Finally, the principals' leadership roles may vary with the special needs that the students bring. Silva et al. (2017) showed that principals may promote social justice through providing emotional education, social cohesion, and support. Future research may explore the impact of catering to special needs of students on the personal and professional lives of principals, and the role of tertiary support systems —such as the Board, NGOs, or educational authorities—in this context.

Yukl (2002) defined leadership as a "social influence process whereby intentional influence is exerted by one person [or group] over other people [or groups] to structure the activities and relationships in a group or organization" (p. 45). There are few other contexts in which the nature, scope, and outcome of such influence is of more importance than in the case of schools. Extensive research in this direction may influence policy actions and organizational development at a desired scale, so that schooling becomes a meaningful experience for all the stakeholders involved.

References

AITSL. (2015). Preparing future leaders effective preparation for aspiring school principals. *Australian institute for teaching and school leadership*. Retrieved from https://www.aitsl.edu.au/docs/default-source/school-leadership/principal-preparation/preparing-future-leaders.pdf.

Anderson, K. L. (2017). *School leadership preparation: Aspiring principal succession*. Doctoral dissertation, Grand Canyon University. Retrieved from https://www.aitsl.edu.au/docs/default-source/school-leadership/principal-preparation/preparing-future-leaders.pdf.

Arani, A. M., & Abbasi, P. (2004). Relationship between secondary school teachers' job satisfaction and school organizational climate in Iran and India. *Pakistan Journal of Psychological Research, 19*(1/2), 37.

Avolio, B. J., Bass, B. M., & Jung, D. I. (1999). Re-examining the components of transformational and transactional leadership using the multifactor leadership. *Journal of Occupational and Organizational Psychology, 72*(4), 441–462.

Avolio, B. J., Walumbwa, F. O., & Weber, T. J. (2009). Leadership: Current theories, research, and future directions. *Annual Review of Psychology, 60,* 421–449.

Azquotes (n.d.). *Eli broad*. Retrieved from http://www.azquotes.com/quote/36517.

Balazs, V. (2007). *Is Japanese management different? History and future for Japanese management methods*. Retrieved from http://www.edamba.eu/userfiles/file/Balazs%20Vaszkun.pdf.

Bass, B. M. (1990). From transactional to transformational leadership: Learning to share the vision. *Organizational Dynamics, 18*(3), 19–31.

Bass, B. M., & Avolio, B. J. (1993). Transformational leadership and organizational culture. *Public Administration Quarterly*, 112–121.

Beck, A. C., & Hillmar, E. D. (1987). *Positive management practices*. San Fransisco, CA: Jossey-Bass.

Beycioglu, K., & Kondakçı, Y. (2017). Understanding leadership practices in a sustainable school model: A case from Turkey. In *Building for a sustainable future in our schools* (pp. 151–169). Springer International Publishing.

Bhatnagar, N., & Das, A. (2014). Regular school teachers' concerns and perceived barriers to implement inclusive education in New Delhi, India. *International Journal of Instruction, 7*(2), 89–102.

Biswas, S. (2009). Organizational culture & transformational leadership as predictors of employee performance. *The Indian Journal of Industrial Relation, 4*(4), 611–627.

Blase, J., & Blase, J. (1999). Principals' instructional leadership and teacher development: Teachers' perspectives. *Educational Administration Quarterly, 35*(3), 349–378.

Blase, J., & Kirby, P. C. (2000). *Bringing out the best in teachers: What successful principals do*. Thousand Oaks, CA: Corwin Press.

Blumberg, A., & Greenfield, W. (1986). *The effective principal: perspectives on school leadership*. MA: Publication Sales, Allyn and Bacon.

Bolman, L. G., & Deal, T. E. (1991). *Reframing organizations*. San Francisco: Jossey-Bass Publishers.

Bolman, L. G., & Deal, T. E. (2017). *Reframing organizations: Artistry, choice, and leadership*. New York, NY: Wiley.

Brauckmann, S., & Pashiardis, P. (2011). A validation study of the leadership styles of a holistic leadership theoretical framework. *International Journal of Educational Management, 25*(1), 11–32.

Bush, T., & Glover, D. (2004). *Leadership development: Evidence and beliefs*. Nottingham, England: National College for School Leadership.

Carrier, L. (2011). *What is instructional leadership and what does it look like in practice? A multicase case study of elementary school principals who have led schools from being identified as under performing to performing*. Doctoral Dissertation. University of

Massachusetts Amherst. Retrieved from http://search.proquest.com/openview/e683224786 3381d5fd0c19a5c768a97e/1?pq-origsite=gscholar&cbl=18750&diss=y.

Cerit, Y. (2010). The effects of servant leadership on teachers' organizational commitment in primary schools in Turkey. *International Journal of Leadership in Education, 13*(3), 301–317.

Chen, Y. G., Cheng, J. N., & Sato, M. (2017). Effects of school principals' leadership behaviors: A comparison between Taiwan and Japan. *Educational Sciences-Theory & Practice, 17*(1), 145–173.

Clayton, J. K. (2014). The leadership lens: Perspectives on leadership from school district personnel and university faculty. *International Journal of Educational Leadership Preparation, 9*(1), n1.

Colon, R. J. (1994). Rethinking and retooling for the 21st century: A must for administrators. *NASSP Bulletin, 78*(564), 84–88.

Conley, D. T., & Goldman, P. (1994). Facilitative leadership: How principals lead without dominating. *OSSC Bulletin, 37*(9), n9.

Cosner, S. (2009). Building organizational capacity through trust. *Educational Administration Quarterly, 45*(2), 248–291.

Daresh, J. C. (2001). *Leaders helping leaders: A practical guide to administrative mentoring*. Thousand Oaks, CA: Corwin Press.

Darling-Hammond, L., Ancess, J., & Ort, S. W. (2002). Reinventing high school: Out-comes of the coalition campus school project. *American Educational Research Journal, 39*(3), 639–673.

Darling-Hammond, L., & Goodwin, A. L. (1993). Progress toward professionalism in teaching. *Challenges and Achievements of American education*, 19–52.

Davis, S., Darling-Hammond, L., LaPointe, M., & Meyerson, D. (2005). Developing successful principals. *Stanford Educational Leadership Institute,* (Ed.).

Deal, T. E., & Peterson, K. D. (2016). *Shaping school culture*. Wiley.

Dimmock, C. (1999). Principals and school restructuring: Conceptualizing challenges as dilemmas. *Journal of Educational Administration, 37*(5), 441–462.

Dimmock, C., & Walker, A. (2005). School leadership in context: Societal and organizational cultures. In T. Bush (Ed.), *The principles and practice of educational management* (pp. 70–85). London: Paul Chapman.

DiPaola, M., & Hoy, W. K. (2013). *Improving instruction through supervision, evaluation, and professional development*. IAP.

Donaldson, G. A. (2001). *Cultivating leadership in schools: Connecting people, purpose, and practice*. New York: Teachers College Press.

Duke, D. L. (1982). Leadership functions and instructional effectiveness. *NASSP Bulletin, 66*(456), 1–12.

Eckman, E. (2017). A case study of the implementation of the co-principal leadership model. *Leadership and Policy in Schools*, 1–15.

Edmonds, R. R. (1982). *Programs of school improvement: An overview*. Retrieved from http://files.eric.ed.gov/fulltext/ED221536.pdf.

Fink, D., & Brayman, C. (2006). School leadership succession and the challenges of change. *Educational Administration Quarterly, 42*(1), 62–89.

Fiore, D. J. (2004). *Introduction to educational administration: Standards, theories, and practice*. Larchmont, NY: Eye on Education.

Freedman, B. (2003, January). *Principal visibility and classroom walk-throughs: Supporting instructional leadership and school improvement.* Paper presented at Annual Conference of the International Congress of School Effectiveness and School Improvement, Sydney, Australia.

Fullan, M. G. (1995). The limits and the potential of professional development. In T. R. Guskey & M. Huberman (Eds.), *Professional development in education: New paradigms and practices* (pp. 253–267). New York: Teachers College Press.

Fullan, M. (2013). *The new meaning of educational change* (3rd ed.). Columbia University, New York, NY: Teachers College.

Gersten, R., & Carnine, D. (1981). *Administrative and supervisory support functions for the implementation of effective educational programs for low income students*. Retrieved from http://files.eric.ed.gov/fulltext/ED208519.pdf.
Glickman, C. (1989). Has Sam and Samantha's time come at last? *Educational Leadership, 46*(8), 4–9.
Goldring, E., Porter, A., Murphy, J., Elliott, S. N., & Cravens, X. (2009). Assessing learning-centered leadership: Connections to research, professional standards, and current practices. *Leadership and Policy in Schools, 8*(1), 1–36.
Greenlee, B. J. (2007). Building teacher leadership capacity through educational leadership programs. *Journal of Research for Educational Leadership, 4*(1), 44–74.
Hall, P., Childs-Bowen, D., Cunningham-Morris, A., Pajardo, P., & Simeral, A. (2016). *The principal Influence: A framework for developing leadership capacity in principals*, ASCD.
Hallinger, P. (1989). Developing instructional leadership teams in secondary schools: A framework. *NASSP Bulletin, 73*(517), 84–92.
Hallinger, P. (1992). The evolving role of American principals: From managerial to instructional to transformational leaders. *Journal of Educational Administration, 30*(3).
Hallinger, P., & Leithwood, K. (1998). Unseen forces: The impact of social culture on school leadership. *Peabody Journal of Education, 73*(2), 126–151.
Hallinger, P., Murphy, J., Well, M., Mesa, R. P., & Mitman, A. (1983). Identifying the specific practices, behaviours for principals. *NASSP Bulletin, 67*(463), 83–91.
Hallinger, P., Shaobing, T., & Jiafang, L. (2017). Learning to make change happen in Chinese schools: Adapting a problem-based computer simulation for developing school leaders. *School Leadership & Management, 37*(1–2), 162–187.
Hargreaves, A., Halász, G., & Pont, B. (2008). The finnish approach to system leadership, a case study report for the OECD improving school leadership activity. *Improving School Leadership, 2*.
Harris, A., Jones, M., Cheah, K. S. L., Devadson, E., & Adams, D. (2017). Exploring principals' instructional leadership practices in Malaysia: Insights and implications. *Journal of Educational Administration, 55*(2), 207–221.
Harvey, J., & Holland, H. (2011). The school principal as leader: Guiding schools to better teaching and learning. *The wallace foundation*.
Heck, R. H., & Hallinger, P. (2010). Collaborative leadership effects on school improvement: Integrating unidirectional- and reciprocal-effects models. *The Elementary School Journal, 111* (2), 226–252.
Hofstede, G. (1991). *Cultures and organizations: Software of the mind*. Maidenhead: McGraw-Hill.
Hoppey, D., & McLeskey, J. (2013). A case study of principal leadership in an effective inclusive school. *The Journal of Special Education, 46*(4), 245–256.
Hoy, W. K., Hannum, J., & Tschannen-Moran, M. (1998). Organizational climate and student achievement: A parsimonious and longitudinal view. *Journal of School Leadership, 8*, 336–359.
Ishikawa, J. (2012). Leadership and performance in Japanese R & D teams. *Asia Pacific Business Review, 18*(2), 241–258.
Jensen, B., Hunter, A., Lambert, T., & Clark, A. (2015). *Aspiring principal preparation, prepared for the Australian Institute for Teaching and School Leadership*. Melbourne: AITSL.
Jones, A. C. (2012). *Becoming a strong instructional leader: Saying no to business as usual*. New York, NY: Teachers College Press.
Kale, P. (1970). The guru and the professional: The dilemma of the secondary school teacher in Poona, India. *Comparative Education Review, 14*(3), 371–376.
Keefe, J. W., Kelley, E. A., & Miller, S. K. (1985). School climate: Clear definitions and a model for a larger setting. *NASSP Bulletin, 69*(484), 70–77.
Khetarpal, I., & Srivastava, R. C. (2000). Management styles grounded in interpersonal roles: Focus on heads of school in India. *International Journal of Educational Management, 14*(2), 74–83.

Kingdon, G. G. (2007). The progress of school education in India. *Oxford Review of Economic Policy, 23*(2), 168–195.
Klein, R. (2014). *These are the countries where kids go to school for the longest*. The Huffington Post. Retrieved from http://www.huffingtonpost.com/2014/07/21/school-life-expectancy-map_n_5599716.html.
Knapp, M. S., Copland, M. A., Honig, M. I., Plecki, M. L., & Portin, B. S. (2010). *Learning-focused leadership and leadership support: Meaning and practice in urban systems*. Seattle, WA: Center for the Study of Teaching and Policy-University of Washington.
Knapp, M. S., Copland, M. A., & Talbert, J. E. (2003). Leading for learning: Reflective tools for school and district leaders. CTP Research Report.
Krajewski, R. J. (2012). *The principal's guide to instructional improvement*. Lanham, MD: Rowman & Littlefield.
Krug, S. E. (1992). Instructional leadership: A constructivist perspective. *Educational Administration Quarterly, 28*(3), 430–443.
Lai, T. T., Luen, W. K., Chai, L. T., & Ling, L. W. (2014). School principal leadership styles and teacher organizational commitment among performing schools. *Journal of Global Business Management, 10*(2), 67.
Lave, J. (1991). Situating learning in communities of practice. *Perspectives on Socially Shared Cognition, 2*, 63–82.
Leithwood, K. (1994). Leadership for school restructuring. *Educational Administration Quarterly, 30*(4), 498–518.
Leithwood, K., Harris, A., & Hopkins, D. (2008). Seven strong claims about successful school leadership. *School Leadership and Management, 28*(1), 27–42.
Leithwood, K., & Jantzi, D. (2005). A review of transformational school leadership research 1996–2005. *Leadership and Policy in Schools, 4*(3), 177–199.
Leithwood, K., Seashore-Louis, K., Anderson, S., & Wahlstrom, K. (2004). *How leadership influences student learning (learning from leadership project executive summary)*. New York: The Wallace Foundation.
Levine, A. (2005). *Educating school leaders*. New York: The Education School Project.
Lezotte, L. W. (2001). Revolutionary and evolutionary: The effective schools movement. Retrieved from https://www.edutopia.org/pdfs/edutopia.org-closing-achievement-gap-lezotte-article.pdf.
Little, J. W. (1988). Assessing the prospects for teacher leadership. In A. Lieberman (Ed.), *Building a professional culture in schools* (pp. 78–108). New York: Teachers College Press.
Liu, S., Hallinger, P., & Feng, D. (2016). Supporting the professional learning of teachers in China: Does principal leadership make a difference? *Teaching and Teacher Education, 59*, 79–91.
Louis, K. S., & Miles, M. B. (1990). *Improving the urban high school: What works and why*. New York: Teachers College Press.
Lunenburg, F. C., & Lunenburg, M. R. (2013). Convergent roles of the school principal: Leadership, managerial, and curriculum-instructional. *International Journal of Education, 1*(1), 1–9.
Lynch, M. (2012). A guide to effective school leadership theories. Routledge.
Macmillan, R. (2000). Leadership succession, cultures of teaching and educational change. *The sharp edge of educational change: Teaching, leading and the realities of reform* (pp. 52–71).
Malloy, J., & Leithwood, K. (2017). Effects of distributed leadership on school academic press and student achievement. In *How school leaders contribute to student success* (pp. 69–91). Springer International Publishing.
Marks, H., & Louis, K. S. (1997). Does teacher empowerment affect the classroom? The implications of teacher empowerment for instructional practice and student academic performance. *Educational Evaluation and Policy Analysis, 19*(3), 245–275.
Marks, H. M., & Printy, S. M. (2003). Principal leadership and school performance: An integration of transformational and instructional leadership. *Educational Administration Quarterly, 39*(3), 370–397.

Marzano, R. J., Waters, T., & McNulty, B. A. (2005). School leadership that works: From research to results. ASCD.
Mei Kin, T., Abdull Kareem, O., Nordin, M. S., & Wai Bing, K. (2017). Principal change leadership competencies and teacher attitudes toward change: The mediating effects of teacher change beliefs. *International Journal of Leadership in Education*, 1–20.
Mertkan, S., Arsan, N., Inal Cavlan, G., & Onurkan Aliusta, G. (2016). Diversity and equality in academic publishing: The case of educational leadership. *Compare: A Journal of Comparative and International Education*, 1–16.
Mitchell, R. M., & Tarter, C. J. (2016). A path analysis of the effects of principal professional orientation towards leadership, professional teacher behaviour, and school academic optimism on school reading achievement. *Societies, 6*(1), 5.
Militello, M., Fusarelli, B. C., Mattingly, A., & Warren, T. (2015). "We do what we're told": How current assistant principals practice leadership and how they wish they could. *Journal of School Leadership, 25*(2).
Mulford, B., & Silins, H. (2011). Revised model and conceptualization of successful school principalship for improved student outcomes. *International Journal of Educational Management, 25*(1), 61–82.
Murphy, J. (2006). *Preparing school leaders: Defining a research and action agenda*. Scarecrow Pr.
Musa, K., & Noor, M. A. M. (2017). School principal holistic leadership: A study in high performance schools in the central zone, Malaysia. *International Journal of Academic Research in Business and Social Sciences, 7*(2), 678–685.
Natarajan, R. (2001). School organizational climate and job satisfaction of teachers: A study. *Journal of Indian Education, 27*(2), 36–43.
Ng, S. W., & Chan, Y. F. (2014). Aspiring principals' perceptions of applicability of acquired leadership capacities in the school context. In *International Studies in Educational Administration (Commonwealth Council for Educational Administration & Management (CCEAM)), 42*(3).
Niece, R. D. (1993). The principal as instructional leader: Past influences and current resources. *NASSP Bulletin, 77*(553), 12–18.
OECD. (2005). *Teachers matter: Attracting*. OECD, Paris: Developing and Retaining Effective Teachers.
OECD. (2006). The teaching workforce: Meeting aspirations and enhancing motivation. *Education Policy Analysis 2005–2006*. Paris: OECD.
Ogawa, R. T., & Bossert, S. T. (1995). Leadership as an organizational quality. *Educational Administration Quarterly, 31*, 224–243.
Paletta, A., Paletta, A., Alivernini, F., Alivernini, F., Manganelli, S., & Manganelli, S. (2017). Leadership for learning: The relationships between school context, principal leadership and mediating variables. *International Journal of Educational Management, 31*(2), 98–117.
Pan, H. W., Nyeu, F., & Chen, J. S. (2015). Principal instructional leadership in Taiwan: Lessons from two decades of research. *Journal of Educational Administration, 53*(4), 492–511.
Pandey, S. (1989). Organizational climate and teacher morale. *Journal of Educational Planning and Administration, 3*(3).
Pashiardis, P. (2014). The conceptualization and development of the Pashiardis-Brauckman holistic leadership framework. In *Modeling school leadership across Europe in search of new frontiers* (pp. 13–46). New York: Springer.
Peterson, K. D. (2002). The professional development of principals: Innovations and oppor-tunities. *Educational Administration Quarterly, 38*(2), 213–232.
Peterson, P. E. (2010). *Saving schools: From Horace Mann to virtual learning*. Harvard University Press.
Pont, B., Nusche, D., & Hunter, M. (2008). *Improving school leadership: Policy and practice* (Vol. 1). OECD publishing.
Purkey, S. C., & Smith, M. S. (1983). Effective schools: A review. *The Elementary School Journal, 83*(4), 427–452.

Reitzug, U. C. (1997). Images of principal instructional leadership: From supervision to collaborative inquiry. *Journal of Curriculum Supervision, 12,* 356–366.
Robinson, V. M., Hohepa, M., & Lloyd, C. (2007). *School leadership and student outcomes: Identifying what works and why* (Vol. 41). Winmalee: Australian Council for Educational Leaders. Retrieved from http://www.peersupport.edu.au/wp-content/uploads/2014/08/Student-leadership.pdf.
Ryabova, G. (2010). Cross-cultural differences in decision-making styles of Thai and foreign principals in Thai and international schools in Bangkok. *Scholar, 2*(1), 30–34.
Sanders, M. G., & Harvey, A. (2002). Beyond the school walls: A case study of principal leadership for school-community collaboration. *Teachers College Record, 104*(7), 1345–1368.
Sergiovanni, T. (2008). *Managing a school, theoretical and practical aspects.* TelAviv: Open University.
Sharma, U. (2001). *The attitudes and concerns of school principals and teachers regarding the integration of students with disabilities into regular schools in Delhi, India.* Doctoral dissertation, University of Melbourne, Faculty of Education.
Sharma, S., Sun, H., & Kannan, S. (2012). A comparative analysis on leadership qualities of school principals in China, Malaysia & India. *International Online Journal of Educational Sciences, 4*(3).
Sheppard, B. (1996). Exploring the transformational nature of instructional leadership. *Alberta Journal of Educational Research, 52,* 325–344.
Silva, P., Slater, C. L., Lopez Gorosave, G., Cerdas, V., Torres, N., Antunez, S., et al. (2017). Educational leadership for social justice in Costa Rica, Mexico, and Spain. *Journal of Educational Administration, 55*(3), 316–333.
Smith, W. F., & Andrews, R. L. (1989). *Instructional leadership: How principals make a difference.* Alexandria: Publications, Association for Supervision and Curriculum Development.
Spillane, J. (2006). *Distributed leadership.* San Francisco, CA: Jossey-Bass.
Stoll, L., Bolam, R., & Collarbone, P. (2002). Leading for change: Building capacity for learning. In K. Leithwood & P. Hallinger (Eds.), *Second international handbook of educational leadership and administration* (pp. 41–73). Dordrecht: Kluwer Academic Publishers.
Tarter, C. J., & Hoy, W. K. (2004). A systems approach to quality in elementary schools: A theoretical and empirical analysis. *Journal of Educational Administration, 42*(5), 539–554.
Truong, T. D., Hallinger, P., & Sanga, K. (2017). Confucian values and school leadership in Vietnam: Exploring the influence of culture on principal decision making. *Educational Management Administration & Leadership, 45*(1), 77–100.
Uhl-Bien, M., Marion, R., & McKelvey, B. (2007). Complexity leadership theory: Shifting leadership from the industrial age to the knowledge era. *The Leadership Quarterly, 18*(4), 298–318.
Vogel, L. R., Weiler, S., & Armenta, A. (2014). Pushing back and forging ahead: Making principal preparation responsive to state and national changes. *Planning and Changing, 45*(1/2), 210.
Waldron, N., & McLeskey, J. (2010). Establishing a collaborative culture through comprehensive school reform. *Journal of Educational and Psychological Consultation, 20*(1), 58–74.
Walker, A., & Hallinger, P. (2015). A synthesis of reviews of research on principal leadership in East Asia.*Journal of Educational Administration, 53*(4), 554–570.
Weberg, D. (2012). Complexity leadership: A healthcare imperative. *Nursing Forum, 47*(4), 268–277.
Whitaker, B. (1997). Instructional leadership and principal visibility. *The Clearing House: A Journal of Educational Strategies, Issues and Ideas, 70*(3), 155–156.
Witcher, A. E. (1993). Assessing school climate: An important step for enhancing school quality. *Nassp Bulletin, 77*(554), 1–5.
Wylie, C. (2007). *School governance in new zealand—How is it working?* New Zealand Council for Educational Research, Wellington. Retrieved from https://www.researchgate.net/profile/Cathy_Wylie/publication/242632582_School_governance_in_New_Zealand_-_how_is_it_working/links/53fd40de0cf22f21c2f7e140.pdf.

Young, M. D. (2002). Ensuring the university's capacity to prepare learning focused leadership. In *Report presented at the meeting of the National Commission for the advancement of educational leadership* (pp. 7–8).

Yu, H., Leithwood, K., & Jantzi, D. (2002). The effects of transformational leadership on teachers' commitment to change in Hong Kong. *Journal of Educational Administration, 40*(4), 368–389.

Yukl, G. A. (2002). *Leadership in organizations*. Upper Saddle River, NJ: Prentice-Hall.

Yukl, G. (2009). Leading organizational learning: Reflections on theory and research. *The Leadership Quarterly, 20*(1), 49–53.

Zaidatol, A. L. P., Afsaneh, B., & Soaib, A. (2014). Entrepreneurial leadership behaviour among school principals: Perspective from Malaysian secondary school teachers. *Pertanika Journal Social Sciences and Humanities, 22*(3), 825–843.

Chapter 18
Towards Positive Schooling, Training, and Motivation: A Teacher Education Model

Vimala Veeraraghavan

Abstract A good school provides practices and activities that would help improve the overall educational climate. Positive learning and teaching environment are essential if students are to succeed in school both in academics, character development, as well as human relations. This chapter focuses on training of teachers to create the required positive climate in the school so that there is effective teaching and learning and inculcation of positive values and attitudes in students. For this to occur, highly trained and motivated teachers with an aptitude for teaching and interacting with children of different age groups from diverse backgrounds are needed. While there are many methodologies to train teachers to make them effective and efficient, the training presently being imparted in Indian colleges and institutions at undergraduate and postgraduate levels is not adequate, either in qualitative terms, or in terms of the large number of teachers needed in government and private schools. In particular, such teachers should be capable of handling students from diverse social, cultural, and economic background and help children achieve their potentials with positive attitudes and values. The chapter also argues for appropriate selection of students for admission to B.Ed. and M.Ed. programmes through entrance examination and assessment by interview. It is important that the selected students should have the aptitude to work with young people and be committed to education and teaching as a full-time vocation. After admission, the trainees should be provided with skills and knowledge that they need in a comprehensive manner. The present training being imparted as part of the B.Ed. and M. Ed. courses should be deepened, with personal supervision and longer periods of guided apprenticeship in good schools. Management and leadership at the school have a key role in promoting positive schooling through school climate and recurrent training, on the lines mentioned above.

V. Veeraraghavan (✉)
Department of Psychology, Delhi University, New Delhi, India
e-mail: vveera2000@gmail.com

V. Veeraraghavan
Department of Psychology, IGNOU, New Delhi, India

S. Deb (ed.), *Positive Schooling and Child Development*,
https://doi.org/10.1007/978-981-13-0077-6_18

Keywords Positive schooling · Teachers · Training · Motivation
Students

Introduction

A recent report in the Hindustan Times, on 8 June 2017, states, on the basis of official data, that about 200,000 students were enrolled in government schools in Delhi in Grade 11 in the year 2014. Out of this, around 133,000 were enrolled in Grade 12 in 2015. Another 15,000 had been re-enrolled in Grade 11; these were the detained students. The remaining, around 45,000, disappeared from the system; they were the drop-outs in grade 11. There will be further drop-outs in Grade 12, as well as a number of failures. Even those who complete Grade 12 successfully may not have the kind of knowledge and skills they need for tomorrow's world. This tremendous waste of human potential is not confined to government schools; except for some very good schools, the same situation will obtain in private schools.

It may be argued that the pass or fail in Grade 12, signifying satisfactory completion of higher secondary education or even high marks obtained in Grade 10 or Grade 12, are not the sole or even the main indicators of effective and successful education. If the system has produced effective learners, who continue their learning through their life, it may be said that education has achieved its purpose. But there are no indicators that this is indeed true. One must therefore conclude that the present system of education is not providing the learning that the youth of today desperately need.

We can hold many factors, both institutional and individual, responsible for this state of affairs, but one single effective reform pertaining to teacher education can dramatically change the situation. Ultimately, the teachers ought to be held accountable for the learning of children. The teacher education reform that is being suggested should include both effective pre-service training and continuing professional development through in-service training and peer group collaborative learning. It will be the teacher's job to create a positive and energizing climate in the school, that will raise the involvement and motivation of all children, in spite of social, economic, cultural, and linguistic diversity. The reform of teacher education suggested in this chapter should be able to equip the teacher to handle such diversities and ensure a positive learning and motivational climate in the school. Studies on this aspect indicate 8 positive school dimensions described below:

1. Positive teacher-student interactions.
2. Students who feel safe, connected, and engaged.
3. Policies promoting social, emotional, ethical, civic and intellectual skills, knowledge, dispositions, and engagement, plus a comprehensive system to address barriers to learning and teaching in order to reengage students who may veer off-track.

4. Clear, appropriate, and consistent expectations and consequences to address disruptive student behaviours.
5. Parental involvement.
6. Collaborative relationships between the school leader and faculty as well as *between* faculty members.
7. Focus on learning and high expectations for student achievement.
8. Decreased teacher turnover and increased teacher satisfaction (the students can see this!) (Rodwell 2015).

The NCF (National Curriculum Framework 2009), reported about the growing problem of psychological pressure on children and parents during examination. Pressure leads to tension, stress, and, in the case of children, stress leads to poor performance and for parents, it creates anxiety in them regarding their child's future. All these pressures, anxiety, and stress can be easily avoided if the climate in the school is positive and healthy in nature. For this, it is important to have well trained, qualified, and motivated teachers who not only use excellent teaching–learning processes but also create a positive innovative climate that would make children relax and perform at their best. Effective learning requires a meaningful, open-ended positive climate which would provide challenging problems for the learners to solve. According to Mishra and Bhaskar (2011), all knowledge is socially constructed and hence, social interaction plays an important role in learning. If students, principal, teachers and parents work together to assess the child's performance over a period of time, it would contribute to better understanding of the child's progress and the problems they face in learning, and thus help them take suitable measures to help children become more innovative, creative as well as original in problem solving, which are all part of a healthy and positive school climate. To create this climate, the teacher-trainee must be given intense training during the B.Ed. and M.Ed. courses. Apart from the pedagogy, the trainee must be trained to create a positive climate, where the students learn adequately and teachers teach effectively (Yadav 2010). In such a positive climate, the foundations are formed of three elements: care, trust, and diversity. This positive climate inspires teachers and students to be effective teachers and learners respectively, and also instils hope in students for a better future. In this positive schooling, students get empowered and consider themselves to be not only a part of the society, but they also believe that they have the potential to change and improve. If students have to succeed in school, they require such a positive learning and teaching environment.

Positive schooling pays attention to safety norms, provides support to academic activities in the school, maintain discipline in students, teachers and staff and make them respect, care and trust each other in addition to making the physical environment attractive, soothing and enjoyable. In course of time, such a climate stimulates in school a norm of trust, care, and respect for each other. Thus, according to the Safe Schools Action Team Report, positive schooling is the "sum total of all of the personal relationships within a school. When these relationships are founded in mutual acceptance and inclusion and also modelled by all, a culture of respect becomes the norm" (2006, 6).

In positive schooling, the teacher-trainee learns to treat each individual student as a unique person. According to Tomlinson (2003), the teacher-trainee learns how to increase or decrease the pace and scope of teaching in line with the fast or slow nature of learning of the student. Also, the trainee should learn to put in place a mechanism for both content and language learning. The trainees also learn to identify difficulties faced by some students, and also the causes for giving up learning in certain other students, and learn the various strategies to bring the students back to the power of learning.

It is well known that past efforts on teacher education reform in India have not met with much success.

The proposal outlined in the curriculum framework for 2-year B.Ed., and 2-year M.Ed. programme by NCTE, can meet the requirement of positive schooling in all its 8 dimensions mentioned above. But the conception of the professional programme must follow the distinction between professional and liberal programme pointed out by NCTE itself in the 2-year M.Ed. Curriculum Framework as under:

> even though both the course designs are almost the same, one difference that emerges between the two is that the M.A. (Ed) does not have much of training or hands on practice in graderoom teaching, whereas the M.Ed. course has these as part of the syllabus.
>
> Furthermore, to make the trainees well equipped in both pedagogy and hands-on practice in teaching, a logical framework must be worked out for the core courses and specialization fields, so that teacher-trainees when they pass out of the college or university are ready to take over various professional roles, including teacher educators, curriculum developers, policy makers, administrators and the like. (NCTE 2014)

These observations are based on the recommendations made by the Justice Verma Commission (JVC) Report which called for a logical balance between theory and field exposure (JVC Report 2012), and pointed out that the professional programme, in addition to critical comprehension of theory and selective reflection obtained in good liberal programmes, have a distinct additional emphasis on hands-on and field-based experiences. It should also provide for deep and protracted reflective practice, development of competencies and skills, particularly those related to the practice of the profession, and inculcation of the ethical principles that characterize a profession.

In the B.Ed. programme (professional course) one should therefore expect a much greater emphasis on imparting the practical competencies and skills as these constitute the core of the teaching profession. The curriculum framework for the 2-year B.Ed. programme (Curricular framework NCTE for B.Ed.), envisages that it shall provide for sustained engagement with the field through establishing close connection between different curricular areas. In the first year, work on the field is envisaged at a minimum of 4 weeks spread over several days throughout the year. It is proposed to include one week of school engagement and 3 weeks of other engagements. In the second year, a minimum of 16 weeks of engagement with the field is envisaged, of which 15 weeks are for school internship and one week for other field engagements. The detailed course outline of NCTE states that a minimum of 20 weeks (4 + 16) shall be allocated over the 2 years for tasks, assignments, and school internship in the field, under the broad curricular area, 'Engagement with the field'. The weightage of internal assessment for engagement with the field shall be 100%.

The curriculum framework for B.Ed. proposes that the internship could be in one school; though it can be split into two parts: one in a government and the other in private school or one at elementary and the other at the secondary level in the same school. Under no circumstances, should the teacher-trainee be sent to more than 2 schools in the internship period. Further NCTE also emphasized that,

> Internship should not be reduced to the delivery of a certain number of lesson plans, but should aim for meaningful and holistic engagement with the learners in the school. Moreover teaching should not be practiced through reductionist approach of micro teaching of isolated skill and simulated lesson (NCTE 2014).

The NCTE further states that the various tasks and projects given to the teacher-trainee would help in substantiating perspective and theoretical framework, studied in the teacher education classroom, with field-based experiences. "These tasks and projects may include collaborative partnerships with the school for developing CCE (Comprehensive Continuous Evaluation) practices, creative ways of tracking learner's progress, establishing Study Circle/Science Clubs/Forums, and the like, for professional development of trainee and in-service teachers" (NCTE 2014).

While the NCTE has thus indeed provided for field practice, it is felt that what is envisaged is grossly inadequate for the teacher-trainees to learn to teach and also learn about creating a positive climate, motivate students, and challenge them at their levels. Also, the 15 week training suggested by the NCTE, at field level in the second year, needs rethinking. In this chapter an alternative model is presented, which is for 320 h (I year = 144 h; and II year = 176 h) of field training in school, covering all aspects such as observation and learning to adopt the method of disciplining children, motivating them to do their best, and so on, by observing the senior teacher in the graderoom. In the first 2 semesters, they could cover disciplining methods, motivating children, the kind of assignments given in the graderoom and for homework, the kind of activities given to children as extra-curricular programmes, identifying children with behaviour problems and how to refer them to the counsellor in the school, learning to deal with parents, and so on. In the II year, the teacher-trainees are involved in teaching the gradees the concerned curriculum as specified by the school supervisor. In addition, the trainee also learns how to set question paper, how to conduct examinations, both internal and external, and how to evaluate, as well as the criteria to be used for the same. During the fourth semester, they are also involved in conducting workshops, managing the classroom, and taking part in some administrative work as the supervisor considers fit.

On completion of the two year theoretical and practical courses, the teacher-trainee should be sent for a one-month internship, when she or he functions as a full-fledged teacher in the classroom. Her/his involvement is complete as regards the school and the students. Responsibilities, if any, given to the intern by the senior teacher or the principal, such as the assessment and evaluation of students, writing of report of the students under his/her care, and so on, may still need some guidance and supervision but not as intensely as it was in the first 2 years of training.

Thus, the whole training is for 2 years, a duration of 496–500 h. Normally, most professional courses in psychology, applied psychology, social work, and similar courses require the teacher-trainee to complete 450 h during the entire course of 2 years including the one-month internship.

While the curriculum framework can be commended for its very high objective, it is important to consider if 15 weeks of internship in one or two schools, and one week of field exposure would be at all sufficient to realize the objective which the NCTE envisages, or whether there are more effective methods of ensuring the objectives of competency and skills in the 8 aspects of school climate noted above.

Mentoring/Supervision of Field Training in Teacher Education

It is also important to examine how exactly the training should be imparted, under whose mentorship and supervision, and how the feedback process will be utilized to assess and raise the level of skill and competencies of the teacher-trainee and if more time will be required to be devoted to practice teaching with supervised feedback (NCTE 2014).

To train the teacher-trainee adequately, there should be a supervisor from the college of education/university, and a supervisor from within the school to which the trainee is attached for field training to acquire teaching skills through hands-on experience.

To begin with, 12 teacher-trainees may be placed in the selected schools with one trainee in each Grade from KG to Grade XI. The school supervisors, who can also be former retired teachers, will be responsible for guiding the students on how to observe a particular lesson being taught, and what to observe in it. The students will also observe and learn how the students are controlled and how they are disciplined and how the focus on the work in the class is being maintained. Following the observation, the students have to write up verbatim all they observed and learnt in the practical notebook.

The school supervisor should evaluate what the students have observed, including what has been missed out, and give comments on the written report, and what more could have been done. They have to point out the errors in the observation and skills in teaching so that, in the next session, the observation could be even better, leading to acquisition of skills to incorporate what was observed into the teaching process.

It is an important function of the school supervisor to make the teacher-trainee understand the various concepts being taught and understand when to use various teaching aids.

The teacher-trainee's attention should be drawn to normal and abnormal behaviours of children in the classroom to make them understand the same in terms of developmental stages and the context in which the behaviour occurs.

The supervisor should draw attention to various cultural and social aspects relating to behaviour, which may not be desirable in the classroom. The trainees should be guided in the handling of such children, with regard to their motivation and the improvement of their standards in academic and other activities.

The supervisor should guide the trainee with regard to the kinds of assignments to be given in the class and for home work. The responsibilities of a mentor/supervisor are enormous and includes modelling, different instructional methodologies, providing regular observation and feedback, working jointly on introduction of new curriculum materials, assisting in classroom actual research, and serving in a resource and consultant role to the teacher-trainee/intern (Portner 2005).

It is obvious that the supervisors have to be trained for such a role. Also, the task of school-based supervision should be distributed amongst teachers, one for elementary, one for the middle and one for the secondary.

Role and Functions of Faculty Supervisors from College/University

Since the objective of the professional teacher-education programme is to ensure the development of requisite teaching–learning skills by the teacher-trainee, and since teachers teach as they learn, it is very important that the practical part of the curriculum is carefully implemented, and an expert's guidance and supervision are provided so as to ensure that the requisite professional skills in the trainees are indeed developed.

Only very good schools should be chosen for imparting practical training. The training will be under the joint supervision of the school where the practical training is imparted and the college of education in which the teacher-trainee is enrolled. The faculty supervisor in the college of education should, of course, have the ultimate responsibility for selecting the school, placing the students, ensuring that the students have an observation class each week at least for one hour, and submit a written report to both faculty supervisor and the school supervisor of his or her observation in the same week. The report must be submitted through the school supervisor who can add his or her own comments and suggestions. The faculty supervisor from the college of education should discuss this report individually with the trainee before the next week's practical observation. Moreover, the faculty supervisor can hold group meetings of all the trainees under him/her. The faculty supervisor will be required to provide written suggestions to the trainee on the report of the students.

Within the school itself, adequate arrangements have to be made to guide the trainee by the school supervisor; it would be ideal if 12 trainees are allotted to a good school for practical training so that one trainee can be placed in each grade (KG to Grade XI). The students could be rotated to different grades, so that they are able to observe the teaching learning process at different grades. Their observations should cover not only what and how the teaching-learning occurs, but should also cover discipline, behaviour, and motivation of students. In particular, they should observe how different students are motivated by teachers, and how socio-cultural and other differences are handled, and especially how undesirable behaviour is handled by the teachers. The teacher-trainees should record their observations in detail soon after their observations of the class. The school supervisor can also draw attention to any gap and also make suggestions for improvement.

One other important point is of evaluating to what extent the teacher-trainee has transformed into a professional teacher, for which there should be a joint supervision and evaluation by the supervisors of both the school and the college of education. It is only by paying closest attention to supervising, and guiding the placement, teaching, and internship, and promoting self-reflection throughout the training period, aided by diary and meetings and discussions with the school and college supervisors, that the skilled practice component of the course can be adequately imparted. This should constitute the core of the teacher-education programme.

It might be said that one is expecting too much from school supervisors and also from the faculty supervisor of the college. There may be a shortage of trained supervisors in both the school and the college of education. This can be overcome if necessary by appointing on a part-time basis, those who have specialized in this kind of supervision who may be available in certain other applied fields, such as in clinical psychology or applied psychology. Another method is to have crash courses for training and development of supervisors at school and faculty levels. The supervision and mentoring by trained and experienced persons is the key factor in the success of any teacher-education programme and hence one should not compromise on depth and quality of such supervision, and the practical training, practical exposure training, internship, and reflection that it entails.

As part of a technical exercise, the Institute of Education, University of London, carried out an assessment (in May 2012), of the curricula as it obtained in selected teacher-training institutions in India (Institute of Education 2012). In their assessment they have expressed a concern that, in many of the teacher training "syllabuses in India, there is a tendency conflate knowledge, skills and dispositions and omit references to teaching and learning approaches which are appropriate for these different elements … if this is not taken into account the teacher trainer is unlikely to teach the knowledge set, or disposition in the most effective way. For example the student-teacher cannot be told how they should operate effectively in the graderoom; they need to be able to perform, however inadequately, in the graderoom and learn by reflecting on the mistakes they have made and subsequently make improvements to their performance" (Institute of Education, London 2012).

In addition, the supervisor, while mentoring the teacher-trainee should make the trainee aware that students model their behaviour after their teachers, and if the teacher expects the students to develop open-minded, inquisitive, and inquiring approaches, the teacher should also demonstrate the same. Also, it is not necessary that the student should know everything, and have all the correct answers, but they need to be encouraged to be curious and wondering about various issues that are taught in the classroom (Barrel 2012).

Mukunda (2009) makes a distinction between conceptual understanding and procedural learning. The latter relates to how to do things and almost everything that one does in schools require some degree of procedural learning. These are 'how to' skills taught through modelling. That is, the teacher demonstrates the skills by doing, whether it is solving equations, parsing sentences, or writing neatly, and the student repeats the same to the best of his/her abilities. These skills are learnt by doing, and practice is needed to perfect the same. Mukunda concludes that, in India, drill is given undue emphasis and conceptual teaching takes a back seat, and what we need is a balance in both types of learning. While this may be true of schools, in teacher-education institutes, there is too much emphasis on theory and conceptual understanding, and too little on practice and skills training.

The list of learning outcomes or curricular standards for an ideal model of pre-service teacher training have been summarized in the Report of Institute of Education, London (Strategy document focusing on published teacher training curricula, May 2012) referred to above, in so far as they pertain to skills and dispositions. Learning outcomes include: (i) Understand how a body of knowledge (which includes cognition, skills and dispositions) can be translated into pedagogic knowledge related to performance, behaviour, communication, and relations with students and develop the capacity to translate the one into the other; (ii) Develop the capacity to undertake action-research projects and to take part in teacher learning community; (iii) Develop classroom teaching dispositions, related to performance, behaviour, communication, and relations with students; (v) Develop capacity to apply knowledge, skills, and dispositions in educational settings; (vi) Understand the ethical dimensions of common situations faced by teachers in school settings, develop and put into operation an appropriate plan of action in the work place in response to the ethical dilemma, and develop the capacity to behave in ethically appropriate ways in different circumstances; (vii) Develop the capacity to apply appropriate professional standards in real life; (viii) Develop the capacity to use appropriate classroom management strategies, with particular reference to discipline maintenance and maintaining a positive learning environment in the school classrooms; (ix) Develop capacity to read and construct educational sets, such as national, state, or district curricula, textbooks, or major documents, where these capacities refer to critical thinking, educational literacy, reconceptualization, contextual application; and (x) Use spoken and written language clearly, fluently, and appropriately to interact in different educational contexts and recognize and appreciate the country's linguistic diversities (Institute of Education, London 2012)

The above "rather long listing of learning outcome/curricular standards for skills and dispositions to be developed in the pre-service teacher education programme, clearly indicate the need for (a) adequate practice (b) time allotment and above all (c) skilled and experienced mentors and supervisors who can indeed guide and help the teacher training".

Here it would also be appropriate to quote from the M.Ed. Programme (Curricular framework: 2-year M.Ed. programme 2016).

> Professional preparation and continuing professional development of teacher in turn need teacher educators who are themselves professional teachers and who have, through a process of critical scrutiny of theory, critical reflection of practice as well as doing research, deepen their understanding … of the nature and structure of knowledge that the learners construct as well as hands on reflective practice (p. 8).

The biggest challenge to implementing an effective programme of teacher education is to identify and develop a cadre of experienced and motivated supervisors, mentors, and other teachers for teacher-education colleges at B.Ed. and M. Ed. levels. The dearth of effective supervisors and mentors in teacher-education colleges, as well as in schools, is indeed the most formidable obstacle in implementation of the programme.

Crash courses and special workshops can overcome this shortage if suitable faculties are identified and intensely trained.

Selection and Motivation

Many issues regarding training of teachers have been discussed so far and perhaps one of the most important aspects is to select and recruit the right type of teachers. In this context, Stronge and Hindman (2006) in their book *Teacher Quality Index*, Association for Supervision and Curriculum Development (ASCD), pointed out that teacher recruitment is a process of providing an adequate number of quality applicants. For any school, hiring, supporting, and sustaining effective teachers is one of the most important responsibilities of school principal and the school's managing committee. For effective teaching–learning process to take place, good teacher selection is absolutely indispensable.

For positive and effective schooling, committed hard working teachers are a must. Commitment and motivation levels amongst teachers can be expected to be along the Bell curve, as indeed with other professions. However, in regard to the teaching profession it is essential to have persons with a different kind of aptitude and different practices to sustain motivation, commitment, and enthusiasm to continue teaching. Too little attention is being given, during recruitment, to the teaching aptitude of the candidates. Perhaps it may be possible to introduce a system of apprentice teachers to judge the suitability of the candidates, so that the teachers themselves may decide whether they should be in this profession at all.

In a country with massive white collar unemployment, and with the teaching profession being considered more as a part-time job and as a dignified employment only for women, it is particularly important to assess teachers for aptitude and hard work, even before admission to B.Ed. courses, so that only those who meet the criteria in this regard are admitted to the B.Ed. course. The government has already initiated steps to close down a number of ineffective B.Ed. colleges in India. Perhaps one can have entry to B.Ed. courses based on academic performance and a National Aptitude Test. And, while recruiting teachers, the candidates could be administered an aptitude test, which must be given higher weightage in selection.

It is also necessary to improve the attractiveness of the teacher-education courses through extrinsic and intrinsic motivation. Teacher Education is a profession in which intrinsic motivation must play a major part; however, extrinsic rewards are equally important to raise the status of teachers as well as attract better calibre teachers.

The recommendation for an All India Education service has been pending for a very long time. Education should be deemed a lifelong career that gives equal if not better opportunities as other sectors. It is important to note that the neglect of the education sector and of the teaching profession is responsible for many of India's problems today.

One of the reasons for the decline of educational standards in India and a relative lack of educational progress at all levels of education is that the leadership in the field of education is are not professionals. Ministers and Secretaries of Education from different states and central institutions are generally non-educationists, who do not quite understand and appreciate the requirements of education. Since the leadership is non-professional—and even experienced and able teachers are not groomed for such positions—teachers do not aspire to senior decision-making and leadership roles/levels in education. Also, it is well known that non-professional leadership has created chaos from ill-thought-out and poor implementations of many suggested reforms. The rapid professionalization of leadership in education is a necessary condition for the progress of teacher education in the country.

Emotional Security and Learning

Mukunda (2009) says that, ideally, schools and teachers should give as much importance to the students' emotional states as they do to their learning. Yet, in a typical school, it may be extremely difficult for the teacher to attend to the emotional needs of the student and thus the importance of emotions is denied in learning, which can be a great mistake. Emotions, according to Mukunda, are inextricably intertwined with motivation and cognition, and the three phenomena form the basis of all school learning (Mukunda 2009).

Mukunda therefore emphasizes that it is important to create a school environment that is affectionate and affirming instead of impersonal and competitive. The supporting educational environment addresses the issue of academic emotions in a holistic way. She points out, on the basis of research studies, that learning is most enjoyed when there is a balance of one's skill level and the challenge level of the activity. She points out that teachers should explore imaginative ways to give more students this correct and appropriate match between ability and talent. She cites studies that report highest level of attention to work when the children were happy and at the activities chosen by them. While fear of punishment for not doing homework, and similar fears, may be a major source of stress for students, the social stress of being rejected by one's peers, or the stress of witnessing conflict between one's parents, are equally, if not more, painful. A healthy positive climate in school and/or positive schooling would be able to help students be happy and participate in the teaching-learning process meaningfully and with higher level of performance.

The practical training of teachers should include a substantial element of understanding and handling of such problems.

Continuing Professional Development

According to the Report of the Institute of Education, University of London (2012), "Current research on teacher development clearly stresses the importance of teacher centred; individualized coaching that takes place in real world institutional setting … Network created through online platform allows teachers to relate to each other beyond the confines of their discipline, level, and school contexts … moreover, the teachers adopt perspectives of the learner in the process, which increases their empathy for the students" (2012).

Since the students have to be lifelong learners, learning from the internet and also from their peers, what better method to demonstrate the same than to practice this approach for continuous improvement of teacher capacity. Enhancing teacher collaboration, sharing of experiences and new knowledge, contextualizing contents, and building of several other capacities through systematic, regular professional teacher-development programmes, and especially encouraging blended learning and teacher communities for this purpose, should become part of the education system. In this connection, attention may be drawn to the commendable pioneering work by ECHO, initiated in collaboration with Ambience Public School, Delhi and several other schools. It provides a platform for sharing of knowledge, skills, and experience on a regular basis.

Role of Management and Leadership

The importance teachers and the principal attach to promotion of a positive climate in the school, and to the training of teachers for the purpose, will depend on the management and leadership of the school. If the management takes its goal seriously, allots requisite budget, provides space and supporting facility, and reviews the situation periodically, while empowering the principal and the teachers, the school is likely to develop effective training arrangements both for the teachers and the teacher-trainees. This would also promote a positive culture of education in the school. Management would be well advised to have a strong agenda for positive schooling and monitor all the arrangements required for the purpose. They should appoint requisite mentors and supervisors, full-time and part-time, and give due weightage to ongoing faculty development in their periodic assessment of teachers and the principal. They should also arrange for periodic or recurring leadership training for the principal and senior functionaries in the school leadership. If the principal gets the requisite support and feels empowered in this regard, it is bound to have a great impact in establishing and promoting positive schooling.

References

Barrel, J. (2012). *How do we know they are getting better? Assessment for 21st century Minds K-8*. California: Corwin (A Sage Company).

Government of India. (2012). *Report of the high powered commission on teacher education constituted by hon'ble supreme court of India*, (JVC) (Vol. 1, August). Government of India, Ministry of HRD, Department of School Education and Literacy.

Hindustan Times. (2017). *Survey of schools in Delhi*. June 8 2017.

International Institute of Education. (2012). *Pre service and in-service teacher training: Strategy document focusing on published teacher training curricula* (p. 3). Institute of Education, University of London.

Mishra, B., & Uday Bhaskar, A. (2011). Knowledge management process in two learning organisations. *Journal of Knowledge Management, 15*(2), 344–359.

Mukunda, K. V. (2009). *What did you ask at school today? A handbook of child learning*. India: Harper Collins Publishers.

NCTE. (2009). *National curriculum framework for teacher education*. New Delhi: NCTE Government of India.

NCTE. (2014). *Curriculum framework: Two year M.Ed. program* (p. 5). New Delhi: NCTE, HansaBhawan.

Portner, H. (2005) (Ed). *Teacher mentoring and induction: The state of the art and beyond*. California, USA: Corwin Press.

Rodwell, P. (2015). 8 aspects of a positive school climate and culture. In *Kickboards's in the effect of school climate and culture on K-12 academic achievement*.

Safe Schools Action Team Report. (2006). *Safe Schools: What is the school climate? Safe schools policy and practice: An agenda for actions* (June, p. 6).

Stronge, J. H., & Hindman, J. L. (2006). The teacher quality index: A protocol for teacher selection. *Association for Supervision and Curriculum Development 1703 N.* Beauregard St., Alexandria, VA, USA.

Tomlinson, C. A. (2003). *Fulfilling the promise of the differential graderoom: Strategies and tools for responsive teaching*. Alexandria, VA: Association for Supervision and Curriculum Development.

Yadav, M. (Ed.). (2010). *Teacher education curriculum*. New Delhi: Kaveri Books.

Chapter 19
Children with Disability in India: Policies, Assessment, and Management

Anjali Gireesan

Abstract The present chapter aims to understand the issue of disability in India in the context of various legislations available to different stakeholders, and its success in addressing the concerns of the population as well as the management of disability. Also, the chapter aims to understand two types of disabilities—intellectual disability and learning disability—with respect to their cardinal symptoms, prevalence, assessment, and intervention to give a broad understanding of the disabilities since these are understood to be the most prevalent in classroom settings. The last section of the chapter includes the results of a primary research conducted in order to understand the knowledge and perception about inclusive education amongst teachers of regular schools. The chapter concludes with effective recommendations that may help in better management of disability across the nation for children.

Keywords Children · Disability · India · Policies · Assessment Management

Introduction

Every individual in this world has a past, present and future. The past shapes the present and the present shapes the future. This is true for the society as well in which we all live. An individual is the basic building block of a society. Unless these single units remain balanced and in synchrony, a society's foundation will always be weak and it will be devoid of progress in any form. Hence, only the progress of these individual units may be translated into the progress of the society.

Disability is an umbrella term covering impairments, activity limitations, and participation restrictions (WHO 2009).

A. Gireesan (✉)
Defence Research and Development Organization (DRDO), New Delhi, India
e-mail: anjali.gireesan@gmail.com

S. Deb (ed.), *Positive Schooling and Child Development*,
https://doi.org/10.1007/978-981-13-0077-6_19

Table 19.1 Prevalence of different types of disabilities across children and adolescents

Type of disability	5–9 years	10–19 years
In seeing	0.28	0.31
In hearing	0.32	0.34
In speech	0.17	0.17
In movement	0.17	0.28
Mental retardation	0.11	0.18
Mental illness	0.02	0.04
Any other	0.33	0.35
Multiple disabilities	0.15	0.16

Source Census of India (2011)

- *Impairment* is a problem in body function or structure.
- *Activity limitation* is a difficulty encountered by an individual in executing a task or action.
- *Participation restriction* is a problem experienced by an individual in involvement in life situation.

Disability, in India, is viewed from multiple perspectives. Constitutionally, disability and disability data are often viewed in terms of the different legislations. Based on these, the census of 2011 depicts that India has a prevalence of 2.21% of population with different kinds of disabilities. The census covers eight types of disabilities which are: disability in seeing, hearing, speech, movement, mental retardation, mental illness, and any other and multiple disability. The highest incidence is found in the seeing and hearing categories (20.2%). Another observation is disability across age groups. All types of disabilities follow a similar trend in which maximum prevalence is found across the elderly population. Since most of the disabilities described in the constitution are in terms of physical disabilities, and elderly population have these problems in a higher ratio, the data should be viewed with caution. Also, the category of 'any other' has a prevalence of 18.2%. Since this category is defined in a vague and ambiguous manner, chances are that the problems of this group remain unaddressed. The data for children (2.68%) and adolescents (1.82%), may not be reliable as there is a tendency to hide disability in this population because of the anticipation of social isolation and stigmatization by the guardians of these children. The census also shows prevalence of disabilities across different categories (Table 19.1).

A child with disability seems to have been deprived of many things that make the childhood the most beautiful time of one's life. From being a pure and innocent bundle of joy, he is instead seen as an unwanted burden in society. They are often alienated and treated indifferently. Sometimes they are deprived of even the unconditional love of parents that every child should enjoy. It turns out that the supposed most wonderful time of their life is filled with memories of hurt, neglect, and isolation. A child needs nurturance and support to realize its potential to the optimum level. Each child is unique. A child with disability should be seen in the light of his myriad of possible abilities, rather than in the context of just one or two apparent disabilities. The fact that disabled children and their families may have different priorities and need different support systems and arrangements to achieve them, does not mean that they should be precluded from participating in ordinary experiences enjoyed by others.

Disability in India is still treated as a social welfare issue rather than from a perspective of violation of rights. The recent Persons with Disabilities Act, 2012 that was drafted has de-emphasized special education and focused upon inclusive education instead. But teachers are not trained and schools don't have the infrastructure to deal with children with disabilities. Neither are paediatric wards of hospitals equipped to deal with them. There is not enough data on the number of children living with disabilities to allow the government to provide the necessary services.[1]

Disability Laws in India

India is a country which is often complimented for its comprehensive legal system. Since this nation has learnt from the positive aspects of different constitutions, like that of United Kingdom and Australia, the constitutional provisions, various legislations and policies are available to the masses. The problem lies at the awareness level of these laws, which often are not utilized to their maximum potential because of ignorance. In a similar context, there are legislations and Government initiatives in the direction of disability as well those which span the areas of education, health, family, income tax and other specific acts which will be discussed in brief here.

Constitutional Provisions

The constitution treats people with disability at par with other population of India. All the fundamental rights are guaranteed to them whether it is right to life and liberty (Article 21), freedom to practice any religion and belong to a culture (Article 25) and Protection from any form of abuse (Article 23). The non-enforcement of fundamental rights is considered to be a serious offence and can be directly taken to the Supreme Court (Article 32). They have the right to equality and non-discrimination (Article 15 (1) and Article 17) in all sectors, whether it be accessibility to various types of infrastructure like shops, restaurants, and other public places and employment (Article 15 (2)) as well as right to own property and the most importantly, the right to vote in elections.

[1]http://www.childlineindia.org.in.

Educational and Health Provisions

Article 29 and Article 45 are directly related to the educational provisions of the constitution. Where Article 29 says that all the citizens, without any discrimination on the basis of caste, creed, and religion, have right to admission in educational institutions, Article 45 provides for free and compulsory education to all children up to 14 years of age. Article 47 makes it the mandatory duty of the Government to do active work in improving the standards of health and nutrition of its people. It means that that the constitution expects that the Government will come up with various initiatives which will be directed towards the development of positive outcomes in all people equally.

Family-Life Provisions

The constitution also ensures that the people with disability have a right to make a family. This is denied only in cases lunacy, mental illness, or when there is a living spouse. These clauses are applicable to all people under the constitution. The various other provisions are mentioned under different marriage acts which need not be discussed in detail in the present context. Similarly, The Indian Succession Act 1925 and The Hindu Succession Act 1956, both provide benefits for owning authority over property and assets by people with disability as well.

Income Tax Concessions

Section 80DD, 80V, and 88B provide for the concession in the tax being paid if there is a medical bill incurred for treatment for a person with disability and the income of a person with disability has further rebate and deduction on the payable amount of the tax.

These were some of the general provisions in the Constitution that attempt to fulfil the basic needs of people with disability. But in reality, it is very difficult to ascertain if these provisions are utilized or if they are efficient in addressing the needs of this section of the population. This situation arises because of many reasons like lack of proper disability statistics on prevalence of different types of disability, the services available for these people, the professional expertise needed to address their concerns, and lack of data on children with disability. In order to address these concerns, we also have specific acts with disability. These acts are as follows.

Persons with Disabilities Act, 1995

This act is considered to be one of the milestones in the legislative framework of India. It is divided into 14 chapters and 74 sections, and has considered seven categories of disability. It provides for their diagnosis, education, employment, health, non-discrimination, research and manpower development, affirmative action, social security and grievance redressal.

Prevention and Early Detection of Disabilities: In order to understand disability, the first step should be identifying the prevalence and etiological factors involved in the area. For this, investigations through surveys are needed and precautionary measures to take care of the pre-natal, peri-natal, and post-natal care of mother and child is also necessary.
Education: Provisions that ease the admission and process of learning like removal of infrastructural barriers, accessibility to various skill development services, training institute for teachers and creation of special schools have been elucidated in this act.
Employment: In all the government sectors, there is 3% reservation for persons with disabilities. Also, there are special provisions for training and welfare of these persons, and it has again been stressed how the environment of the organization should be reconstructed to make it disability-friendly.
Affirmative Action: This includes provisions for accessibility to instruments and assistive devices that will enhance the existing potential of people with disabilities. It also includes measures of providing land to these people, for purposes like establishing recreation houses and special schools.
Research and Manpower Development: Government has mandated research in the field of disability, and also financial assistance towards projects which help in making this data richer as well as create more awareness in the community. Also, grants have been given to universities and institutes that take disability as their core research area.
Social Security: Both financial and insurance benefits are mentioned under this act for the employed person with disabilities, and unemployment allowance is also mentioned for people with disabilities who have been registered with employment exchange for a period of more than one year.
Grievance Redressal: In the case of provisions not being allotted appropriately, Chief Commissioner of Persons with Disabilities can be approached at the central government level and Commissioner of Persons with Disabilities can be approached at the state government level.

Though this act is very comprehensive in itself, it has major issues like General policy issues, Sectorial policy issues, implementation of the act, political commitments between states, and Awareness of PWD Act (World Bank Report 2007; Math and Nagaraja 2008). Since Awareness is the most important factor that decides the effective utilization of any programme intended for welfare of community (Vijaykumar and Singh 2004), this act is not able to fulfil its potential. Various services for persons with disabilities in India are short on supply and do not cover even more than one percent of the population (Sharma and Vashisht 2002). Medicalization of disability is another problem where everyone tries to find a cure for the condition but the truth is that disability can only be managed, which requires a long-term plan of execution and cooperation from different stakeholders (Addlakha and Mandal 2009; Bhanushali 2007). The Act is unclear on the issues of special school-integration and special education-inclusion (Bhattacharya 2010). Specific learning disability is not included in the Act (Unni 2012). Only one percent of funds under the *Sarva Shiksha Abhiyan* are spent on inclusive education (Anbalagan 2011). Lack of funds for teacher training, the allocation of which should have been a part of this Act, creates a paradox in the context of basic provisions of this act.

Mental Health Act, 1987

This is an act which ensures that a mentally less sound person has every right to get treatment either on voluntary basis or on the consent of guardians taking care of this person. There are also provisions which state that, if this person does not have financial protection to undergo the treatment procedures, the state government shall incur the costs. Also, it is prohibited under this act to deny any kind of entitled pay, pension, or gratuity to a person with mental illness. If the person is not able to manage funds, there are provisions for appointment of guardians for both care taking and financial guardianship.

National Trust Welfare Act, 1999

This act has mainly come into force with objectives of setting up a welfare trust with different board members that will look into the financial requirements of people with disability. Those people who are registered with this trust are taken care of, by not only providing monetary benefits but also appointment of guardians and removal of them if there is a misappropriation of funds or property. Lack of resources that people with disabilities often face, can be addressed through the provisions of this Act. This act that vouches for empowerment of persons with disability is criticized for its clause for appointing guardians for effective decision making (Math and Nagaraja 2008), thus making an individual dependent rather than independent.

Rehabilitation Council of India Act, 1992

This act basically ensures that the identification, diagnosis, and intervention for disability are carried out by trained and qualified professionals. The educational institutes that provide training to these professionals also need to be certified under this act. Also, it is mentioned that there should be a periodic evaluation of both the professionals and the institutes in order to ensure that minimum standards of care-providing and support services are maintained by them. The failure of this mandates the council to cancel the registration of these bodies.

What is notable in the discussion above is that the PWD Act, 1995 emerges to be the most studied legislation in the context of disability. The other acts, which aim at making the support services efficient, have not been studied in detail and their follow-up has also been poor. Such provisions need to be brought into public notice so that their implementation can be evaluated and norms can be revised as per the requirement of this population.

Developmental Disorders

Developmental disorders are a heterogeneous group of conditions that show their effect in one or more areas of developmental patters whether it be physical, cognitive, or social in nature. DSM-V has renamed this group of conditions as Neurodevelopmental disorders. This is an umbrella term which includes intellectual disability, learning disability, Autism spectrum disorder, Attention Deficit Hyperactive disorder, and Developmental coordination disorder.

- *Intellectual disability* is a term used to refer to a condition where the individual has compromised cognitive development and is lower than that of their counterparts of the same age.
- *Learning disability* is a group of conditions where the problem lies in specific areas of language like reading, writing, spellings, and mathematics.
- *Autism spectrum disorders* are a group of conditions where the social communication and development of an individual is compromised and is characterized by behavioural difficulties.
- *Attention deficit hyperactive disorder* is a condition where an individual is impulsive, not able to focus attention and hyperactive in natures. These three conditions might occur simultaneously or in isolation in the individual.
- *Developmental and coordination disorder* is motor disability where the problems occur in integrated motor movements and thus the individual might experience problems in both gross and fine motor skill development.

All the developmental disabilities have both organic and social basis. In order to manage these in an effective manner, it is imperative that both of these are considered and included in the diagnosis as well as the intervention procedures.

As observed, the developmental disorders are different in terms of the developmental areas affected in a person. But there are some commonalities between them. Though two individuals might be diagnosed with the same disability, their diagnosis and intervention will be different because of difference in the degree of severity and the nature of co-morbidity might be varied. These are lifelong conditions and can be managed but cannot be cured completely. In the following sections, two types of disabilities that are most often seen in classroom settings are discussed. These are Intellectual disability and Learning disability.

Intellectual Disability

Intellectual disability is a condition in which the person shows cognitive delays and is unable to perform different activities in accordance with one's age norms. This disability is viewed in the context of four categories:

- Mild (Educable): The persons having this condition are educable, and can live a normal functioning life with adequate social support.
- Moderate (Trainable): This group of people may not be able to complete their education, but may be trained to live independently. But for certain activities, they might be dependent on others.
- Severe (Manageable): This group can be taught only activities of daily living and for that, too, they are dependent on the social support of others.
- Profound (Restricted): This group is severely restricted and is completely dependent on others for their survival. Most of them do not live a long life American Psychiatric Association (2013).

Intellectual disability is divided into different categories on the basis of IQ assessment. The normal IQ range spans from a score of 90 to 110. Any person with a score below 70 is categorized as having intellectual disability. This is then further divided into different categories as stated above. Children with intellectual disabilities have been observed to have more of behavioural and emotional problems —compared to children without intellectual disabilities—like anxiousness, delinquent and aggressive behaviour, and attention problems (Dekker et al. 2002). Thus, a combination of lower IQ and marked behavioural issues may be prescribed for a screening of this disability. It is important to perform early intervention for this disability. The probability of positive prognosis increases with early intervention for intellectual disability. Thus, it is necessary for teachers and parents to be aware about these symptoms so that delays may be avoided. Depending on the research method being used, and the region, the prevalence of this disability varies from 1/1000 to 32/1000 in India (Girimaji and Srinath 2010). This indicates that, across the nation, there is a requirement for a more uniform procedure and categorization of the disability so that management interventions for the disability may be more streamlined. The major aspects that are included in the management plan of children with intellectual disability are:

- **Special Education**: These are curricula designed keeping in mind the individual special needs of a child. The methods used in this type of education are more nuanced, slower paced, and employ integration of different senses that makes the education easier as compared to the modalities adopted in regular education.
- **Behavioural Management**: Behavioural management becomes important for this group of children as the learning and understanding process of social norms that are relatively automatic for their peers, has to be made a conscious and explicit process for children with intellectual disabilities. For example, the expression of attraction towards opposite gender needs to be taught and managed, which is not often the case with children without any disabilities. The same applies for many other emotional and behavioural issues like aggressive behaviour, feelings of isolation and somatic complaints. These first need to be documented and then subsequently addressed.
- **Medications**: Children with intellectual disability may also have other medical complications, like a weaker immune system which makes them more susceptible to diseases, metabolic disorders, and somatic complaints like pain in various body parts. The child needs to have periodic health check-ups and the medications need to take into consideration the level of intellectual disability.
- **Diet**: Children with intellectual disabilities have often been observed to have co-morbid conditions of obesity because of certain compromising physical restrictions. Hence, special attention needs to be paid to their diet.

Learning Disability

Learning disorders or disabilities are a heterogeneous group of disorders. According to DSM-V, they are defined as "disorders that are diagnosed when the individual's achievement on individually administered, the standardized tests in reading, mathematics, or written expression is substantially below that expected for age, schooling, and level of intelligence". There are four categories of this disorder: Dyslexia (Reading disorder); Dyscalculia (Mathematics disorder); Dysgraphia (Writing disorder); and learning disorders not otherwise specified. The prevalence of these disorders in India is difficult to ascertain because the research studies are very few and scattered and when it comes to children, the statistical support is not adequate. In other countries, like the United States of America and the United Kingdom, these studies have been more systematic and are able to give prevalence in different contexts, like comparing prevalence across race and ethnicities, early childhood longitudinal studies, and prevalence trends of children in various intervention programmes (Boat et al. 2015).

Dyslexia, also known as the reading disorder, is the most widely studied learning disorder with a prevalence rate of 7% (Vasudevan and Iyer 2015). In India, this prevalence has been explored in a few studies. In a study by Rao et al. (2017), the prevalence of dyslexia was studied in a group of 400 students in Mysore, and the rate was found to be 13.67%. In another study, Arun et al. (2013) attempted to study the prevalence of specific learning disabilities in students of Class VII to XII in Chandigarh. This was a large study, with a sample of 1301 from Government schools and 1101 from private schools. The rate was found to be 1.58%. In another cross-sectional study, with a large sample size of 1314, in Belgaum (Karnataka), the prevalence rate of dyslexia was found to be 11.2% (Mogasale et al. 2012). Dyslexia has been shown to have very strong brain basis, where there is a difference in the pattern of activation in three areas: Broca's area, the Parieto-temporal region, and the Occipito-temporal regions. The indicators of dyslexia can be observed in pre-school, primary, and secondary school children, which include symptoms like mispronouncing words, slow effortful reading, and fear of reading aloud (Thambirajah and Ramanujam 2016).

Dyscalculia, on the other hand, is the mathematical disorder, where the individual faces problems while attempting mathematical operations. The overall prevalence rate of this disability has been observed to be 6% (Wilson 2012). In India this rate ranges between 5.5 and 6% (Ramaa and Gowramma 2002; Karande and Kulkarni 2005). This disorder also has a brain basis, which includes bilateral horizontal segments of the intra-parietal sulcus (HIPS), an area that contains spatial representation of numbers, and fusiform gyrus, which gets activated when numerical tasks are performed. Dyscalculia has a genetic cause and is observed to run in families.

Dysgraphia is the disorder where an individual basically faces problems in the context of written expression. Globally, the prevalence of this disability is at 5%. There are limited studies on dysgraphia in India. One such study is based in rural Jaipur, where the rate was found to be 22.30% (Dhanda and Jagawat 2013), while another study was based in Belgaum, where the rate was found to be 12.5%. In yet another study, based in three districts of Telangana state, this prevalence was found to be 15% (Indira and Vijayan 2015). Since there are only a few studies here, it is difficult to generalize about the prevalence rate of dysgraphia in India. The brain basis of dysgraphia include supraspinal networks, cerebellum, and certain cortical regions (Van Hoorn et al. 2013).

Interventions

Disability is an area which, if managed at the correct and appropriate time, can have a good prognosis. A very important part of this procedure is the assessment phase. Testing and assessment are, many a time, used interchangeably but there is a basic difference between the two terms. While testing gives one a measurement of a particular trait or entity, assessment is more holistic in nature. It is a battery of different methods, undertaken to understand the problem and hence arrive at a solution. There are basically three categories of initial assessment followed when looking at disability. These are: interviews; Psychometric testing; and situational and functional assessment. All of them have their own advantages and disadvantages and more often than not, they are used in combination with each other. Assessment becomes important in the following ways:

- Behavioural prediction
- Helps in acquiring the knowledge of personality and support systems
- To gauge the existing potential and abilities in an individual
- To understand the organic basis of the condition
- To evaluate the efficacy of an intervention

The efficacy of these different types of assessment does not only depend on their robustness, but on the professionals involved in the administration and interpretation of these tests as well. A well-established test, if handled by a not-so-well-equipped professional, will not be beneficial in understanding the condition of individuals. An ability to understand the condition involves theoretical understanding of disability, expertise to individualize the assessment procedures, and sensitivity to cultural and social factors that surround the individual. Only a combination of the above-mentioned factors can lead to successful and efficient assessment.

There are a lot of tests that are employed in understanding the level of disability for children with learning disabilities. These differ on the basis of the degree and type of disability that the child has. There are mainly three types of learning disability viz., (1) Dyslexia or reading disability; (2) Dyscalculia or mathematical disability; and (3) Dysgraphia or writing disability. We will now discuss the different tests and interventions used for each of these types.

Dyslexia

The classic symptoms that have been mentioned earlier, are the first indication that a child might be having this learning disability. There are multiple tests that need to be conducted for reading which are: tests of performance, tests of phonological awareness, tests of decoding, and test of reading speed (Thambirajah and Ramanujam 2016). The major psychological tests used in the assessment procedure are Wechsler individual achievement test, wide range achievement test and comprehensive test of phonological processing. Two important things that need to be noted here are that: (1) Intelligence tests are seldom used as an assessment procedure for dyslexic children; and (2) The tests of phonological awareness are of special significance in case of dyslexic children. Some of the Indian tests used in this procedure are as follows:

- **Dyslexia Screening Test Junior, Indian Edition**: This is a comprehensive test used to screen dyslexic children. It now has 13 subtests with addition of new subtests like spoonerisms and Non-verbal reasoning. It provides a holistic assessment as well being able to shed light on the problem areas in reading ability (Fawcett and Nicolson 1995). This test has been used in research endeavours like integrating dyslexia and music (Overy 2003), computer based reading intervention (Nicolson et al. 2000), and in devising learning strategies (Kirby et al. 2008).

- **NIMHANS Neuropsychological Battery of Tests for Children**: This battery is one of the few robust psychological tests used with Indian population and has norms for children as well. For children with learning disability, this battery gives effective scores for reading, writing, as well as mathematical abilities. More often than not, children have multiple learning disabilities rather than having specific learning disability. In such a scenario, this test proves to be quite useful. This test has been used for assessing cognitive development in children (Kar et al. 2008), as well in understanding other psychological disorders in children like Obsessive and Compulsive disorders (Rao et al. 2008).

Dyscalculia

This type of disability relates to the mathematical difficulties experienced by children. As in dyslexia, this type of learning disability is also assessed through multiple tests. The mathematical components include counting, quantity knowledge, and approximate estimation, number facts, arithmetic operations, mathematical reasoning, and the language used in mathematics. A child might be facing problems in either one of these areas or a combination of different components. In the assessment procedures, the non-formal strategies include analyzing the error patterns—for example, addition might be correct but subtraction might be wrong—and what are the strategies adopted by children when they are solving a mathematical problem. The standardized assessments of mathematical ability are as follows:

- **Key Math 3 Diagnostic Assessment** (Connolly 2007): This is a comprehensive test to ascertain the understanding of basic concepts of Mathematics, operations and application of this understanding in solving different problems. This test is divided into 14 subtests. Although it has been advised that all the subtests should be administered, these can be administered individually as well, if the problem areas have been identified initially.
- **Test of Early Math Ability** (Ginsburg and Baroody 2003): This test has been devised to test the mathematical abilities of children in the age group of 3–9 years. This test is a little different from Key Math 3 in the aspect that it also measures pre-counting, counting, formal, and informal mathematics. In this age group, understanding of numbers is considered to be more important than performing operations with them. Hence, there is more emphasis on these skills rather than the concept and operational understanding of the subject. This test has been used in different researches concerning cultural differences in early mathematical learning (Huntsinger et al. 1997), achievement tests (O'Neill et al. 2004), and inhibitory controls (Fuhs and McNeil 2013).

The intervention for children with dyscalculia have been shown to be effective and promising (Chodura et al. 2015). There are numerical as well as non-numerical deficits involved in mathematical disability. Thus, it is advocated that the interventions should focus on both of these. While mathematical strategies include cognitive strategies and use of visual representations, non-numerical interventions include behavioural and psychological interventions, non-invasive brain stimulation, and pharmacological interventions (Furlong et al. 2016). Work on remedial instruction programmes in India emphasize individualized teaching programmes for these children, verbalizing the problems and practice sessions of mathematical concepts (Gowramma 2005).

Dysgraphia

This is writing disability and, as in the case of previous types, this skill is also composed of different components like legibility of writing, spelling, and composition. These are assessed through both formal and informal ways of assessment. An informal method of assessment can be carried out by teachers to understand if the child is suffering from dispositional symptoms or whether it is just because of situational factors. Apart from the battery of tests mentioned in dyslexia, there are other standardized tests to assess the writing ability of a child. These are as follows:

- **Test of Early Written Language (TEWL-3)**: This is a robust test which assesses the writing ability of a child which is split into two components: the basic writing ability of the child and the contextual writing ability of the child. This test is for the age group 4–10 years of age. The basic writing test looks at a child's ability to use language and its tools, like grammar, whereas contextual writing involves how a child is able to articulate the writing skills when given a situation like describing a picture. A combination of both the scores gives the score for overall writing.
- **Test of Written Language (TOWL-4)**: This test is used for an older age-group of children, when the writing is assumed to have been more developed and sophisticated. The writing of a child becomes more differentiated and it is articulated better by the child. Consequently, as compared to TEWL, TOWL has more components and is divided into different subtests. The two bases of assessment are writing components and assessment format. The three writing components are: conventional, linguistic, and conceptual. Two assessment formats are contrived and spontaneous.
- **Detailed Assessment of Speed Handwriting**: This is a test that evaluates different aspects of handwriting speed, identify the difficulties, and thus contribute to making a framework of intervention to remedy the situation. The five subtests are aimed at studying the level of dexterity the child has, ability to reproduce known material quickly, maintain time between two writing tasks and the speed with which the child is able to write something original.
- **Single Word Spelling Test**: This is a test which exclusively looks at the pattern of spelling errors made by the child. It has nine tests for spelling and each series has about thirty to fifty words. It is used for the age group of 5–14 years.

The errors are then analyzed to identify the components which are posing a problem for the child.

Interventions for dysgraphia have been shown to be successful. Since these children find it difficult to learn from the usual errorful learning techniques, one of the ways to handle the situation is by promoting errorless learning strategies in the initial stages of intervention (Raymer et al. 2010). In errorless learning children are provided with feedback on every correct response. This prompt prevents children from making errors. On the other hand, in errorful learning, children learn by the method of trial and error. Once the child understands the concepts, then the training is given to adopt errorful learning strategies again, because both therapies have been shown to have better outcomes in general (Whiteside et al. 2012; Thiel and Conroy 2014). These strategies lend themselves to modification according to the needs of an individual. Thorough writing practice, with explicit instructions for promoting different skills, and use of mnemonics for better memory of rules of writing, also enhance the writing skills of a child (Thambirajah and Ramanujam 2016).

Perception of Teachers on Inclusive Education

Children with disability require resources and understanding at a different level from various social agents. In this section, the results of one study, which was conducted to understand the knowledge and perception of inclusive education of teachers, are discussed. The sample consisted of hundred and twenty three teachers across six schools in the Ernakulum district of Kerala.

Inclusive education is a very broad term, the implementation of which requires understanding, resources, and commitment at the physical, psychological, social, and economic levels. Merely admitting a child with disability into a regular school does not serve the purpose of implementing compulsive inclusive education in schools. It requires removal of barriers that hinders the education of a child, as well as change in the organizational environment down to the policy level (De Beco 2014). In this study, this kind of understanding of inclusive education was observed to be prevalent in very few teachers, which, in turn, would affect the quality of care and education being provided to these children. Most of them also feel that educating children with disabilities is a developmental issue rather than just a welfare or a charity issue. This is a positive observation because then education in appropriate terms will be treated as a right-based issue rather than just another social service. They advocated that these children are part of society, equal to other children, should be respected, and have a right to learn as the other children have. Such an opinion may become a key factor in implementing the policies that are mentioned in the UN Convention adopted right-based education policy. Right-based education will ensure both identification of students with disability, their management, and the revisions that are required to promote this step in a progressive direction. Since teachers can become very effective leaders in this direction, their training, knowledge, and concerns need to be taken into consideration.

The qualification of teachers and educators is of special significance in case of children with disability. Although a majority of the current sample of teachers have a Bachelor of Education degree as their educational qualification, they do not have professional training in the field of disability. But, as per the government and constitutional requirement, their institute is bound to practice inclusive education by law. Here comes the major discrepancy, where the policy is there but the resources and instruments needed to implement the same are seriously lacking. The current Bachelor of Education programme has no separate module for dealing with children with disability in a regular classroom setup. Those who wish to deal with these children may pursue a different degree which is known as Bachelors in Special Education. It is, therefore, unrealistic to advocate inclusive education in regular schools when there is a basic distinction being between the professionals employed who take care of these children, which are also being implemented by the same education system. This professional lacuna may also result in the experience of frustration and burnout when regular teachers engage with children with disability in a regular classroom, because they are not fully equipped to understand the course of action that needs to be devised for these children. The trained professionals, in comparison, experience better adjustment because of their knowledge and training (Boujut et al. 2016).

The good point here is that the educators and teachers understand that this kind of teacher training is a basic necessity of inclusive education, because most of them have advocated for the same. Lack of trained professionals has also been identified as one of the challenges in implementing inclusive education. The other areas that they have given are also important and a necessary part of inclusive education which include: infrastructure, syllabus revision, availability, and accessibility to trained professionals like psychologists and special educators, social support and compassion. Teachers emphasized on a very holistic perspective on these necessities, where not only individual factors (skill development and compassion), but also environmental factors (Infrastructural changes and social support) have also been considered. These necessities are observed to be not fulfilled because most of the educators say that they perceive that all these factors are lacking in many ways. Since the basic requirement of inclusive education is not taken care of, as per the responses of teachers, the success of policy implementation is improbable. Unless the basic necessities are taken care, it would be futile to expect advanced progress in this field.

The suggestions given by the teachers were basically in the line of the challenges elucidated by them. Awareness about various issues like prevalence of different types of disability, the procedures to identify the condition, and a dynamic platform of the stakeholders, need to be strongly advocated and brought into force. Such programmes would also ensure participation from parents and better pooling of resources. Encouraging social and family support for children will safeguard the children from discrimination and isolation, which directly affects the mental well-being of children. At this period in their life, they have a constant need of approval and encouragement from their family, society, and friends. A withdrawal of such opportunities from them, at this stage, may result in life-long role confusion according to Erikson's theory of psychosocial development. The need to bring special education into mainstream schools is one of the most contentious suggestions. Though initially, this might be difficult, such steps have been shown to have long-term positive outcome for children with disability in regular schools (Grindle et al. 2012). Social network analysis is one such method which can augment the process of bringing special education into mainstream schools (Charlotte et al. 2015). Here cultural and structural aspects of the institution are studied in detail, and an individualized assessment is provided, thus making the implementation of special education in an organization more specific. As far as improvement in government and legal support measures are concerned, they are underutilized by all stakeholders, mostly because they are not aware about the provisions already being given. They need to be first practiced, and then can a conclusion be reached about whether the policies are effective in bringing about changes or if they need to be revised. There needs to be a system which can evaluate these policies, which again will not take effect unless there is some amount of active utilization of these policies.

Teaching children with disability is not an easy task. Moreover, there have been many studies which document that this field has always had high rate of attrition (Cook and Cook 2013; Feng and Sass 2013; Johnson and Semmelroth 2013; Brunsting et al. 2014). Hence, it was asked, in this study, as to what can be the motivating factors to retain more teachers in the field of inclusive education. A majority of the teachers said that it is the intrinsic motivation of individuals that brings and increases the chances of retention in this field. Thus, programmes that enhance altruistic intention of professionals can be used to decrease the attrition rates. Altruism is an important psychological concept. According to Social exchange theory, people are more likely to help when their perceived input is less and perceived rewards are more. So, if a professional has expertise and experience of dealing with a child with disability, he or she is more likely to stay in the profession as compared to someone who does not have adequate expertise, and thus is always under stress. Other factors like financial incentives and accessibility to other resources further add to this paradigm. On the other hand, the empathy-altruism hypothesis states that if we feel empathy towards a person, then our tendency of altruism increases. Activities that promote radical listening, deepen understanding of human nature, and inculcate curiosity can help in increasing empathy in people. With empathy emerging to be a very actively researched topic in Positive Psychology, there is a scope of increasing the emotion among people.

Another interesting observation in this study was that the teachers of rurally situated schools had a better mean score on attitude towards including children with disability in regular classrooms, compared to both urban and semi-urban areas. There are advantages of teaching in rural areas. Not only does one has a smaller class size and better parental involvement, but also the degree of position and authority perceived is higher when compared to other communities (Berry and Gravelle 2013; Provasnik et al. 2007). The teachers of schools in urban and semi-urban setup complained that teacher-student ratio is too big for them to cater to the individual needs of a child, and the probability of frequent interaction with parents is also less because, more often than not, both parents will be professionally occupied. This also indicates that teacher preparedness to include children with disability in regular classrooms has a chance of being enhanced by reducing the class size, and ensuring that they get support from other social agents like parents and school management.

In conclusion, though teachers may lack specialized training in the field of disability and may not have appropriate understanding of inclusive education, they are aware of the basic necessities and challenges of the same field. They have a positive attitude towards including these children in the regular classrooms and can be motivated to become a part of this system with good professional training which will enhance their knowledge base and skills, as well as timely and appropriate incentives in different forms like money and recognition.

Recommendations

Care and support services to children with disabilities involve resources and revisions at multiple levels. This needs help from many stakeholders, apart from the main care givers, like communities around, local bodies of the Government and other organizations that can provide infrastructural, economic, and legal aids to these children. This study included only some stakeholders in the study. There is a need to understand the other variables as well in order to provide children with optimum services.

Intervention Programmes

Intervention programmes need to be more streamlined for children with learning disabilities. IQ assessments, academic assessments, and special education are given to these children in their respective centres and the professionals offering these services are doing a good job in management of the conditions of these children. However, the services being offered are currently concentrating only on academic needs of the child. There needs to be periodic evaluation of the services being offered, and how they facilitate the social well-being of the children as well. More people should be employed in order to address this need, as periodic evaluation is not possible without adequate professional manpower. Life skill training and special sessions on social skills need to be introduced, as these have been evidenced to improve self-esteem and perception of belongingness in children. Interventions should also focus on preparing children to enter inclusive education classrooms, so that when the opportunity comes, children can shift to regular schools. A monthly involvement of parents in the intervention programme in school premises will bring positive outcomes for children. This will also facilitate interaction between parents of children with learning disabilities by providing a dynamic platform for interaction among parents, which will further reinforce social support for them. Though yoga and meditation are included in the curriculum of most special schools, it is important that parents participate in some sessions as well so that this practice can be continued at home as well.

Policy Level Revisions Are Needed

The legislations and laws that are available for addressing the concerns of people with disabilities have been discussed. But there is a need to revisit the legislations and make needful amendments in these laws. The definition of disability needs to be revised to include all neuro-developmental disorders. Uniformity needs to be brought to the issuing of learning disability certificates. There need to be appropriate and well-specified legislations for children with learning disabilities and slow learners, as they are a largely ignored group in terms of provisions by law. Legal recognition needs to be given to these conditions. The services being offered to people with disability also need the services of paediatricians. Their role in disability management also needs to be clearly stated. Most of the legislations concentrate on revisions in tangible resources. There need to be reforms that concentrate on improving mental resources as well. Inclusive education related legislations need to be reformed. Integrated education and inclusive education need to be separately and specifically defined. There are schools which can easily implement integrated education but may not be able to provide reforms for inclusive education. There should also be sources mentioned which can facilitate the appropriate reforms in school to implement inclusive education.

Intervention should also include an active programme for preparing the children to enter inclusive education in regular schools, which is advocated by our laws and legislations.

Role of Community Needs to Be Reinforced

The community has been observed to be a passive stakeholder in the context of disability. This needs to be reconstructed. The community can play a very important role by giving social support to the service providers, parents, and children with disabilities. As observed, most of the stakeholders view lack of social support as one of the constraints in delivering effective services. Involvement of communities, by employing local people as administrative staff of the school, outsourcing monitoring jobs to local bodies, and arranging door-to-door campaigns to create awareness in communities is one way of bringing the community closer to these children. This process will definitely bring some change in the perception of communities.

Training Needs of the Professionals

In this study, it was observed that, apart from the service providers, both teachers of regular schools and the paediatricians lacked training in the field of disability. Service providers also affirmed the need for further training in the field of disability. As all these professions encounter cases of disability on a regular basis; this training needs to be included in their professional degrees itself. Pursing a special course for disability is often viewed as an additional task. Inclusion of this in regular courses will reduce this burden.

References

Addlakha, R., & Mandal, S. (2009). Disability law in India: Paradigm shift or evolving discourse? *Economic and Political Weekly*, 62–68.

American Psychiatric Association. (2013). *Diagnostic and statistical manual of mental disorders* (5th ed.). Washington, DC: Author.

Anbalagan, C. (2011). Challenges and prospects of Indian higher educational services—A global view. *International Journal of Research in Management & Technology (IJRMT), 1*(2).

Arun, P., Chavan, B. S., Bhargava, R., Sharma, A., & Kaur, J. (2013). Prevalence of specific developmental disorder of scholastic skill in school students in Chandigarh, India. *The Indian Journal of Medical Research, 138*(1), 89.

Berry, A. B., & Gravelle, M. (2013). The benefits and challenges of special education positions in rural settings: Listening to the teachers. *The Rural Educator, 34*(2).

Bhanushali, K. (2007). Changing face of disability movement: From charity to empowerment. In *National Seminar on Revisiting Social Work in the Field of Health—A Journey from Welfare to Empowerment*, February 20–21, 2007.

Bhattacharya, T. (2010). Re-examining issue of inclusion in education. *Economic and Political Weekly*, 18–25.

Boat, T. F., Wu, J. T., Sciences, S., & Sciences, T. N. A. (2015). *Prevalence of learning disabilities*.

Boujut, E., Dean, A., Grouselle, A., & Cappe, E. (2016). Comparative study of teachers in regular schools and teachers in specialized schools in France, working with students with an autism spectrum disorder: Stress, social support, coping strategies and burnout. *Journal of Autism and Developmental Disorders*, 1–16.

Brunsting, N. C., Sreckovic, M. A., & Lane, K. L. (2014). Special education teacher burnout: A synthesis of research from 1979 to 2013. *Education and Treatment of Children, 37*(4), 681–711.

Chodura, S., Kuhn, J. T., & Holling, H. (2015). Interventions for children with mathematical difficulties: A meta-analysis. *Zeitschrift für Psychologie, 223*(2), 129.

Connolly, A. J. (2007). *KeyMath 3: Diagnostic assessment*. San Antonio, TX: Pearson.

Cook, B. G., & Cook, S. C. (2013). Unraveling evidence-based practices in special education. *The Journal of Special Education, 47*(2), 71–82.

De Beco, G. (2014). The right to inclusive education according to Article 24 of the UN Convention on the rights of persons with disabilities: Background, requirements and (remaining) questions. *Netherlands Quarterly of Human Rights, 32*(3), 263–287.

Dekker, M. C., Koot, H. M., Ende, J. V. D., & Verhulst, F. C. (2002). Emotional and behavioral problems in children and adolescents with and without intellectual disability. *Journal of Child Psychology and Psychiatry, 43*(8), 1087–1098.

Dhanda, A., & Jagawat, T. (2013). Prevalence and pattern of learning disabilities in school children. *Delhi Psychiatry Journal, 6*(2), 386–390.

Fawcett, A. J., & Nicolson, R. I. (1995). The dyslexia early screening test. *The Irish Journal of Psychology, 16*(3), 248–259.

Feng, L., & Sass, T. R. (2013). What makes special-education teachers special? Teacher training and achievement of students with disabilities. *Economics of Education Review, 36,* 122–134.

Fuhs, M. W., & McNeil, N. M. (2013). ANS acuity and mathematics ability in preschoolers from low-income homes: Contributions of inhibitory control. *Developmental Science, 16*(1), 136–148.

Furlong, M., McLoughlin, F., McGilloway, S., & Geary, D. (2016). Interventions to improve mathematical performance for children with mathematical learning difficulties (MLD). *The Cochrane Library.*

Ginsburg, H. P., & Baroody, A. J. (2003). *Test of early mathematics ability*. Austin, TX: PRO-ED.

Girimaji, S. C., & Srinath, S. (2010). Perspectives of intellectual disability in India: Epidemiology, policy, services for children and adults. *Current Opinion in Psychiatry, 23*(5), 441–446.

Gowramma, I. P. (2005). *Development of remedial instruction programme for children with dyscalculia in primary school*. Mysore, India: Chethana Publishers.

Grindle, C. F., Hastings, R. P., Saville, M., Hughes, J. C., Huxley, K., Kovshoff, H., Griffith, G. M., Walker-Jones, E., Devonshire, K., & Remington, B. (2012). Outcomes of a behavioral education model for children with autism in a mainstream school setting. *Behavior Modification*. 0145445512441199.

Huntsinger, C. S., Jose, P. E., Liaw, F. R., & Ching, W. D. (1997). Cultural differences in early mathematics learning: A comparison of Euro-American, Chinese-American, and Taiwan-Chinese families. *International Journal of Behavioral Development, 21*(2), 371–388.

http://www.childlineindia.org.in.

Indira, A., & Vijayan, P. (2015). A study of identification and assessment of children with dysgraphia in Telangana State. *Asian Journal of Research in Social Sciences and Humanities, 5*(10), 37.

Johnson, E., & Semmelroth, C. L. (2013). Special education teacher evaluation: Why it matters, what makes it challenging, and how to address these challenges? *Assessment for Effective Intervention*. 1534508413513315.

Kar, B. R., Rao, S. L., & Chandramouli, B. A. (2008). Cognitive development in children with chronic protein energy malnutrition. *Behavioral and Brain Functions, 4*(1), 1.

Karande, S., & Kulkarni, M. (2005). Specific learning disability: The invisible handicap. *Indian Pediatrics, 42*(4), 315–319.

Kirby, J. R., Silvestri, R., Allingham, B. H., Parrila, R., & La Fave, C. B. (2008). Learning strategies and study approaches of postsecondary students with dyslexia. *Journal of Learning Disabilities, 41*(1), 85–96.

Manual, I. *Census of India 2011*.

Math, S. B., & Nagaraja, D. (2008). Mental health legislation: An Indian perspective. *Mental Health Care and Human Rights*, 49.

Mogasale, V. V., Patil, V. D., Patil, N. M., & Mogasale, V. (2012). Prevalence of specific learning disabilities among primary school children in a South Indian city. *The Indian Journal of Pediatrics, 79*(3), 342–347.

Nicolson, R., Fawcett, A., & Nicolson, M. (2000). Evaluation of a computer-based reading intervention in infant and junior schools. *Journal of Research in Reading, 23*(2), 194–209.

O'neill, D. K., Pearce, M. J., & Pick, J. L. (2004). Preschool children's narratives and performance on the peabody individualized achievement test–revised: Evidence of a relation between early narrative and later mathematical ability. *First Language, 24*(2), 149–183.

Overy, K. (2003). Dyslexia and music. *Annals of the New York Academy of Sciences, 999*(1), 497–505.

Provasnik, S., Kewal Ramani, A., Coleman, M., Gilbertson, L., Herring, W., & Xie, Q. (2007). *Status of education in rural America (NCES 2007–040)*. Washington, DC: National Center for Educational Statistics, Institute for Education Sciences, U.S. Department of Education.

Ramaa, S., & Gowramma, I. P. (2002). A systematic procedure for identifying and classifying children with dyscalculia among primary school children in India. *Dyslexia, 8*(2), 67–85. https://doi.org/10.1002/dys.214.

Rao, N. P., Reddy, Y. J., Kumar, K. J., Kandavel, T., & Chandrashekar, C. R. (2008). Are neuropsychological deficits trait markers in OCD? *Progress in Neuro-Psychopharmacology and Biological Psychiatry, 32*(6), 1574–1579.

Rao, S., Raj, A., Ramanathan, V., Sharma, A., Dhar, M., Thatkar, P. V., & Pal, R. (2017). Prevalence of dyslexia among school children in Mysore. *International Journal of Medical Science and Public Health*, Online First: August 29, 2016. https://doi.org/10.5455/ijmsph.2017.05082016592.

Raymer, A., Strobel, J., Prokup, T., Thomason, B., & Reff, K. L. (2010). Errorless versus errorful training of spelling in individuals with acquired dysgraphia. *Neuropsychological Rehabilitation, 20*(1), 1–15.

Sharma, A. K., & Vashisht, P. (2002). Community based rehabilitation in primary health care system. *Indian Journal of Community Medicine*, 3.

Thambirajah, M. S., & Ramanujam, L. L. (2016). *Essentials of learning disabilities and other developmental disorders*. New Delhi: Sage publications India, Pvt. Ltd.

The World Bank. (2007). *People with disabilities in India: From commitments to outcomes*. South Asia region: Human Development Unit.

Thiel, L., & Conroy, P. (2014). A comparison of errorless and errorful therapies for dysgraphia after stroke. *Neuropsychological Rehabilitation, 24*(2), 172–201.

Unni, J. C. (2012). Specific learning disability and the amended "persons with disability act". *Indian Paeditrics, 49*, 445–447.

Van Hoorn, J. F., Maathuis, C. G., & Hadders-Algra, M. (2013). Neural correlates of paediatric dysgraphia. *Developmental Medicine and Child Neurology, 55*(s4), 65–68.

Vasudevan, N., & Iyer, A. (2015). *Developmental dyslexia—Its prevalence and treatment in India*.

Vijaykumar, S., & Singh, U. (2004). PWD act: Awareness among beneficiaries and members of rehabilitation team. *IJPMR, 15*, 12–16.

Whiteside, S. P., Inglis, A. L., Dyson, L., Roper, A., Harbottle, A., Ryder, J., et al. (2012). Error reduction therapy in reducing struggle and grope behaviours in apraxia of speech. *Neuropsychological Rehabilitation, 22*(2), 267–294.

Chapter 20
Children's Rights to Healthy Development and Learning in Quality Early Childhood Education and Care in Australia

Ann Farrell

Abstract Increasing international attention is focused on children's rights to participation, protection, and provision, in contexts that promote children's healthy learning and development. Optimizing children's life chances by promoting children's health and safety, and physical and psychological well-being is being prioritized by governments and national agencies in a range of countries. An example is Australia's National Quality Framework, a legislative and policy vehicle driving a significant national reform agenda for the health, well-being, and learning of young children in Australia. Established in 2012, the National Quality Framework was designed to raise quality and drive continuous improvement and consistency in Australian ECEC (long day care, family day care, preschool/kindergarten, and outside schools hours care services). This chapter examines Australia's national agenda for optimizing children's life chances for health development and learning. It considers empirical evidence and policy initiatives that focus on children's health, safety and development, and the promotion of their growing competence, confidence, and independence. The chapter considers the Australian Government's national resource, the 'Get up and Grow Guidelines' (for children's health and well-being), based on the national Healthy Eating Guidelines and the Physical Activity recommendations for children in ECEC contexts. In considering strategies for achieving national goals, the chapter identifies key enablers and barriers to optimizing children's life chances for health development and learning.

Keywords Children · Rights · Healthy development · Learning
Australia

A. Farrell (✉)
School of Early Childhood and Inclusive Education, Faculty of Education,
Queensland University of Technology, Brisbane, Australia
e-mail: a.farrell@qut.edu.au

S. Deb (ed.), *Positive Schooling and Child Development*,
https://doi.org/10.1007/978-981-13-0077-6_20

Introduction

Internationally, there is increased focus on young children's rights to participation, protection, and provision in contexts that promote their healthy development and learning (cf. United Nations Convention on the Rights of the Child 1979). Across a range of countries, governments and apex bodies are prioritizing children's health and safety, and their physical and psychological well-being (Organization for Economic Cooperation and Development [OECD] 2017a, b, c; United Nations Children's Fund [UNICEF] 2008, 2015). Such commitments are exemplified in the United Nations Sustainable Development Goals (2015).

So too, international policy attention has turned to Early Childhood Education and Care (ECEC), the sector catering for children birth to age eight, prioritizing quality health and learning outcomes and optimizing children's life chances, now and into the future (Camilli et al. 2010; OECD 2001, 2006, 2012, 2017a, b, c; UNICEF 2015). UNICEF's Executive Board Special Session on Equity (2015) avowed that "Investing in the most disadvantaged children is our greatest hope of breaking the intergenerational cycle of inequity that affects billions of people" (5).

The OECD's International Early Learning and Child Well-being Study (IEL) was launched in 2017. This was a survey across three to six countries, designed to assess children's learning and well-being at five years of age and to identify key enablers and barriers to early learning in both home and ECEC settings. According to the IEL, ECEC settings denote an (officially registered) ECEC setting that caters for children of five to five-and-a half years of age, and provides an educational programme for at least two hours per day and 100 days per year. Domains include cognitive, social, and emotional development, with skills in language and literacy, numeracy and mathematics, and self-regulation. The IEL has attracted both commendation and concern, for its focus on comparative international data on children's early learning in the vein of the Programme for International Student Assessment (PISA), the triennial international assessment of the skills and knowledge of 15-year-olds.

For at least a decade, ECEC in Australia has been a national investment priority, a strategic agenda to redress inequity and to improve access to, and participation in, quality ECEC services (Irvine and Farrell 2013). The Australian Government's Productivity Commission (2016) identified ECEC and school education as key contributors to the "well-being and quality of life of young Australian as well as the capabilities and productivity of Australia's future labour force" (3). In short, ECEC is a prime agenda for national investment and policy.

A prime example of Australia's commitment to ECEC is its National Quality Framework, a legislative and policy vehicle designed to drive a significant national reform agenda for the health, well-being and learning of young children in Australia (Australian Children's Education and Care Quality Authority [ACECQA] 2012). Established in 2012, the National Quality Framework was designed to raise quality and to drive continuous improvement and consistency in Australian ECEC (in long day care, family day care, and preschool/kindergarten and outside schools hours care services).

This chapter examines Australia's national agenda for optimizing children's life chances for healthy development and learning. It considers policy initiatives and empirical evidence that focus on children's healthy development and learning. The chapter examines two national resources for the early years in Australia: (i) Belonging, Being And Becoming: The Early Years Learning Framework for Australia (known as the *Early Years Learning Framework*, Council of Australian Governments [COAG]) (2009), Australia's first-ever national curriculum framework for children birth to five years; and (ii) the Get Up and Grow Guidelines for children's health and well-being, based on the national Healthy Eating Guidelines and the Physical Activity (2013) recommendations for children in ECEC contexts. In considering strategies for achieving national goals for young children, the chapter identifies key enablers and barriers to optimizing young children's life chances for healthy development and learning.

Australia's National Quality Framework

Australia's legislated National Quality Framework (NQF) (ACECQA 2012) documents the national standard for ECEC and the qualifications of educators. In Australia, children under 5 years of age are increasingly participating in ECEC services. Most recent statistics show that in excess of 50% of 2- to 3-year-olds, and 85% of 4- to 5-year-olds participate in a recognized ECEC service, with an average time of 18 h per week being spent by each child in such a service (Australian Bureau of Statistics 2014). In June 2014, of the 3.8 million children aged 0–12 years, 48% (1.8 million) usually attended some type of childcare compared to 52% in 2011.

In 2009, all Australian governments, through the Council of Australian Governments (COAG), agreed to a partnership to establish a National Quality Framework for Early Childhood Education and Care ('National Quality Framework') (cf. ACECQA 2017a, b, 7–8). The partnership was based on a shared understanding of the importance of the early years to ensure the well-being of children throughout their lives and to lift the productivity of the nation as a whole. The NQF aimed to raise quality and continuous improvement in ECEC through:

- the National Quality Standard for Early Childhood Education and Care and School Age Care ('National Quality Standard')
- a national quality rating and assessment
- streamlined regulatory arrangements
- the establishment of ACECQA to oversee the system (ACECQA 2017a, b).

The NQF is underpinned by the Education and Care Services National Law ('National Law') and Education and Care Services National Regulations ('National

Regulations'). Together they set the National Quality Standard (NQS) and the regulatory framework for most long day care, preschool/kindergarten, family day care and outside school hours care services in all states and territories. The guiding principles of the NQF (ACECQA 2017a, b) are:

- the child's rights and best interests
- the notion the child is a successful, competent and capable learners
- equity, inclusion and diversity
- the valuing of Aboriginal and Torres Strait Islander cultures
- respect and support for parents and families
- best practice in ECEC

The NQS drew significantly on the work of the OECD in identifying quality in ECEC services, particularly with respect to structural quality, interactions between educators and children and targeted services for particular families and communities. The NQS acknowledged that children learn from birth and that learning occurs in a range of settings. Both the EYLF (2009) and the national framework for school age care, My Time, Our Place: Framework for School Age Care In Australia (Australian Government 2011) document practices designed to support and promote children's learning. The EYLF, for example, guides educators in developing quality programmes for children from birth to 5 years and in their transition to school. The framework for school-age care, in turn, extends the principles, practices, and outcomes of the EYLF to cater to children and young people who attend school, and to ensure that children in school age care are provided opportunities for leisure and play-based experiences that are responsive to their changing interests and needs.

Within the NQF, individual ECEC services are assessed and rated by their respective state or territory regulatory authority, against the NQS in a cycle of 1–3 years in the 7 quality areas (below), and 18 standards with 2–3 standards in each quality area (58 elements in total):

1. "Educational programme and practice
2. Children's health and safety
3. Physical environment
4. Staffing arrangements
5. Relationships with children
6. Collaborative partnerships with families and communities
7. Leadership and service management"

Each ECEC service is required to display their rating at their service, and ratings are published on the national register and the *Starting Blocks* and *My Child* websites. From February 2018, a revised NQS, enacted by national law, stands to provide clearer language and a reduction in the number of elements and standards. Currently, overall ratings are:

- "Excellent Rating, awarded by ACECQA
- Exceeding National Quality Standard

- Meeting National Quality Standard
- Working Towards National Quality Standard
- Significant Improvement Required" (Fig. 20.1)

Since its introduction in 2012, the NQS has been the focus of empirical attention and scholarly critique (Hunkin 2016; Jackson 2015; Logan et al. 2012; Logan and Sumsion 2010; Roberts 2015). The 'E4Kids' longitudinal study of the quality of ECEC services in Australia, for example, found that Australian ECEC averaged in the medium range on most of the measured components of quality (using CLASS and subscales of the ECERS-R), with the exception of personal care routines and

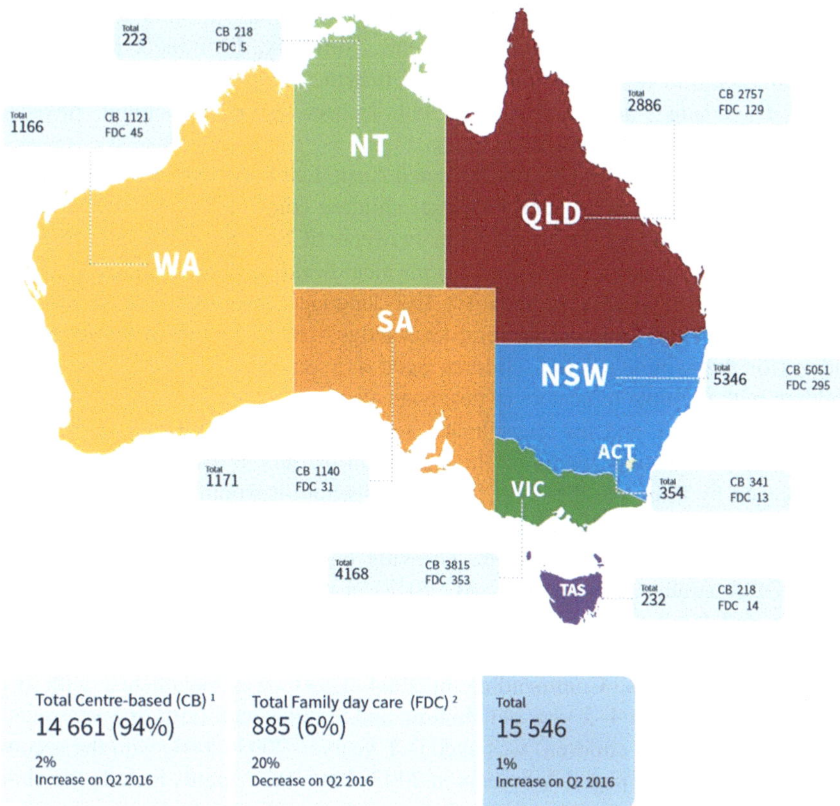

Fig. 20.1 Number of ECEC services in Australia (ACECQA 2017b, 5) NB. (1) A centre-based service is an education and care service other than a family day care service. This includes most long day care; preschool and outside school hours care services that are delivered at a centre. It does not include preschools in Tasmania or Western Australia out of scope of the NQF, as well as other services that aren't regulated under the National Law. (2) A family day care service (FDC) is an education and care service delivered through the use of two or more educators to provide education and care for children in residences, whether or not the service also provides education and care to children at a place other than a residence. They are sometimes known as family day care schemes and they are administered and supported by central coordination units

instructional support (Tayler et al. 2013). Tayler et al. (2013) found, however, that the average quality of ECEC varied according to service type, with kindergarten having significantly higher quality than long day care, a pattern akin to that found in the United States and the United Kingdom.

Linked to service type is socio-economic status. A study by Cloney et al. (2016) showed that there is no guarantee that children from low socio-economic status (SES) backgrounds are able to access quality services. Their study of 2,494 children enrolled in 1,427 ECEC settings (controlled for a range of child, family, home and community-level background factors), showed that children from lower SES background were more likely to attend lower quality programmes, the largest quality gap being in prior-to-kindergarten contexts. Cloney et al. (2016), in turn, argued for targeted ECEC programmes in lower SES areas, in order to ameliorate children's differential SES quality gradients. Similarly, Ishimine's (2011) case study of ECEC in urban Australia showed that the community's social and economic disadvantage impacted quality with respect to the curriculum, physical environment, and adult-child interactions.

Drawing upon data from the teacher-rated Australian Early Development Census (AEDC), using a full population cohort of children commencing school, Goldfeld et al. (2016) examined the relationship between ECEC and children's developmental outcomes across 5 domains: "(i) physical health and well-being; (ii) social competence, (iii) emotional maturity; (iv) language and cognitive skills; and (v) communication skills and general knowledge" (p. 42). Using a Disadvantage Index (for the sample's 3,615 children aged 4–5 years), the research found that children with multiple indicators of disadvantage were less likely than their peers to be using preschool, and for fewer hours, and were more likely to be in exclusive parental care. The study identified the significant barriers to participation in ECEC experienced by those children and families for whom it would most benefit.

Another study of disadvantaged children's access to quality ECEC conducted by Wong et al. (2014) used data from 'Growing up in Australia: The Longitudinal Study Of Australian Children' (LSAC 2017), a representative sample of 10,000 children and families from urban and rural areas in all states and territories of Australia, capturing the diversity of social, economic and cultural contexts of children and families. Commending in 2004, LSAC was established with two cohorts (families with 4–5 year old children and families with birth to 1 year olds), the first cohort (5000 children) was aged 0–1 years in 2003–2004, with the second cohort (5000 children) aged 4–5 years in 2003–2004. Participants include the child (at an appropriate age) and parents (both resident and non-resident), carers and teachers. Conducted in conjunction with the Department of Social Services, the Australian Institute of Family Studies and the Australia Bureau of Statistics, LSAC focuses on individual, family, and wider social and environmental factors, that contribute to developmental trajectories, with a view to informing policy debate and decision making in ECEC.

Considerations of the NQS have also included critiques of 'quality'; for example, the critique of Logan et al. (2013) noted little mention of 'quality' for the period 1972–2009 and the COAG launch of the Early Years Learning Framework.

The researchers posited the Child Care Act 1972 as a critical juncture in the development of Australian ECEC policy and the emerging quality improvement agenda.

As noted, the Australian Government introduced two related frameworks, the Early Years Learning Framework (COAG 2009) and the Get Up and Grow Guidelines (Commonwealth of Australia 2009) to tackle disadvantage and social inequity experienced by Australia's children and families. The chapter now turns to the Early Years Learning Framework.

Early Years Learning Framework

Australia's first national learning framework for early childhood educators was developed with the support of the Council of Australian Governments (COAG) to extend and enrich children's learning from birth to 5 years, and through transition to school. COAG's commitment was that, "all children [should] have the best start in life to create a better future for them and for the nation" (COAG 2009, 5). The EYLF makes explicit the importance of play-based learning, communication, and language (literacy/numeracy), and social and emotional development. Designed for everyday use by educators operating in partnership with families, the EYLF was informed by the 2008 State, Territory, and Commonwealth Ministers of Education meeting, and the Ministerial Council on Education, Employment, Training, and Youth Affairs' commitment in the Melbourne Declaration on Educational Goals for Young Australians (2008). Moreover, the framework draws upon the United Nations Convention on the Rights of the Child (1979) that all children have the right to an education that lays a foundation for the rest of their lives, maximizes their ability, and respects their family, cultural and other identities and languages; and that recognizes children's right to play and be active participants in all matters affecting their lives (COAG 2009).

The EYLF comprises five Learning Outcomes:

- "Children have a strong sense of identity
- Children are connected with and contribute to their world
- Children have a strong sense of well-being
- Children are confident and involved learners
- Children are effective communicators" (COAG 2009, 8)

It comprises three inter-related elements: Principles, Practice, and Learning Outcomes; all three elements central to early childhood pedagogy and curriculum decision-making. Within the EYLF, curriculum as an ongoing cycle encompasses all the interactions, experiences, routines, and events, planned or intentional and unplanned that occurs in the learning context. Curriculum involves educators—drawing upon their professional in-depth knowledge of each child—and working in partnership with families. Pedagogy involves the educator's professional practice in cultivating nurturing relationships, curriculum decision-making, and teaching and learning.

In relation to health and well-being, the EYLF (2009) is concerned with "children's developing resilience and their ability to take increasing responsibility for self-help and basic health routines in order to foster a sense of independence and confidence" (2009, 30). Children's learning about healthy lifestyles—including nutrition, personal hygiene, physical fitness, emotions, and social relationships—is seen to be integral to their well-being and self-confidence. As children become more independent, and their motor skills and independence develop, they can take greater responsibility for their health, hygiene, and personal care, and become mindful of their own and others' safety. Within the EYLF, routines provide opportunities for children to learn about health and safety, to experience a range of healthy foods and to learn about food choices from adults and each other.

Get up and Grow Guidelines

Along with the EYLF, Australia developed the 'National Healthy Eating Guidelines and Physical Activity Recommendations for Early Childhood' (Get up & Grow Guidelines [GUG], 2013) to advance children's healthy eating and exercise in early childhood as a key strategy to curb childhood obesity and to promote healthy development and learning for children in Australia. ECEC services were identified as key contexts for promoting healthy eating practices and obesity prevention, with educators identified as key players in modelling and integrating healthy practices across the curriculum. The national GUG agenda focused on the knowledge and skill that educators bring to the health and well-being of children in ECEC contexts. In practical terms, ECEC services are required to meet the NQS standard 2.2: 'healthy eating and physical activity are embedded in the programme for children' and the desired learning outcome that "children take increasing responsibility for their own health physical" well-being (Early Years Learning Framework 2009, 32).

Within the national GUG agenda, various jurisdictions have developed their own programmes to assist the implementation of the guidelines within their ECEC services. Programmes include: 'Munch and Move' (Hardy et al. 2010; New South Wales Government 2017), 'Kids—Go for your life', instigated in Victoria (de Silva-Sanigorski et al. 2010) and LEAPS (Learning Eating Active Play and Sleep 2016) in Queensland. The LEAPS programme, for example, was funded by the Queensland Government between 2013 and 2016 to deliver a free professional learning programme (>1700 educators participated), designed to increase and strengthen educator knowledge and skills to support the implementation of the GUG guidelines in ECEC services throughout Queensland. The LEAPS state-wide evaluation (cf. LEAPS Report 2016) showed that educators increased their knowledge of nutrition and physical activity guidelines, and planned to implement changes in their practices as a result. Overall, the LEAPS professional development programme exemplified the need for evidence-based healthy environments for children's development and learning.

A challenge inherent in such programmes, however, is the currency of the knowledge and skill of educators since their pre-service education. The NQF stipulates a minimum qualification requirement for educators, and each of the qualifications approved is to include a component on healthy eating and physical activity (ACECQA 2013a, b). In Queensland, however, 25% of educators have worked in this setting for 5–9 years, while another 29% have worked in the sector for 10 or more years (Department of Education Training and Employment 2014), thus reducing the likelihood of uniform qualifications and currency of knowledge in relation to healthy eating and physical activity.

Challenges also include ECEC educator use of 'everyday' knowledge rather than specialist knowledge in integrating health guidelines across the early year's curriculum. A recent study of educator knowledge and skills conducted by Cole et al. (2017) found that educators in long day care services relied upon personal knowledge, experience, and 'common sense' when determining the nutritional adequacy of the food consumed by those in their care. Despite confidence in providing nutrition advice to parents/careers, educators showed a lack of awareness use of current regulatory requirements and nutrition guidelines.

Research conducted by Pagnini et al. (2007) with staff from 8 preschools and long day care services in New South Wales showed that, while educators saw the promotion of healthy eating and active play as their core responsibility, they reported being constrained by external factors such as social expectations and commercial influences.

While the research of Cole et al. (2017) focused on educators, other work focused on children, in particular their health and eating practices. A systematic review conducted by Finch et al. (2016), for example, examined centre-based childcare interventions for increasing child physical activity. Their data sources included: Cochrane Central Register of Controlled trials, MEDLINE, EMBASE, PsycINFO, ERIC, CINAHL, SCOPUS and SPORTDISCUS. Overall, Finch et al. (2016) found that interventions significantly improved child physical activity, with significant effects for interventions that included structured activity delivered by experts. A case-in-point was the child-focused quasi-experimental study conducted by Wiseman et al. (2016) with 82 children aged 3–5 years. It found that exposure to a setting-based healthy lifestyle programme influenced knowledge and preference of food and physical play in preschool children.

Another related yet distinct service type is family day care; that is, the care and education of children in the home setting of the carer. Temple and O'Connor (2005) identified carer reports of the barriers and enablers to meaningful physical movement for children in family day care. Despite general agreement amongst family day care educators that physical activity is an important part of young children's lives in family day care, there was little support for structured or programmed physical activity in family day care. This is an area for further policy attention.

Another study in relation to sleep/rest in ECEC, a key component of the NQS, identified tensions in the NQS's provision for children's sleep, rest, and relaxation in ECEC (Staton et al. 2015). While the NQF requires everyday opportunities for learning and physical health and for the agency of each child and their family to make everyday decisions, Staton et al. (2015) found that the scheduling of a standard sleep time in ECEC remains a common practice, even in rooms catering for older children, for whom daytime sleep may no longer be necessary. Their work calls for reconsideration of sleep/rest practices as part of continuous quality improvement in ECEC in Australia.

Another topical area within the GUG guidelines is television viewing, now more broadly seen as 'screen time'. The Australian Communications and Media Authority (ACMA) (2017) report on the viewing habits of Australian children in the context of their multi-screen environments, showed that, on average, a child in Australia uses 3.2 devices and 2.9 different platforms to watch children's programmes. Daily use is most frequent for free video-on-demand (VOD) content through YouTube (27%), with multi-tasking (children doing other activities on another device while catching TV) being a feature of children's viewing practices. The ACMA report found that only 16% of children use one device to watch children's programmes, with the majority of these children (85%) doing so via a TV set, and that the prevalence of use of multiple devices increases with age, with 38% of children aged 0–4 using multiple devices, increasing to 74% of children aged 10–14 years. The related Australian Child Health Poll (2017), commissioned by the Royal Children's Hospital Melbourne, revealed that screen use is common among Australian children (television being the most frequently used screen-based device), with the majority of children, across all age groups, exceeding national guidelines for screen time. Younger children were found to spend a significant time using screens at home; infants and toddlers averaged 14 h, the two- to five-year-olds 26 h, and the six- to 12-year age group averaged 32 h per week. Moreover, 36% of pre-schoolers were found to own their own mobile screen-based device.

Garvis and Pendergast (2011) undertook research with parents in response to a GUG recommendation to ban children from watching television until they turn 2 years old, and limiting viewing to one hour per day for children from 2 to 5 years. Parent responses to these recommendations showed six themes: television as an educator; television as a babysitter; television as a motivator for increasing physical exercise; policy as a challenge to parental rights; age appropriateness; and viewing standards. The responses provide insights into children's viewing habits and the ways in which television is used in the family household. Findings also showed that parents accepted that television programmes labelled as 'educational' were a positive influence on their child's learning, and did not scrutinize the content beyond this assumption.

A more recent study by Edwards et al. (2013) of children, parents, and teachers, addressed the links between young children's digital viewing behaviour and their health, sustainability choices, and play. Instead of focusing on digital literacy or healthy eating, the researchers advocated children's play as a basis for raising questions about health and sustainability consequences of the decisions that are associated with their activity. Such work provides fertile ground for further research, particularly as children's worlds are increasingly digital.

While this chapter focuses on initiatives for healthy development and learning in prior-to-school ECEC in Australia, other work focuses on similar initiatives in school contexts (Ardzejewska et al. 2013; Bruce et al. 2012; Hardy et al. 2016; Hesketh et al. 2005; Shepherd et al. 2006). There is a similar corpus of complementary research in primary health care provision, as distinct from ECEC contexts (Cross et al. 2007; Hearn et al. 2008; Pagnini et al. 2009), as well as a growing body of research in health and well-being initiatives for young children in other countries, such as Canada (cf. Chow and Humbert 2011, 2014; Tremblay et al. 2012; Tucker et al. 2011) and the United Kingdom (cf. Mooney et al. 2008).

Enablers and Barriers to Young Children's Healthy Development and Learning

Australian policy contends that facilitating change through quality ECEC can break the cycle of disadvantage and transform the lives of the individual children, their families, and the wider community. So what are the enabler and barriers of achieving such laudable policy goals?

A study conducted by Roberts (2015) identified that the key enabler was access to services located in a place where families felt safe and empowered, non-judged by the community, and supported by quality frameworks. Barriers were social, cognitive, developmental and language vulnerabilities, lack of transport and financial constraints in accessing services.

Disadvantage is particularly pronounced for children and families from culturally and linguistically diverse (CALD) backgrounds. Cyril et al. (2017) examined the barriers to and facilitators of the engagement of CALD families in health practices and obesity prevention initiatives. Their work with 39 participants from Vietnamese, Burmese, African, Afghani, and Indian origins living in disadvantaged areas of Victoria, Australia, showed that CALD parents identified key barriers as: competing priorities in the post-migration settlement phase; language, cultural, and programme accessibility barriers; low levels of food and health literacy; junk food advertisement targeting children; and lack of mandatory weight checks for schoolchildren. Key facilitators were: the work of bicultural playgroup leaders; ethnic community groups; and school-based healthy lunch box initiatives.

Wolfenden et al. (2015) examined whether certain factors are associated with the implementation of healthy eating and physical activity policies and practices in ECEC services. Their cross-sectional survey of Service Managers of ECEC services assessed operational characteristics, policy, and practice implementation. They found that 41% of surveyed services were fully implementing healthy eating and physical activity policies and practices targeted by a region-wide obesity prevention programme. Such evidence points to the importance of leadership at the service level in ensuring that policy and practice support healthy development and learning.

Yoong et al. (2016) examined the implementation of healthy practices in ECEC, in New South Wales for the period 2006–2013, to ascertain how services changed their physical activity and nutrition-promoting practices, in light of socioeconomic status and locality. Supervisors reported on their service's adoption of six practices: "(i) having written nutrition and physical activity policies; (ii) staff trained in physical activity and nutrition in the past year; (iii) scheduled time for fundamental movement skills and (iv) outdoor play; (v) weekly or less screen time opportunities; and (vi) serving only non-sweetened beverages" (p. 767). They concluded that Government investment in obesity prevention programmes can equitably improve childcare service's adoption of healthy eating and physical activity promoting practices.

In summary, the enablers and barriers of children's healthy development and learning relate to factors that are structural (societal), systemic (institutional/sectorial) and local (family/community). Ensuring that children and their families have access to structural and systemic opportunities, and ensuring that programmes at the local level engender authentic participation and engagement, will facilitate rather than thwart their chance of moving towards healthy development and learning. This, in turn, calls for authentic structural, systemic, and local initiatives, working cooperatively with children, families, and communities.

Conclusion

This chapter has focused on Australia's National Quality Framework as a vehicle for promoting ECEC for children's healthy development and learning and for setting children's life-course trajectories and enhancing their life chances. Despite the claims of quality outcomes as children's rights, researchers such as Cumming and Mawdesley (2013) warn that the rhetoric of the 'best interests of the child' as enshrined in the United Nations Convention on the Rights of the Child (1979) may still be under-valued in Australian legislation and policy pertaining to education and education provision. In conclusion, the chapter calls for a focus on children's rights, informing policy and practice decisions relating to the healthy development and learning of each and every child.

References

Ardzejewska, K., Tadros, R., & Baxter, D. (2013). A descriptive study on the barriers and facilitators to implementation of the NSW (Australia) healthy school canteen strategy. *Health Education Journal, 72*(2), 136–145. https://doi.org/10.1177/0017896912437288.

Australian Bureau of Statistics. (2014). *Childhood education and care, Australia*. Available from: http://www.abs.gov.au/ausstats/abs@.nsf/mf/4402.0.

Australian Child Health Poll. (2017). *Screen time. What's happening in our homes?* Melbourne: Royal Children's Hospital Melbourne.

Australian Children's Education and Care Quality Authority (ACECQA). (2012). *National quality framework*. Government, Canberra, ACT: Author.

Australian Children's Education and Care Quality Authority (ACECQA). (2013a). *Guide to the national quality framework*. Canberra, ACT: Author.
Australian Children's Education and Care Quality Authority (ACECQA). (2013b). *Guide to the national quality standard*. Sydney, NSW: ACECQA.
Australian Children's Education and Care Quality Authority (ACECQA). (2017a). *Guide to the education and care services national law and the education and care services national regulations 2011*. Sydney, NSW: Author.
Australian Children's Education and Care Quality Authority (ACECQA). (2017b). *National quality standard snapshot*. Sydney, NSW: Author.
Australian Communications and Media Authority. (2017). *Children's television viewing and multi-screen behaviour. Analysis of 2005–16 OxTAM audience data and 2017 survey of parents, careers and guardians*. Melbourne, VIC: Author.
Australian Government. (2009). *Healthy eating and physical activity guidelines for early childhood settings*. Canberra: Australian Government.
Australian Government. (2013). *Get up and grow: Healthy eating and physical activity for early childhood*. Canberra, ACT: Author.
Australian Government Department of Education, Employment and Workplace Relations for the Council of Australian Governments. (2011). *My time, our place: Framework for school age care in Australia*. Canberra, ACT: Author.
Australian Government Productivity Commission. (2016). *National education evidence base. Productivity commission inquiry report. Overview and recommendations*. Canberra, ACT: Author.
Australian Institute of Family Studies. (2017). *Longitudinal study of Australian children*. Melbourne: AIFS.
Bruce, E., Klein, R., & Keleher, H. (2012). Parliamentary inquiry into health promoting schools in Victoria: Analysis of stakeholder views. *Journal of School Health, 82*(9), 441–447. https://doi.org/10.1111/j.1746-1561.2012.00720.
Camilli, G., Vargas, S., Ryan, S., & Barnett, S. W. (2010). Meta-analysis of the effects of early education interventions on cognitive and social development. *Teachers College Record, 112* (3), 579–620.
Chow, A. F., & Humbert, L. (2011). Physical activity and nutrition in early years care centers: Barriers and facilitators. *Canadian Children, 36*(1), 26.
Chow, A. F., & Humbert, M. L. (2014). Perceptions of early childhood educators: Factors influencing the promotion of physical activity opportunities in Canadian rural care centers. *Child Indicators Research, 7*(1), 57–73. https://doi.org/10.1007/s12187-013-9202.
Cleland, P., & Gallegos, D. (2016). *LEAPS Report*. Brisbane: Queensland University of Technology.
Cloney, D., Tayler, C., Hattie, J., Cleveland, G., & Adams, R. (2016). The selection of ECEC programmes by Australian families: Quality, availability, usage and family demographics. *Australasian Journal of Early Childhood, 41*(4), 16–27.
Cole, A., Vidgen, H., & Cleland, P. (2017). Food provision in early childhood education and care services: Exploring how staff determine nutritional adequacy. *Nutrition & Dietetics, 74*(1), 105–110. https://doi.org/10.1111/1747-0080.12310.
Council of Australian Governments (COAG). (2007). *Council of Australian governments' meeting, Melbourne Communiqué*. Canberra, ACT: Commonwealth of Australia. http://www.coag.gov.au/sites/default/files/Communique%2020%20December%202007.pdf.
Council of Australian Governments (COAG). (2008). *National partnership agreement on early childhood education*. Canberra, ACT: Commonwealth of Australia. http://rti.cabinet.qld.gov.au/documents/2009/nov/national%20quality%20agenda%20for%20early%20childhood%20ed%20and%20care/Attachments/national_partnership_on_early_childhood_education.pdf.
Council of Australian Governments (COAG). (2009). *National early childhood development strategy: Investing in the early years*. Canberra, ACT: COAG.
Cross, D., Miller, M., & Hearn, L. (2007). Engaging primary health care providers in the promotion of healthy weight among young children: Barriers and enablers for policy and

management. In N. Glasgow & L. Naccarella (Eds.), *Australian Journal of Primary Health, 13* (2), 66–79.

Cumming, J., & Mawdesley, R. (2013). Australia, quality education and the 'best interests of the child'. *Australasian Journal of Education, 57*(3), 292–309.

Cyril, S., Nicholson, J. M., Agho, K., Polonsky, M., & Renzaho, A. M. (2017). Barriers and facilitators to childhood obesity prevention among culturally and linguistically diverse (CALD) communities in Victoria, Australia. *Australian and New Zealand Journal of Public Health, 41* (3), 287–293. https://doi.org/10.1111/1753-6405.12648.

de Silva-Sanigorski, A., Elea, D., Bell, C., Kremer, P., Carpenter, L., Nichols, M., Smith, M., Sharp, S., Boak, R., & Swinburn, B. (2011). Obesity prevention in the family day care setting: Impact of the Romp & Chomp intervention on opportunities for children's physical activity and healthy eating. *Child: Care, Health and Development, 37*(3), 385–393.

de Silva-Sanigorski, A., Prosser, L., Carpenter, L., Honisett, S., Gibbs, L., Moodie, M., et al. (2010). Evaluation of the childhood obesity prevention programme Kids-'Go for your life'. *BMC Public Health, 10*(1), 288.

Department of Education Training and Employment. (2014). *Early childhood education and care services census 2013, regulated education and care services in Queensland*. Brisbane: Author.

Edwards, S., Skouteris, H., Rutherford, L., & Cutter-Mackenzie, A. (2013). 'It's all about Ben10™': Children's play, health and sustainability decisions in the early years. *Early Child Development and Care, 183*(2), 280–293. https://doi.org/10.1080/03004430.2012.671816.

Fenech, M., Giugni, M., & Bown, K. (2012). A critical analysis of the national quality framework: Mobilizing for a vision for children beyond minimum standards. *Australasian Journal of Early Childhood, 37*(4), 5–14.

Finch, M., Jones, J., Yoong, S., Wiggers, J., & Wolfenden, L. (2016). Effectiveness of center-based childcare interventions in increasing child physical activity: A systematic review and meta-analysis for policymakers and practitioners. *Obesity Reviews, 17,* 412–428. https://doi.org/10.1111/obr.12392.

Garvis, S., & Pendergast, D. (2011). Warning-television viewing may harm your child's health: Parent perceptions of early childhood viewing habits. *Australasian Journal of Early Childhood, 36*(4), 22–28.

Goldfeld, S., O'Connor, E., O'Connor, M., Sayers, M., Moore, T., Kvalsvig, A., et al. (2016). The role of preschool in promoting children's healthy development: Evidence from an Australian population cohort. *Early Childhood Research Quarterly, 35*, 40–48. https://doi.org/10.1016/j.ecresq.2015.11.001.

Hardy, L. L., Hector, D., Saleh, S., & King, L. (2016). Australian Middle Eastern parents' perceptions and practices of children's weight-related behaviors: Talking with parents' study. *Health and Social Care in the Community, 24*(5), 63–71. https://doi.org/10.1111/hsc.12247.

Hardy, L. L., King, L., Kelly, B., Farrell, L., & Howlett, S. (2010). Munch and move: Evaluation of a preschool healthy eating and movement skill programme. *International Journal of Behavioral Nutrition and Physical Activity, 7*(1), 80.

Hearn, L. A., Miller, M. R., & Campbell-Pope, R. (2008). Review of evidence to guide primary health care policy and practice to prevent childhood obesity. *The Medical Journal of Australia, 188*(8), S87–S91.

Hesketh, K., Waters, E., Green, J., Salmon, L., & Williams, J. (2005). Healthy eating, activity and obesity prevention: A qualitative study of parent and child perceptions in Australia. *Health Promotion International, 20*(1), 19–26. https://doi.org/10.1093/heapro/dah503.

Hunkin, E. (2016). Deploying foucauldian genealogy: Critiquing 'quality' reform in early childhood policy in Australia. *Power and Education, 8*(1), 35–53. https://doi.org/10.1177/1757743815624114.

https://www.childhealthpoll.org.au/polls/screen-time-whats-happening-in-our-homes/.

https://www.acma.gov.au/theACMA/kids-tv-viewing-and-multi-screen-behaviour.

http://www.curriculum.edu.au/verve/_resources/National_Declaration_on_the_Educational_Goals_for_Young_Australians.pdf.

Irvine, S., & Farrell, A. (2013). Are we there yet? Early rears reform in Queensland: Stakeholder perspectives on the introduction of funded preschool programmes in long day care services. *International Journal of Early Childhood, 45*(2), 221–236.

Ishimine, K. (2011). Quality in early childhood education and care: A case study of disadvantage. *The Australian Educational Researcher, 38*(3), 257–274. https://doi.org/10.1007/s13384-011-0028-6.

Jackson, J. (2015). Constructs of quality in early childhood education and care: A close examination of the NQS assessment and rating instrument. *Australasian Journal of Early Childhood, 40*(3), 46–50.

Logan, H., Press, F., & Sumsion, J. (2012). The quality imperative: Tracing the rise of 'quality' in Australian early childhood education and care policy. *Australasian Journal of Early Childhood, 37*(3), 4–13.

Logan, H., & Sumsion, J. (2010). Early childhood teachers' understandings of and provision for quality. *Australasian Journal of Early Childhood, 35*(3), 42–50.

Logan, H., Sumsion, J., & Press, F. (2013). The Child Care Act 1972: A critical juncture in Australian ECEC and the emergence of 'quality'. *Australasian Journal of Early Childhood, 38*(4), 84–91.

Ministerial Council on Education, Employment Training and Youth Affairs. (2008). *Melbourne declaration on educational goals for young Australians.* Canberra, ACT: Author.

Mooney, A., Boddy, J., Statham, J., & Warwick, I. (2008). Approaches to developing health in early years settings. *Health Education, 108*(2), 163–177. https://doi.org/10.1108/09654280810855603.

New South Wales Government. (2017). *Munch and move.* https://www.healthykids.nsw.gov.au/home/site-map.aspx.

Organization for Economic Cooperation and Development (OECD). (2001). *Starting strong.* Paris: OECD.

Organization for Economic Cooperation and Development (OECD). (2006). *Starting strong II.* Paris: OECD.

Organization for Economic Cooperation and Development (OECD). (2012). *Starting strong III. A quality toolbox for ECEC.* Paris: OECD.

Organization for Economic Cooperation and Development (OECD). (2017a). *Key OECD indicators on early childhood education and care.* Paris: OECD. https://doi.org/10.1787/9789264276116-en.

Organization for Economic Cooperation and Development (OECD). (2017b). *International early learning and child well-being study (IEL).* Paris: OECD.

Organization for Economic Cooperation and Development (OECD). (2017c). *Programme for international student assessment.* Paris: OECD. http://www.oecd.org/pisa/.

Pagnini, D., King, L., Booth, S., Wilkenfeld, R., & Booth, M. (2009). The weight of opinion on childhood obesity: Recognizing complexity and supporting collaborative action. *International Journal of Pediatric Obesity, 4*(4), 233–241. https://doi.org/10.3109/17477160902763333.

Pagnini, D., Wilkenfeld, R., King, L., & Booth, M. (2007). Early childhood sector staff perceptions of child overweight and obesity: The weight of opinion study. *Health Promotion Journal of Australia: Official Journal of Australian Association of Health Promotion Professionals, 18*(2), 149–154.

Roberts, W. (2015). Enabling change through education for children and their families experiencing vulnerability and disadvantage: The understandings of early childhood professionals. *Australasian Journal of Early Childhood, 40*(2), 49–56.

Shepherd, J., Harden, A., Rees, R., Brunton, G., Garcia, J., Oliver, S., et al. (2006). Young people and healthy eating: A systematic review of research on barriers and facilitators. *Health Education Research, 21*(2), 239–257.

Staton, S., Irvine, S., Pattinson, C., Smith, S., & Thorpe, K. (2015). The sleeping elephant in the room: Practices and policies regarding sleep/rest time in early childhood education and care. *Australasian Journal of Early Childhood, 40*(4), 77–86.

Tayler, C., Ishimine, K., Cloney, D., Cleveland, G., & Thorpe, K. (2013). The quality of early childhood education and care services in Australia. *Australasian Journal of Early Childhood, 38*(2), 13–21.

Taylor, C., & Thorpe, K. (2012). Assessing the quality of Australian child care and kindergartens. *E4Kids: Effective Early Educational Experiences Research Bulletin, 2*, 1–6. http://web.education.unimelb.edu.au/E4Kids/news/pdfs/E4Kids_Research_Bulletin_Issue2.pdf.

Temple, V., & O'Connor, J. P. (2005). Constraints and facilitators for physical activity in family day care. *Australian Journal of Early Childhood, 30*(4), 1–9.

Tremblay, L., Boudreau-Larivière, C., & Cimon-Lambert, K. (2012). Promoting physical activity in preschoolers: A review of the guidelines, barriers, and facilitators for implementation of policies and practices. *Canadian Psychology/Psychologie Canadienne, 53*(4), 280–290. https://doi.org/10.1037/a0030210.

Tucker, P., van Zandvoort, M. M., Burke, S. M., & Irwin, J. D. (2011). Physical activity at daycare: Childcare providers' perspectives for improvements. *Journal of Early Childhood Research, 9*(3), 207–219. https://doi.org/10.1177/1476718X10389144.

United Nations. (1979). *Convention on the rights of the child*. New York: UN. http://legal.un.org/avl/ha/crc/crc.html.

United Nations. (2015). *United Nations sustainable development goals*. New York: UN. http://www.un.org/sustainabledevelopment/sustainable-development-goals/.

United Nations Children's Fund (UNICEF). (2008). *Innocenti report card. The child care transition. A league table of early childhood education and care in economically advanced countries*. Florence: UNICEF Innocenti Research Centre.

United Nations Children's Fund (UNICEF). (2015). *A fair chance for every child. UNICEF Executive Board special session on equity*. New York: UNICEF.

Wiseman, N., Harris, N., & Lee, P. (2016). Lifestyle knowledge and preferences in preschool children: Evaluation of the get up and grow healthy lifestyle education programme. *Health Education Journal, 75*(8), 1012–1024. https://doi.org/10.1177/0017896916648726.

Wolfenden, L., Finch, M., Nathan, N., Weaver, N., Wiggers, J., Yoong, S. L., et al. (2015). Factors associated with early childhood education and care service implementation of healthy eating and physical activity policies and practices in Australia: A cross-sectional study. *Translational Behavioral Medicine, 5*(3), 327–334. https://doi.org/10.1007/s13142-015-0319-y.

Wong, S., Harrison, L., Rivalland, C., & Whiteford, C. (2014). Utilization of early childhood education and care services in a nationally representative sample of Australian children: A focus on disadvantage. *Australasian Journal of Early Childhood, 39*(2), 60–69.

Yoong, S. L., Finch, M., Nathan, N., Wiggers, J., Lecathelinais, C., Jones, J., et al. (2016). A longitudinal study assessing childcare services' adoption of obesity prevention policies and practices. *Journal of Pediatrics and Child Health, 52*(7), 765–770. https://doi.org/10.1111/jpc.13252.

Chapter 21
The Right to Free and Compulsory Elementary Education in India and Positive Schooling in the Context of the Right Against Sexual Exploitation

Lina Acca Mathew

Abstract The Right to Education for children between the ages of six to fourteen has been declared as a fundamental right under the Constitution of India. This has been translated into a legal right by virtue of the Right of Children to Free and Compulsory Education Act 2009 (called in short, the Right to Education Act or RTE). With the promulgation of the Protection of Children against Sexual Offences Act, 2012, increased sexual exploitation of children in Indian schools is being reported. This chapter discusses the main highlights of the Right to Education Act, and the relevant literature regarding sexual exploitation of children in schools. The necessity for further measures to ensure positive schooling free from sexual exploitation of children is highlighted in this chapter.

Keywords Education · India · Positive schooling · Right to education
Sexual exploitation

Introduction

The Right to Education is an internationally recognized right which ought to be made available for everyone. Article 26 of the Universal Declaration of Human Rights, and Articles 13 and 14 of the International Covenant on Economic, Social, and Cultural Rights (ICCPR), specifies this right. According to Article 13 (2) of the ICCPR, the State has a responsibility to provide free and compulsory basic education for individuals who have not completed primary education, an obligation to introduce free secondary education accessible to all in a progressive manner, as well as an obligation to develop equitable access to free higher education in a progressive manner.

L. A. Mathew (✉)
Government Law College, Calicut, Kerala, India
e-mail: linamathew@gmail.com

S. Deb (ed.), *Positive Schooling and Child Development*,
https://doi.org/10.1007/978-981-13-0077-6_21

It includes an obligation to avoid discrimination at all levels of the educational system, to set minimum standards, and to improve the quality of education. Availability, accessibility, acceptability, and adaptability of education are needed in order to enjoy such a right in a meaningful manner.

The Right to Education also includes a responsibility to provide fundamental education for individuals who have not received or completed the whole period of their primary education. In addition, the Right to Education encompasses also the obligation to eliminate discrimination at all levels of the educational system, to set minimum standards, and to improve quality.

At the international level, Article 26 of the UDHR provides that everyone has a right to education, and that Elementary education shall be free and compulsory. Article 13 of the International Covenant on Economic, Social and Cultural Rights, 1966 provides that: primary education shall be compulsory and available free to all; secondary education, which includes technical and vocational secondary education, shall be generally available and accessible to all, and progressively made free; higher education shall be made equally accessible to all on the basis of capacity, and progressively made free; fundamental education shall be encouraged for those persons who have not received or completed the whole period of their primary education, and schools and fellowships systems shall be developed which include improvement of the material conditions of teaching staff.

Most importantly, the UN Convention on the Rights of the Child, 1989 (UNCRC), to which India acceded on 11 December 1992, reiterates this right to education in Article 28. It also exhorts the State parties to prevent various kinds of exploitation of children. These are detailed in Articles 32–35, namely: economic exploitation, trafficking in narcotic drugs and psychotropic substances, sexual abuse and exploitation, the abduction of, the sale of, or traffic in children for any purpose or in any form, and all other forms of exploitation prejudicial to any aspects of the child's welfare.

Though the word 'child' has not been defined under the Constitution of India, the Constitution-makers were conscious of the fact that the children require special treatment on account of their physical and mental immaturity. This was reflected under various articles of the Constitution:

Article 15 empowers the state to make special provision for children.
Article 23 guarantees the fundamental right against exploitation, and guarantees the right of children against trafficking for sexual exploitation and bonded labour.
Article 24 of the Constitution of India prohibits child labour below the age of 14 years in any factory or mine, or engagement in any other hazardous employment.
Articles 39(e) and 39(f) of Part IV of the Constitution of India put an obligation on the State for protection of children and youth from exploitation, and from moral and material abandonment, as a Directive Principle of the State Policy.

Formerly, Article 45 of the Constitution of India, which is a non-justifiable right under Part IV (Directive Principles of State Policy), obliged the State to endeavour to provide, within a period of ten years from the commencement of the Constitution, for free and compulsory education for all children until they complete the age of fourteen years. However, this directive was not fulfilled within the stipulated time. Education is a subject of the Concurrent List in the Indian Constitution[1]; hence, both Central as well as State governments can make laws regarding this subject.[2] However, in case of conflict between central and state laws, it is the Central law that will prevail, unless the State law has been assented by the President.[3] After Indian Independence, almost all the Indian States and Union Territories enacted their own primary education statutes in the absence of a Central enactment.

In the case of *Miss Mohini Jain v. State of Karnataka and Others*,[4] a two-judge bench of the Supreme Court held that the right to education at all levels is a fundamental right to life, of the citizen under Article 21 of the Constitution of India. It held that charging higher fees, known as capitation fee, for admission to educational institutions is illegal and amounts to denial of a citizen's right to education. Capitation fee makes the availability of education beyond the access of the poor. Such a fee is arbitrary, unfair, and unjust and hence is also in violation of Article 14 of the Constitution. The fundamental right to speech and expression under Article 19 of the Constitution cannot be fully enjoyed unless the citizen is educated and conscious of his individualistic dignity. The honourable judges opined that education in India has never been a commodity for sale.

The Supreme Court examined the correctness of the decision in *Mohini Jain* in the case of *Unnikrishnan* v. *State of Andhra Pradesh*.[5] The five-bench Supreme Court in a 3:2 majority partly overruled the *Mohini Jain* decision, holding that the right to free education is available only to children until they complete the age of fourteen years. After this age, the obligation of the State to provide education is subject to the limits of its economic capacity and development. The obligations created by Articles 41, 45, and 46, under the Directive Principles of State Policy[6] can be discharged by the State either by establishing its own institutions or by aiding, recognizing, or granting affiliation to private institutions. The Supreme

---

[1]Entry 25, List III—Concurrent List, Seventh Schedule, Constitution of India.

[2]Article 246, Constitution of India.

[3]Article 254, Constitution of India.

[4](1992) 3SCC 666.

[5](1993) 1SCC 645.

[6]Article 41 of the Constitution of India embodies the right to work, to education and to public assistance in certain cases. The State shall, within the limits of its economic capacity and development, make effective provision for securing the right to work, to education and to public assistance in cases of unemployment, old age, sickness and disablement, and in other cases of undeserved want.

Article 45 directed provision for childhood care and education to children below the age of fourteen years. This was amended in 2002. Article 46 aims to promote educational and economic interests of Scheduled Castes, Scheduled Tribes, and other weaker sections of the people from social injustice and all forms of exploitation. All these rights are non-justiciable, which means that they cannot be enforced in a court of law.

Court interpreted Article 45 in Part IV of the Constitution to be read in "harmonious construction" with Article 21 (Right to Life) in Part III, as the Right to Life would be meaningless if it is without access to knowledge. By this judgment, the Supreme Court decreed that "free and compulsory education" of all children up to 14 years of age (including children below six years of age) is a fundamental right. Thereafter, the Saikia Committee (1997) recommended an amendment of the Constitution making education for children under 14 a fundamental right.

The Law Commission of India, in its 165th Report in 1998, titled 'Free and Compulsory Education in India', recommended enactment of a Central legislation on this subject. In 2002, the 86th Amendment of the Constitution of India was passed, adding a new provision, Article 21A, to enshrine as a fundamental (justifiable) right the right of all children to free and compulsory education between the ages of six and fourteen, in such manner as the State may, by law, determine. Article 45 of the Constitution of India was amended to state that the State shall now endeavour to provide early childhood care and education for all children until they complete the age of six years. A new clause (k) was also added to Article 51A, which created a fundamental constitutional duty for parents/guardians to provide opportunities for education to his child/ward between the age of six and fourteen years.

Thereafter, the Right of Children to Free and Compulsory Education Act 2009 (RTE) was enacted to provide a legal right to free and compulsory education to all children between the ages of six to fourteen. Now, Section 11 of RTE directs the appropriate government to provide for free pre-school education of children between the ages of three to six years.

Salient Features of the RTE

Section 3 (1) of RTE

This section provides for the legal right to free and compulsory education for all children in the 6–14 age-group, in a neighbourhood school, until the completion of elementary education.[7]

This means that no child shall be liable to pay any kind of fee or charges or expenses which may prevent him or her from pursuing and completing elementary education.[8] The term 'elementary education' is defined as education from first class to eighth class.[9] 'Compulsory education' means an obligation of the appropriate

[7]Section 3(1), *RTE.*

[8]Section 3(2), *RTE.*

[9]Section 2(f), *RTE.*

Government to provide free elementary education to every child between the ages of 6 and 14 years, and to ensure compulsory admission, attendance, and completion of elementary education by every such child.[10]

Section 4 of RTE

This section provides for admission of children above six years of age, who have not been admitted to any school or who have not completed elementary education, in an age-appropriate class till completion of elementary education beyond 14 years, with right to facilities for special training.[11]

Specification of Duties of Appropriate Government, Local Authorities, and Parents

The government and the local authority have the duty to establish schools,[12] the Central and State Governments have concurrent responsibility to provide funds and share financial and other responsibilities[13] and parents/guardians have the duty to admit their child/ward for elementary education in the neighbourhood school.[14] The duties of the appropriate government, in addition to providing free and compulsory elementary education are to ensure availability of a neighbourhood school with requisite infrastructure, teachers, and learning equipment, to ensure admission, attendance, and completion of elementary education for every child, to ensure that children belonging to disadvantaged or weaker section are not discriminated against and prevented from pursuing or completing elementary education on any ground, to provide special training facilities to out-of-school children admitted to age-appropriate class, to provide training facility for teachers, to ensure timely prescribing of curriculum and course of studies, and to ensure quality education conforming to standards specified in the Schedule of the Act.[15]

[10]Explanation to Section 8 (a), *RTE.*

[11]Section 4, *RTE.*

[12]Section 6, *RTE.*

[13]Section 7, *RTE.*

[14]Section 10, *RTE.*

[15]Section 8, *RTE.*

Specification of Responsibilities of Schools and Teachers

The extent of the school's responsibility for free and compulsory education is specified clearly.[16] The Act prohibits collection of capitation fee and subjecting the child/parents/guardian to any screening procedure.[17] Age proof of child is not necessary for admittance to elementary education in school.[18] Detention in any class or expulsion from school is prohibited until the completion of elementary education.[19] The Act prohibits physical punishment or mental harassment in schools.[20] It prohibits the running of unrecognized schools,[21] the deployment of teachers for non-educational purposes,[22] or any engagement in private tuition activities by teachers.[23] Provisions are laid down for appointment of appropriately trained teachers with requisite entry and academic qualifications.[24] Duties of teachers are laid down with regard to maintenance of regularity and punctuality in the school, completion of entire curriculum within a specified time, assessment of the learning ability of each child and provision of supplementary additional instruction if required, holding regular meetings with parents and apprising them of regularity in attendance, learning abilities, progress and other issues concerning the child, and so on.[25]

Other Responsibilities and Specifications

Specifications regarding the curriculum are to be laid down by the State Government.[26] No child is required to pass any board examination till the completion of elementary education. Every child completing elementary education shall be awarded a certificate.[27]

The bodies entrusted by RTE to advise the State Government regarding the implementation and enforcement of the provisions of the Act are the National Commission for Protection of Child Rights and the State Commissions for

---

[16]Section 12, *RTE*.
[17]Section 13, *RTE*.
[18]Section 14, *RTE*.
[19]Section 16, *RTE*.
[20]Section 17, *RTE*.
[21]Section 18, *RTE*.
[22]Section 27, *RTE*.
[23]Section 28, *RTE*.
[24]Section 23, *RTE*.
[25]Section 24, *RTE*.
[26]Section 29, *RTE*.
[27]Section 30, *RTE*.

Protection of Child Rights,[28] the National Advisory Council[29] and the State Advisory Council.[30]

Specification of the norms and standards for fixed pupil-teacher ratio, buildings and infrastructure, minimum number of working days/instructional hours in an academic year, minimum number of working hours in a week for a teacher etc have been laid down in the statute.[31]

Applicability of RTE to Different Categories of Schools: Constitutionality of Section 12, RTE

RTE was promulgated to include all recognized schools imparting elementary education.[32]

Section 2 (n) RTE defines the term 'school' to mean any recognized school imparting elementary education and includes:

- a school established and controlled by the appropriate government[33] or local authority,[34]
- an aided school receiving aid or grants from the appropriate government or local authority,
- a school belonging to a specified category,[35]
- an unaided school not receiving any aid or grant from the appropriate government or local authority.

Clause 1 of section 12 of RTE lays down that a school established and controlled by the appropriate government or local authority, as per sub clause (i) of clause (n) of section 2, shall provide free and compulsory elementary education to all children admitted therein. An aided school receiving aid or grants from the appropriate government or local authority, as per sub clause (ii) of clause (n) of

[28]Section 31, *RTE.*

[29]Section 33, *RTE.*

[30]Section 34, *RTE.*

[31]Schedule, *RTE.*

[32]As per section 2(f) of *RTE*, this means education from classes 1 to 8.

[33]As per section 2 (a) of *RTE*, this includes schools owned or controlled by the Central government or the government of a Union Territory having no legislature, or within the territory of a state government or the government of a Union Territory having a legislature.

[34]As per section 2 (h) of *RTE*, this includes a Municipal Corporation or a Municipal Council or a Zila Parishad or a Nagar Panchayat or Panchayat, and any such other authority/body having administrative control over the school or empowered by or under any law for the time being in force to function as a local authority in any city, town or village.

[35]As per section 2 (p) of *RTE*, this means any school having a distinct character which may be specified by the appropriate government by notification, like Kendriya Vidyalaya, Navodaya Vidyalaya and Sainik School.

section 2, shall provide free and compulsory elementary education to such proportion of children admitted therein as its annual recurring aid or grants so received, bears to its annual recurring expenses subject to a minimum of 25%.

A school belonging to a specified category, as per sub clause (iii) of clause (n) of section 2 of RTE, and an unaided school not receiving any aid or grant from the appropriate government or local authority, as per sub clause (i) of clause (n) of section 2 of RTE, shall admit in class 1, to the extent of at least 25% of the strength of that class, children belonging to weaker section[36] and disadvantaged group[37] in the neighbourhood and provide free and compulsory elementary education till its completion.

Clause (1) of section 12 of RTE provides also for the application of these provisions regarding free and compulsory education for admission to pre-school education in such schools defined in section 2 (n).

Clause (2) of section 12 of RTE lays down that unaided schools, specified in section 2 (n) (iv), shall be reimbursed by the State for the expenditure incurred for the child. Proviso to this clause states that where any such unaided school specified in section 2 (n) (iv) is already under an obligation to provide free education to a specified number of children on account of it having received any land, building, equipment or other facilities, either free of cost or at a concessional rate, such school shall not be entitled for reimbursement to the extent of such obligation.

In 2012, a three-judge bench of the Supreme Court, in *Society for Un-aided Private Schools of Rajasthan* v. *U.O.I. & Another*,[38] upheld the constitutional validity of the Right of Children to Free and Compulsory Education Act, 2009 by a majority of 2:1. The Court stated that judicial decisions have read the right to education into the right to life in Article 21 of the Constitution of India. When a child is denied right to access education, he is not only deprived of his right to live with dignity under Article 21, but also deprived of his right to freedom of speech and expression enshrined in Article 19(1) (a) of the Constitution of India. The RTE seeks to remove all barriers, including financial and psychological barriers, which a child belonging to the weaker and disadvantaged group has to face while seeking admission. The Court added that it is clear from the scheme of Article 21A of the Constitution of India and the RTE that the primary obligation is of the State to provide for free and compulsory education to children between the age of 6 and 14 years and, particularly, to children who are likely to be prevented from pursuing and completing the elementary education due to inability to afford fees or charges.

---

[36]Section 2 (e) of *RTE* defines the term "child belonging to weaker section" to mean a child belonging to such parent or guardian whose annual income is lower than the minimum limit specified by the appropriate Government, by notification.

[37]Section 2 (d) of *RTE* defines the term "child belonging to disadvantaged group" to mean a child belonging to the scheduled caste, the scheduled tribe, the socially and educationally backward class or such other group having disadvantage owing to social, cultural, economical, geographical, linguistic, gender or such other factor, as may be specified by the appropriate Government, by notification.

[38](2012) 6 SCC 1.

The Supreme Court mandated government/aided/and non-minority unaided schools to reserve 25% of the seats for these children. Hence, this decision excluded unaided minority schools which are protected under Article 30 (1) of the Constitution of India, from the ambit of Section 12 of RTE.[39] So such unaided minority schools do not have to reserve 25% of their seats for the free elementary education of children belonging to weaker section and disadvantaged group in the neighbourhood.

This decision of the Supreme Court was held to be incorrect by the five-judge bench of the Supreme Court in *Pramathi Educational and Cultural Trust & Others* v. *Union of India & Others*,[40] which unanimously ruled that RTE is not applicable to any minority institution, whether aided or unaided.

This judgment is criticized as having failed to notice that, besides the 25% quota in Section 12(1) (c) of RTE, the Act also has provisions on infrastructural norms, pupil-teacher ratio, prohibition on screening tests, and capitation fee and ban on corporal punishment. Instead of annihilating the 'minority character' of such institutions, these provisions would benefit both students and community. This judgment also did not consider the fact that the government-aided minority schools stand on a different footing from their unaided counterparts and are more amenable to regulations than the latter (Sangai 2016).

The RTE is criticized as an opportunity for the government to legitimize rampant commercialization of the education that it had promoted during the previous two decades of its so called economic reforms (Teltumbde 2012). Questions have been raised on how much it actually contributes to ensuring the quality of education (Mehendale 2014). This chapter identifies the dire need for schools to ensure the right against sexual exploitation, as this has been omitted from the ambit of Section 17 of RTE which only prohibits physical punishment or mental harassment in schools. The issue of sexual harassment in schools is not addressed in RTE, and there is lack of governmental rules to prevent this problem when victimization of elementary students occurs within the school premises or when the person in a position of trust or authority is connected with the child's elementary educational institution.

The Right Against Sexual Exploitation

Article 34 of the UNCRC provides that state parties undertake to protect the child from all forms of sexual exploitation and sexual abuses, through appropriate national, bilateral, and multilateral measures. These forms of sexual exploitation and sexual abuses are enumerated as three types, namely:

---

[39]Article 30 (1) of the Constitution of India states that all minorities, whether based on religion or language, shall have the right to establish and administer educational institutions of their choice.
[40]AIR 2014 SC 2114.

(a) The inducement or coercion of a child to engage in any unlawful sexual activity;
(b) The exploitative use of children in prostitution or other unlawful sexual practices;
(c) The exploitative use of children in pornographic performances and materials.

This protection is reiterated in the Optional Protocol on the Sale of Children, Child Prostitution and Pornography of 2002, which was signed by India on 15 November 2004 and ratified on 16 August 2005.

The World Health Organization Report on the Consultation on Child Abuse Prevention (1999) defines child sexual abuse as the involvement of a child in sexual activity that he or she does not fully comprehend, is unable to give informed consent to, or that violates the laws or social taboos of society. Child sexual abuse is evidenced by this activity between a child and an adult or another child who by age or development is in a relationship of responsibility, trust, or power, the activity being intended to gratify or satisfy the needs of the other person. This may include but is not limited to the inducement or coercion of a child to engage in any unlawful activity, the exploitative use of a child in prostitution or other unlawful sexual practices, and the exploitative use of children in pornographic performances and material.

The Pinheiro Report on Violence against Children in 2006 included a cross-sectional survey of schools in Goa published by the National Medical Journal of India. This study of eight schools in Goa, covering 811 students, revealed that one third of the students had experienced at least one type of sexual abuse in the previous 12 months and 6% reported that they had been forced to have sex. The most common perpetrators were older students or friends (53%). Parents or relatives accounted for 8%, and teachers for 4% of the perpetrators.

A study on child sexual abuse carried out by NGOs, Save the Children and Tulir, in 2006 looked at the prevalence and dynamics of child sexual abuse among school-going children in Chennai, India. 2,211 respondents were examined. The study included children from various socio-economic strata of society. The prevalence of sexual abuse in upper and middle class was found to be proportionately higher than in lower and lower middle class (the criteria used for stratification: family income less than Rs. 6,000 per month = lower and lower-middle class; between Rs. 6,000 and Rs. 12,000 per month = middle class; higher than Rs. 12,000 per month = upper class). This study found that 42% of children had faced at least one form of sexual abuse, of which 48% were boys and 39% were girls. The prevalence of sexual abuse in upper and middle class was found to be proportionately higher than in lower or lower middle class. The majority of the abusers were people known to the child. Those close to the child used tactics like trickery, and making the children feel special, in order to abuse them and intimidate them to keep that abuse a secret. These tactics indicated the carefully thought-out path that an abuser often takes in order to first prepare a child for abuse and later to maintain the abuse. This context usually made it difficult for the child to say "no" to acts of abuse, and the abuser was also often successful in giving the child the impression that s/he is a participant in those activities, and/or that these activities must be kept a secret.

In a survey of 350 school girls in New Delhi, by the NGO called Sakshi in 1997, 63% had experienced child sexual abuse at the hands of family members, and 25% of the girls had either been raped, made to masturbate the perpetrator, or engage in oral sex.

A Study on Child Abuse in India in 2007 by the Ministry of Women and Child Development (Kakkar et al. 2007) defined sexual abuse as inappropriate sexual behaviour with a child. It includes fondling a child's genitals, making the child fondle an adult's genitals, sexual assault (intercourse, incest, rape, and sodomy), exhibitionism, and pornography. To be considered child abuse, these acts have to be committed by a person responsible for the care of a child or related to the child (for example, a babysitter, parent, neighbour, relatives, extended family member, peer, older child, friend, stranger, or a day-care provider).

This study identified children between the ages of 5 and 18 on the basis of five categories of children: children in family environment, not attending school; children in schools[41]; children in institutional care; working children; and street children.

This study reported that 5- to 12-year-old children are in the high-risk category of all kinds of abuses, and 70% children have not reported this to anyone. This report stated that 53% of children reported having faced one or more forms of sexual abuse; 22% of children had faced severe forms of sexual abuse; and 50% abusers are persons known to the child or in a position of trust and responsibility. Among the five different evidence groups, the highest percentage of children who faced sexual abuse were those at work (61.61%), followed by children on the streets at 54.51% and children in family environment not going to school, at 53.18%. Children in schools reported 49.92% sexual abuse and children in institutional care reported 47.08%. Most children did not report the matter to anyone.

After the publication of this report, the government became convinced of the need for such legislation. The Protection of Children against Sexual Offences Act 2012 (POCSO) provides a comprehensive list of sexual offences against children.

---

[41]In this report, the data collected from children who go to schools showed that the total percentage of children going to government schools was 55.54%, private schools was 26.29%, NGO-run schools 14.91%, and 3.26% in other schools (namely, schools run by charitable organizations and religious bodies). Out of the total child respondents, 25.41% were children in schools, of which 49.76% were boys and 50.24% were girls. Across the states, the sample size of boys and girls was approximately 50:50 with a 10% variance. 41.54% of children in this evidence group were in the age group of 5–12 years, while 32.98% of children were in the age group of 13–14 years and 25.48% of children were in the age group of 15–18 years. In the age group of 5–12 years, 50.61% children were girls, while 55.80% of children in the age group of 13–14 years, and 42.43% of children in the age group of 15–18 years, were girls.

Offences and Punishments Under POCSO

These are as follows:

Penetrative Sexual Assault and Punishment (Sections 3 and 4 POCSO)

Five types of penetrative acts constitute this offence under section 3: penile penetration; insertion of any object or body part into the body of the child; manipulation of any part of the body of a child so as to cause penetration; into vagina, mouth, urethra or anus of the child or making the child to do so with such person or any other person; or oral application to the penis, vagina, anus, urethra of the child; or making the child to do so to such person or any other person. This offence is punishable under section 4 by imprisonment of either description from seven years to life and fine.

Aggravated Penetrative Sexual Assault and Punishment (Sections 5 and 6 POCSO)

Commission of this offence is based on the class of perpetrators, certain types of acts, and certain types of victims. This is laid down in section 5 *POCSO*.

When persons in certain positions of trust and responsibility commit the act of penetrative sexual assault, then they get aggravated punishment under sections 5 and 6 *POCSO*. Those who come under this category of are:

- Police officers
- Members of the armed forces/security forces
- A public servant or the management/staff of a jail, remand home, protection home, observation home, other place of custody or care and protection
- Management/staff of a hospital (both government-run as well as private hospitals)
- Management/staff of an educational institution or religious institution
- A relative of the child through blood/adoption/marriage/guardianship/in foster care/domestic relationship with parent/living in same or shared household
- Anyone having ownership or management or staff of any institution providing services to the child
- Anyone, being in a position of trust or authority of a child in an institution or home
- Anyone, who knows the child is pregnant and commits penetrative sexual assault on a child

Certain types of acts qualify for aggravated punishment. They are:

- Committing gang penetrative sexual assault on a child
- Use of deadly weapons, fire, heated/corrosive substance for committing penetrative sexual assault on a child
- Causing grievous hurt/bodily harm/injury to sex organs of child
- Physically incapacitating a child or
- Causing a child to become mentally ill
- Causing impairment of child temporarily or permanently
- Making a female child pregnant
- Infecting the child with HIV or other life threatening disease
- Committing penetrative sexual assault more than once or repeatedly on a child
- Attempting to murder the child while committing penetrative sexual assault on a child
- Committing penetrative sexual assault on a child in the course of communal or sectarian violence
- Committing penetrative sexual assault on a child who has been previously convicted of offence under this Act or any sexual offence punishable under any other law for the time being in force
- Committing penetrative sexual assault upon a child and making the child to strip or parade naked in public.

When a child belongs to a certain category of victims, committing penetrative sexual assault on a child would qualify for the commission of the offence of aggravated penetrative sexual assault:

- Mentally or physically disabled children
- A child below 12 years of age.

Punishment under section 6 for the offence of aggravated penetrative sexual assault is rigorous imprisonment for a term not less than ten years, to imprisonment for life and a fine.

Sexual Assault and Punishment (Sections 7 and 8 POCSO)

Two elements need to be present in an act in order to come within the ambit of this offence: physical contact without penetration and sexual intent.

The following acts by a person would qualify under section 7 *POCSO*:

- Touching the vagina, penis, anus, or breast, of a child with sexual intent.
- Making a child touch the vagina, penis, anus, or breast, of such person or any other person.
- Doing any other act with sexual intent which involves physical contact without penetration.

The punishment under section 8 POCSO for sexual assault is imprisonment from three years to five years and fine.

Aggravated Sexual Assault and Punishment (Sections 9 and 10 POCSO)

When persons in certain positions of trust and responsibility commit the act of sexual assault, then aggravated punishment under sections 9 and 10 *POCSO* apply. Those who come under this category of offenders are:

- Police officers
- Members of the armed forces/security forces
- A public servant or the management/staff of a jail, remand home, protection home, observation home, other place of custody or care and protection
- Management/staff of a hospital (both government-run as well as private hospitals)
- Management/staff of an educational institution or religious institution
- A relative of the child through blood/adoption/marriage/guardianship/in foster care/domestic relationship with parent/living in same or shared household
- Anyone having ownership or management or staff of any institution providing services to the child
- Anyone, being in a position of trust or authority of a child in an institution or home
- Anyone, who knows the child is pregnant and commits penetrative sexual assault on a child

Certain types of acts qualify for aggravated punishment:

- Committing gang sexual assault on a child
- Using deadly weapons, fire, heated/corrosive substance for committing sexual assault on a child
- Causing grievous hurt/bodily harm/injury to sex organs of child
- Physically incapacitating a child
- Causing a child to become mentally ill
- Causing impairment of child temporarily or permanently
- Making a female child pregnant
- Inflicting a child with HIV or other life threatening disease
- Committing sexual assault more than once or repeatedly on a child
- Attempting to murder the child
- Committing sexual assault on a child in the course of communal or sectarian violence
- Committing sexual assault on a child when previously convicted of any offence under the *POCSO* or any sexual offence punishable under any other law for the time being in force
- Committing sexual assault on a child and making the child to strip or parade naked in public.

When a child belongs to a certain category of victim, then committing sexual assault on such a child would qualify for the commission of the offence of aggravated penetrative sexual assault:

- Mentally or physically disabled children
- A child below twelve years of age.

The punishment under section 10 *POCSO* for aggravated sexual assault is imprisonment for a term not less than five years up to seven years and fine.

Sexual Harassment and Punishment (Sections 11 and 12 POCSO)

One essential element of all acts of sexual harassment is that there should be sexual intent. Various acts such as uttering words, making sounds or gestures, exhibiting objects or body parts, making a child exhibit his body, showing pornography to a child, stalking a child, blackmailing a child and enticing or giving gratification for pornographic purposes come under the ambit of the definition of sexual harassment.

The following acts with sexual intent would constitute sexual harassment under Section 11 *POCSO*:

- Utterance of any word
- Making any sound or makes any gesture or exhibits any object or part of body with the intention that such word or sound shall be heard or such gesture or object or part of body shall be seen by the child
- Makes a child exhibit his body/any part
- Showing any object to a child in any form or media for pornographic purposes
- Repeatedly or constantly following or watching or constantly contacting a child either directly or through electronic, digital or any other means
- Threatening to use in any form of media, a real or fabricated depiction through electronic, film or digital or any other mode, of any part of the body of the child or the involvement of the child in a sexual act
- Enticing a child for pornographic purposes or giving gratification therefore.

The punishment under section 12 *POCSO* shall be imprisonment up to three years and fine.

Using a Child for Pornographic Purposes and Punishment (Sections 13 and 14 POCSO)

Section 13 POCSO punishes anyone who uses a child in any form of media (including program or advertisement telecast by television channels or internet or any other electronic form or printed form, whether or not such program or advertisement is intended for personal use or for distribution) for the purposes of sexual gratification, which includes: representation of the sexual organs of a child; usage of a child engaged in real or simulated sexual acts (with or without penetration); and the indecent or obscene representation of a child.

An explanation is appended to section 13 *POCSO* regarding the expression "use a child". This expression shall include involving a child though any medium like print, electronic, computer or any other technology for preparation, production, offering, transmitting, publishing, facilitation and distribution of the pornographic material. Punishments are many and varied, and have been extensively laid down in section 14 POCSO as follows:

- For mere usage of a child for pornographic purposes, the punishment is imprisonment of either description up to 5 years and fine. In the event of subsequent conviction, punishment shall be imprisonment of either description up to 7 years and fine (section 14(1) POCSO).
- If a person uses the child for pornographic purposes coupled with penetrative sexual assault, by directly participating in the pornographic act, such person shall be liable for not less than ten years imprisonment of either description to life imprisonment and fine. If a person uses a child for pornographic purposes coupled with aggravated penetrative sexual assault, by directly participating in the pornographic act, the punishment is rigorous imprisonment for life and fine (section 14(2) POCSO).
- If any person uses a child for pornographic purposes coupled with sexual assault, by directly participating in the pornographic act, the punishment shall be imprisonment of either description for a term which is not less than 6 years imprisonment up to 8 years and fine (section 14(3) POCSO).
- If any person uses a child for pornographic purposes coupled with aggravated sexual assault, by directly participating in the pornographic act, the punishment shall be imprisonment of either description for a term of not less than 8 years imprisonment up to 10 years and fine (section 14(4) POCSO).
- If any person commits the offence abetment of any offence under the POCSO, the punishment shall be as provided for the actual commission of the offence. If any person attempts to commit an offence under the POCSO, punishment is imprisonment for a term up to one half of the imprisonment for life or one half of the longest term of imprisonment provided for that offence or with fine or with both (section 14(5) POCSO).

Punishment for Storage of Pornographic Material Involving Child (Section 15 POCSO)

Section 15 POCSO states that if any person, for commercial purposes, stores any form of child pornography, such person shall be punished with imprisonment of either description for a maximum period of three years or with fine or with both.

Abetment of an Offence and Punishment (Sections 16 and 17 POCSO)

A person abets an offence, when that person instigates any person to do that offence or engages in any conspiracy to do that offence, or intentionally aids the doing of that offence is said to aid the doing of that offence (Section 16 *POCSO*). Punishment for abetment is the punishment for that offence.

Punishment for Attempt to Commit an Offence (Section 18 POCSO)

Attempt is punishable with imprisonment of any description provided for in the offence, for a term which may extend to one-half of the imprisonment for life or as the case may be, one-half of the longest term of imprisonment provided for that offence or with fine or with both.

Punishment for Failure to Report (Section 21 POCSO)

This Act has also introduced a legal system of mandatory reporting for the first time in India. As a result of this, teachers, doctors, nurses etc. are now legally obliged to report suspected cases of child sexual abuse. According to section 19 of the Act, any person, including a child, who has apprehension that such sexual offence is likely to be committed or who has knowledge that such offence has been committed, he shall inform the police. Section 21 goes on to add that if any person fails to report the commission of such offence, he shall be punished with either simple or rigorous imprisonment for a period up to six months or with fine or with both imprisonment and fine.

Is There a Right Against Sexual Exploitation of Children in Schools?

Mandatory reporting in the Indian context is problematic, as personnel who come into contact with children who are sexually abused may not be aware of how to handle such information, or be aware about the current legal implications of suppressing such information, which may take place in order to protect the traditionally-assumed ‘larger interest of the child’ or in order to shield the school from legal action, or to avoid interface with the criminal justice system in India, which is notorious for its lack of people-friendliness. Belur and Singh (2015) point out that the lack of training for professionals—doctors, teachers, psychologists, social workers, counsellors—working with children, on how to deal with knowledge of sexual activity and to respond appropriately can be an additional problem.

However, current news reports repeatedly relate horrific stories of elementary school children being sexually assaulted by teachers and other personnel in schools in many parts of India. In this context, Ashok (2017) rightly laments that there is no culture of research which is necessary to study the child sex offender and the patterns and motives governing these crimes, so that such people are identified and adequately treated. He unerringly points out the reality that no campaign so far has demanded that the Indian government institute a program on the lines of the Behavioural Sciences Unit of the Federal Bureau of Investigation in the USA.

Sharma et al. (2015) advocate a 'systems approach' to assuage sexual violence, which consists of augmenting professional competence in victim care and modernizing post-rape protocols/procedures. They urge the Government of India to engage in deployment of forensic nurses/examiners, invest in forensic and rape-crisis facilities, and sensitize professionals to facilitate evidence collection and victim counselling in order to assuage sexual violence. They believe that extreme under-reporting (85% in 2011) and acute shortage of physicians are strong reasons for inclusion of every healthcare professional in victim-care surveillance teams.

Sharma et al. (2015) document the existence of various anti-sexual violence schemes in western countries. The largest anti-sexual violence organization in the USA is called Rape, Abuse, and Incest National Network (RAINN). This network has 1100 local rape treatment hotlines, helping around 1.5 million victims with around-the-clock free confidential victim-care supports, and provides statistics to policy makers, public health centres, and educational institutions. There are 650 sexual assault response teams in the USA, with representatives from health care, forensic, local rape crisis centres, law enforcement and prosecution units. Sharma et al. (2015) quote the National Crime Victimization Survey 2006–2010 Report of the U.S Department of Justice in 2012, which states that these methods have helped the USA to reduce rapes by 60% since 1993, preventing around 2,546,420 rapes in 10 years. A similar European organization, called Rape Crisis Network (RCNE), operates in 30 member countries by collecting data, conducting research, offering counselling, legal advice, and assisting policy makers for educational and legal reform. RCNE's English and Welsh chapters also assist their respective governments similarly.

Section 39 of POCSO directs State governments to prepare guidelines for use of NGOs, professionals and experts or persons having knowledge of psychology, social work, physical health, mental health, and child development to be associated with the pre-trial stage and trial stage to assist the child, subject to rules made on this behalf. Section 44 states that the National Commission for Protection of Child Rights and the State Commissions for Protection of Child Rights shall monitor the implementation of this Act. Rule 9 of the Protection of Children against Sexual Offences Rules states that the National Commission for Protection of Child Rights and the State Commissions for Protection of Child Rights shall be in charge of monitoring the formation of guidelines under Section 39 of *POCSO* and monitoring the application of these guidelines.

It is evident from a reading of the provisions of the POCSO Act, 2012, and its Rules that there is no specific prohibition of child sexual abuse within school environments, nor are measures laid down to prevent and protect children in schools from sexual abuse by persons in positions of trust and authority in schools.

Later studies by Deb and Walsh (2012) cite findings that reveal that 18.1% students experienced sexual violence in their home environment. A 2014 study by Krishnakumar et al. among adolescent school children also report sexual advances which occurred during travel situations in a bus or train.

Review of existing literature on sexual abuse of school children reveal that there are not enough studies that document how school children are sexually exploited within the school environment, or by teachers or helpers in their schools who exploit them outside the school environment. Hence, there is lack of clarity regarding data regarding sexual exploitation of school children by people in positions of trust and authority in schools in India. In response to the case where a seven-year-old Class II student was sexually assaulted and murdered in the toilet of a school by the school bus conductor, the Central Board of Secondary Education (CBSE) issued a circular to the heads of all schools affiliated to the CBSE containing provisions to be strictly followed by all such schools, failing which appropriate action would be taken, which would include the disaffiliation of the school.[42] These provisions are:

- The school must obtain a security/safety audit of its premises and personnel from their respective police station and follow their security related advice. This must be reported on the CBSE website within two months of receipt of this circular.
- CCTV cameras must be installed at all vulnerable areas of the school premises.
- Schools must get police verification and psychometric evaluation of all staff, including detailed evaluation of bus drivers, conductors, peon, and other support staff.
- Support staff must be employed only from authorized agencies and proper records are to be maintained.
- To constitute a parent-teacher-student committee for safety needs of students.
- Controlled access of outsiders to school building and monitoring of visitors.
- To provide training and development for staff.
- There should be separate committees for redressal of public/staff/parents students' grievances, Internal Complaints committee on sexual harassment and committees under the POCSO. The information of these committees must be displaced on the notice board and in the school website.

Conducting security audit of school premises and personnel, and psychometric evaluation of staff are being introduced for the first time by the CBSE. Such kind of

[42]Circular No. 19/2017 dated 12/09/2017.

premise safety check and personnel audit are unique to the Indian school system, and a step in the right direction. However, how such checks are to be conducted has not been specified. Though the CBSE has risen to the occasion, this is not the case with regard to government schools, and government aided schools which are not affiliated to the government. It is clear that there is a glaring lacuna in law and policy regarding protection of the right against sexual exploitation of children who are imparted free and compulsory elementary education in schools in India.

Conclusion

The Indian Government has taken upon itself the positive obligation to ensure the right to free and compulsory elementary education for every child in India between the ages of six and fourteen. By virtue of the RTE, the Government has bound itself to take upon the responsibility, which comes along with this commitment, to develop strong measures to ensure that every child is educated in a safe environment that is free from physical abuse and mental harassment. However, the obligation to provide measures to prevent sexual harassment in school environments was omitted from the ambit of RTE. In the light of India's international commitments under the UNCRC, as well commitment to the objectives of the national legislation on POCSO, new norms must be laid down to ensure that the educational environment is free from persons perpetrating sexual violence, who seem to increasingly be in positions of trust and responsibility in Indian schools today.

References

Ashok, G. V. (2017). *Why Child Rights campaigns in India have failed to stop incidents like Ryan school murder.* http://www.wionews.com/india-news/why-child-rights-campaigns-in-india-have-failed-to-stop-incidents-like-ryan-school-murder-20115.

Belur, J., & Singh, B. B. (2015). Child sexual abuse and the law in India: A commentary. *Crime Science, 4*, 26 https://doi.org/10.1186/s40163-015-0037-2.

Deb, S., & Walsh, K. (2012). Impact of physical, psychological, and sexual violence on social adjustment of school children in India. *School Psychology International, 33*(4), 391–415.

Kakkar, L., Varadan, S., & Kumar, P. (2007). *A study on child abuse: India 2007.* Ministry of Women and Child Development, Government of India. http://www.childlineindia.org.in/pdf/MWCD-Child-Abuse-Report.pdf.

Krishnakumar, P., Satheesan, K., Geeta, M. G., & Sureshkumar, K. (2014). Prevalence and spectrum of sexual abuse among adolescents in Kerala, South India. *Indian Journal of Pediatrics, 81*, 770–774.

Law Commission of India. (1998). *Free and compulsory education in India.* 165th Report. New Delhi. http://lawcommissionofindia.nic.in/101-169/report165.pdf.

Mehendale, A. (2014). The question of quality in education—Does the *RTE* Act provide an answer. *CICE Hiroshima University, Journal of International Cooperation in Education, 16*(2): 87–103. https://clix.tiss.edu/wp-content/uploads/2017/03/The-Question-of-%E2%80%9CQuality%E2%80%9D-in-Education.pdf.

Pinheiro, P. S. (2006). *World report on violence against children*. Geneva, Switzerland: United Nations Secretary-General's Study on Violence against Children.

Sangai, A. (2016). Harmonizing RTE with minority schools. *The Hindu*, July 05, 2016 02:01 IST. http://www.thehindu.com/opinion/op-ed/Harmonising-RTE-with-minority-schools/article14472702.ece.

Sharma, P., Unnikrishnan M. K., & Sharma, A. (2015). Sexual violence in India: addressing gaps between policy and implementation. *Health Policy and Planning, 30*(5), 656–659. https://doi.org/10.1093/heapol/czu015.

Teltumbde, A. (2012). *Supreme court judgment on right to education: Much ado for nothing*. http://www.countercurrents.org/teltumbde130512.htm.

Tulir. (2006). Research on prevalence & dynamics of child sexual abuse among school going children in Chennai. *TULIR—CPHCSA and Save the Children Sweden*.

World Health Organization. (1999). Report of the consultation on child abuse prevention. Geneva, March 29–31. Document WHO/HSC/PVI/99.1 at p. 62.

Chapter 22
Two Visions of Positive Schooling

Sridipa Sinha and Sutripta Banerjee

Abstract Positive schooling refers to an education system that is based on positive psychology which focuses on individual well-being. Learning is a cooperative act where teacher, student and community share positive emotions, support each other, and work together for the general well-being of society. Rabindranath Tagore from Asia (India) and Maria Montessori from Europe (Italy) were leading spokespersons for compassionate humanism and culture in India and the world. This paper seeks to look into the educational features of the schools established by Rabindranath Tagore and Maria Montessori. The paper also tries to identify the various features of positive schooling as reflected in their institutions. The understanding of the practices of Rabindranath Tagore and Maria Montessori institutions will pave the way for creating a positive climate in school of the present era.

Keywords Rabindranath Tagore · Maria Montessori · Positive schooling
India · Italy

Introduction

School is a formal institution designed to transmit knowledge and skills children need to be productive members of society. Schooling refers to the process of being taught in school. The word positive is an adjective, meaning hopeful or certain. Positive Schooling refers to a schooling which is full of hope or certainty of all round development of the child through a joyful learning experience. School is a complex social system where there are students, teachers, classroom, relationships, and social cultural context. Positive schooling takes into account all these factors and makes sure that each and every member of the school is happy and feels proud

S. Sinha (✉)
Department of Education, University of Calcutta, Kolkata, India
e-mail: dr.sridipa.sinha@gmail.com

S. Banerjee
Saheed Nurul Islam Mahavidyalaya, Tentulia, West Bengal, India

S. Deb (ed.), *Positive Schooling and Child Development*,
https://doi.org/10.1007/978-981-13-0077-6_22

to be a part of it. A positive schooling experience focuses on the training of heart and mind. Students not only gain knowledge in this type of schooling but they also develop skills to understand their own well-being as well as others well-being. In positive schooling, the student discovers himself through the teacher's guidance and peer collaboration. In positive schooling, a sense of commitment develops among the teachers, students and the community for holistic development of society.

Modern education stresses on child-centrism. Today, the child occupies the key place in education. Development of mind, body, and spirit of the child are reflected in the program and planning of education. The course of study, syllabi, and teaching methods are framed in accordance with the demands and interests of the children. It aims at the all-round development of children.

The main features of child-centric education are freedom, activity, spontaneous development, and experience based education. In positive schooling, all these features are taken into account.

Positive schooling encourages student independence and stresses on developing problem-solving skills of the students. Constructivism is a new approach of the teaching process that has made the learning process in the modern world more activity-oriented and learner-centric. The Constructivist setting of the school environment is associated with many benefits like developing academic motivation, critical thinking, social and moral maturity, and positive attitudes towards the school. Positive schooling also stresses on all these characteristics among children. So the constructivist approach directly contributes to the concept of positive schooling.

Relationships are another important factor of positive schooling. Positive relationships need to be developed among the teacher and students, among the peers, between the teacher and the parents, between the administrator and the teachers, and lastly the administrators and the parents. Building strong relationships among the student, teachers, administrators, and parents should be given priority in schools. Schools can increase the parent involvement by fostering personal parent–teacher relationships, building bridges between the home culture and school culture, and involving parents in school governance.

Rabindranath Tagore and Maria Montessori have contributed greatly towards the advancement of modern educational ideas and practices. Rabindranath Tagore's experience with conventional instruction was not a really pleasant one, so he devoted his life to establish an alternative course of education at Santiniketan. It aimed at promoting social and environmental harmony. Maria Montessori developed the Montessori Method of training through various experiments. Her method spread and gained popularity throughout the world. She was not just a pioneer, but went on to become one of the leading educators of the globe. The educational visions of the two educators complemented each other and paved the path for a more integrated and a better balanced educational system. Their education system reflects certain important characteristics of positive schooling. First, let us explore the major features of the schools established by both the educators.

The Main Features of Tagore's Santiniketan School

Rabindranath Tagore had established an alternative arrangement of education at Santiniketan, which was later renamed as the Patha Bhavan in 1925. He took a leading role in articulating the program of education based on the spirit of cooperation, brotherhood, and Universalism.

Learning in Nature

Nature occupied an important place in Tagore's concept of education. His concept of nature was based on his childhood experiences, Indian philosophy, the writings of Kalidasa, Vaishnava poetry, and western romanticism. In *Reminiscences*, he writes how he was bounded inside the mansion and he yearned for the outdoor world through the window pane. He saw nature as his companion and a symbol of limitless joy and freedom. In his school, he tried to provide education in a natural setting. Santiniketan was an ideal location in a natural setting which had associations of physical and mental freedom for Rabindranath. Here, children are able to come directly in contact with nature. Tagore believed that education given in a natural setting developed intimacy with the world. It is therefore essential not only to know nature, but to live in nature. 'School' according to him, is like a large home in which the children and teachers with their family lived together, sharing a common life of high aspirations, planning to bring a noble effort in contact with nature on one hand and with the spirit of joy on the other. The children in Santiniketan sat beneath the trees on the mats. Children were free to move around the nature in between the classes. Besides this, the spring festival (*Basant Panchami*) and the rain festival (*Barsha Mangal*) were celebrated at Santiniketan. Children were able to explore the nature and gain knowledge about his surroundings.

The Guru Model

Rabindranath Tagore wanted his students to live in close association with dedicated teachers. A 'Guru' is a teacher who devotes his whole mind and spirit to the service of students "to put life into his pupils with his own life, light their lamps with his own learning, and make them happy with his affection" (Tagore 1961). Rabindranath Tagore derived an example from his life, regarding his brother Jyotindranath as a model. Tagore also set himself as an example. He was affectionately called *Gurudev* by the students. He provided an inspiring role model with his multifaceted talent. He could spontaneously create an atmosphere of games, play, and songs to engage the students. He created a family atmosphere as he also brought in members of his own family, like his brother Dwijendranath Tagore and his nephew Dinendranath Tagore. From outside, teachers like Satish Chandra Ray, Ajit Chakrabarti, Nandalal Bose, Mukul De, C. F. Andrews, and W. W. Pearson, taught at Shantiniketan.

Spiritual Integration

The first syllabus for Santiniketan stated that Tagore's principle in starting his school was to give the students a spiritual culture. "We rely more upon the subconscious influence of nature, of the associations of the place and the daily life of worship that we live, than on any conscious effort to reach them" (Tagore 2012). Tagore believed that the recitation of the *Gayatri Mantra* helped the children realize the connection of the individual with the world around. He believed that the work of education was to connect man to man with love and friendship. The aim of education, according to him, was to help the child to realize the universal whole. The child must have a love for everything and realize the harmony relationship between himself and the world around him. He stressed on humanity and community work in his institution so that the children are able to locate the truth about themselves and the world around.

Aesthetic Education

Tagore gave importance to the development of the aesthetic senses. Music, literature, art, dance, and drama formed an important part of the daily life of the school. He pointed out that "we felt we would try to test everything" and that "no achievement seemed impossible… we wrote, we sang, we acted, we poured ourselves out on, every side" (Tagore 1962). At Santiniketan, creative activities were encouraged among the students. A stimulating atmosphere was maintained in the school where creativity could flourish. Students came out with their own publications. Magazines contained poetry, prose, illustration of painting and drawing of students. Dramas written by Rabindranath Tagore were enacted at Santiniketan, and pupils were actively involved in both the performance and production of the dramas. Children at Santiniketan were encouraged to realize the truth and beauty of nature through the creation of new things in the form of art, music, dance, and drama. Tagore advocated these activities as essential part of his institution.

Education in Mother Tongue

Rabindranath Tagore was in favour of imparting education through the mother tongue. His view was strengthened and consolidated by his personal experiences acquired in different progressive countries of the world, including Germany, France, Japan, and America. He was of the opinion that proper grounding in mother tongue helps to learn foreign languages.

At Santiniketan, the medium of instruction at the primary level was Bengali, with English as a second language. One of Rabindranath Tagore's concerns from an early age was the development of Bengali resources. He tried to enrich the language by writing poems, plays, novels, essays, and text books on language and science. The first criterion in Tagore's vision for relevant education was its local relevance, but at the same time, its conclusion with the larger world.

Kinaesthetic Education

Rabindranath placed great importance on kinaesthetic education; that is, learning through feeling. He believed that children should be given the opportunity to give expression to their feelings through perfect body movement. Tagore emphasizes the importance of education to exercise and enrich the power of sensitivity inherent in everyone which paves the way for free human development. Like the naturalist, he stressed on the training of gateways of learning. He said that:

> If the education of the body does not go on simultaneously with the education of the mind, the mind itself is not properly stimulated. The reason why many boys seem dull is class in that the claims of their bodies are not being met in their education (Tagore 2012).

Activities which were conducive to develop sensory awareness were chosen. Children were taught to take care of their body so that the body became aware and sensitive. Sports of different types like gymnastics, *lathi* play, ju jitsu, and dance were included in the curriculum which provided physical and practical training. So, primary importance in education was given to exercise, and to enrich the powers of sensitivity inherent in everyone which paved avenues to human development and all round excellence of the child.

Education for Freedom

Rabindranath Tagore's concept of freedom was given shape at Santiniketan. An atmosphere of joy and freedom prevailed in Tagore's school where the pupil learnt lessons under the trees in the lap of nature. *Mukti* or freedom is the central idea of Tagore's educational thought. But this freedom does not mean uncontrolled freedom, but freedom with the disciplinary code of conduct of the students. The discipline was self-discipline that came from within. He said that in his institution he tried to make provision of three aspects of freedom-freedom of mind, freedom of heart and freedom of will. Tagore states

> I tried my best to develop in the children of my school the freshness of their feeling for Nature, a sensitiveness of soul in their relationship with the human surroundings, with the help of literature, festive ceremonials and also the religious teaching which enjoins us to come to the nearer presence of the world through the soul, thus to gain it more can be measured- like gaining an instrument in truth by bringing out its music (Tagore 2002).

Tagore wanted freedom for the integrated growth and development of the child. This freedom he believed could be attained by regulating impulses, developing mental abilities through aesthetic performance, cooperation, and community work. The open air classes under the trees provided the ideal environment for the spontaneous and joyful self-expression.

Education for Social Responsibility

Rabindranath Tagore sought a balance between the development of the personality and improvement of the society. Students were made aware of social responsibility. Fellow feelings among the students and seniors, assistance to the neighbours in distress, friendliness towards other sects and communities were encouraged in the institution. Festivals like *Raksha Bandhan* was celebrated in Santiniketan to promote community spirit. Senior students helped junior ones in crises; this illustrated the empathy that the students had among themselves. *Ashrama Sammilani*, a student council, played a vital role. Weekly *Sahitya Sabha* (Literary meeting), *Dan Sangrha* (collection of donation), *Gram Paridarshan* (visit to villages) *Van bhojan* (Annual Picnic) formed a part of co-curricular activities.

Major Features of Montessori's Children's House or *Casa dei Bambini*

Montessori was able to trial her ideas in the Children's Houses. Montessori combined ideas of Rousseau, Pestalozzi Froebel, ltard, and Seguins' educational principles with the games of practical life and the education of senses and the experiences she gained at Orthophrenic Institute. Montessori focused on the physical and mental needs of the children through a sensory motion approach. She also tried to meet their social and emotional needs. Montessori introduced various activities which allowed for a much greater degree of independence in individual activity. By constantly watching the children and learning from them, she experimented with different types of materials and activities. Montessori developed her method by keeping only those activities that the children enjoyed the most. The major features of the Montessori school were as follows.

The Prepared Environment

Montessori believed that the children absorb unconsciously from their environment. The first Montessori school was a tenement room in the Quarter of San Lorenzo. She designed an environment to meet their needs, interests, abilities, and development. A delightful environment was prepared for them. Little pieces of furniture were made and they were coloured with bright colours. The main room was utilized for 'intellectual work'. The room was larger than the customary classrooms with child-sized tables and chairs; small rugs for children were spread on the floor to work on, and it allowed freedom of movement around the furniture Montessori suggested that a playground and a garden should adjoin the classroom so that the children may be free to go and come as they like, throughout the day. Everything placed in the room was in proportion to the child. Besides the physical environment, the prepared environment contained various types of activities and materials. The materials included sensorial materials, materials for acquisition of culture, and the activities included practical life exercises. Montessori also stressed on order in the environment.

The aim of the prepared environment was to make the child independent. That is, it is placed where he can do things for himself/herself—live his/her own life—without the immediate help of adults. Standing (1998) pointed out that one adult—the directress—is, in a sense, a part of the child's environment, but the function of both directress and environment is to assist the child to attain perfection through its own efforts.

So the prepared environment gave a learning atmosphere to the children without destroying the freedom and spontaneity of the child. At the same time, the prepared environment would become useless without a trained directress. The Directress or the teacher was the link between the child and the environment.

Didactic Apparatus

The materials used in the school were known as the 'didactic apparatus'. They were designed to the self-correcting. Through trial and error, the child rectified his own mistakes, until, he succeeded in his work. The apparatuses were

1. Dressing-frames; Purpose: Finger gymnastics.
2. Solid geometric insets Nail board; Purpose: Visual perceptions.
3. Series of blocks; Purpose: Auto-education.

4. Sandpaper strips for rough bodies of various degrees and smooth polish and resistance; Purpose: Development of tactile sense.
5. Stuffs-fabrics; Purpose: Quality through touch.
6. Colour boxes assorting of coloured cards in pairs; Purpose: Visual discriminations.
7. Plane geometric insets, Plane geometric figures fitted; Purpose: Adjustment of fine movements' knowledge of form.
8. Cylindrical sound boxes; Purpose: Discrimination of auditory perceptions
9. Alphabet boxes—sand paper and cardboard; Purpose: Teaching reading and writing (Hardy 1917).

Thus, each didactic material had a purpose. Children took an active part in the activities. They enjoyed the challenges presented to them. They repeated the activities and explored the didactic apparatus with joy and pleasure. The teacher only guided the children. The role of the teacher was of a facilitator. Children learned to recognize different patterns, shapes, and colours through these activities.

The Child as the Master

The child was the master of the Montessori House. Children themselves choose the activities. The classroom was decorated in such a way that the children could move around independently. The chairs and tables were light enough so that the children could carry them from one place to another. Basins were low enough for the children. Different types of materials, including pets, were kept at different corners to make the learning joyful and develop curiosity among children and help them in learning. She focused on learning different skills and practices that were useful in life. The principle of learning by doing and, at the same time, exploration and creation of own world by the children were given importance by Montessori. She created a child-friendly environment to facilitate this process.

Liberty of the Pupil

The "liberty of the pupil" was fundamental to the Montessori Method. This liberty, according to Montessori should "permit a development of individual, spontaneous manifestations of the child's nature" (Montessori 1964). Her belief in the liberty of the child was based on Montessori's conviction that a child was striving for order in his or her life to match the "inherent order and structure in nature" (Spock and Hathaway 1967). Montessori's liberty was always defined in relation to the didactic materials, directress, and prepared environment. Gardner (1966) pointed out that Montessori's approach was to encourage students to be aware of external reality, rather than comprehend only the personalized motives and fantasies of the child. As her biographer Kramer (1988) said that the ultimate aim of education was to be in control of oneself. Montessori achieved it in her own life and she wanted to achieve it in her own school. So Montessori concluded that all children were looking for an organized structure or order, and the best way to achieve it was to provide liberty to the children so that they could reach the goal in their own way.

Discipline

The children as a whole in the *Casa Dei Bambini* gave an impression of extraordinary discipline. They were given freedom to choose their activities. They worked quietly with full concentration. They went about walking quietly to get fresh work or to put back things in place. It was spontaneous self-discipline that came from within. Montessori felt that this natural discipline would provide the foundation for all other forms of discipline in every aspect of life. This showed how discipline was closely related to freedom. Maria Montessori also spelled out clearly the responsibilities of the parent. A set of rules was drawn up and pasted in the Casa Dei Bambini.

> The parents who wish to avail themselves of the advantages of the Casa dei Bambini pay nothing. They must, however assume these binding obligations:
>
> a) To send their children to the Casa dei Bambini at the appointed time, clean in body and clothing and provided with a suitable apron.
>
> b) To show the greatest respect and deference towards the Directress herself in the education of the children. Once a week at least, the mothers may talk with the Directress giving her information, concerning the home life of the child and receiving helpful advice from her.
>
> Students shall be expelled from the Casa dei Bambini:
>
> a) Those children who present themselves unwashed or in soiled clothing.
>
> b) Those who show themselves to be incorrigible.
>
> c) Those whose parents fail in respect to the persons connected with the Casa dei Bambini or who destroy through bad conduct the educational work of the institution. (Kramer 1988)

So we can see that the parents were made liable for maintaining discipline in the school. This helped to maintain a close parent–teacher relation in the school. She emphasized the need of maintaining a close contact with the parents. Parents had certain responsibilities and they were required to follow the directions laid down by Montessori. Parents were also given the liberty to observe the financial planning of the various programs adopted by the school. This provided a sense of parental ownership.

Auto Education

Montessori also believed in auto education. The main concept of auto education is that no teacher is necessary and the child will realize his or her inadequacies through the didactic apparatus which controls every error and the child is able to correct himself. The principle of auto education, as well as the doctrine of liberty, implies the non-intervention of the teacher. E. M. Standing (1998) in one sense the Montessori teacher is helping the child every moment, i.e. indirectly in so far as she has provided for him the whole prepared environment which contains the means at once to stimulate and to sustain the child's creative self-activity. She must also at the proper line help the child directly, in order to imitate him into the proper use of the materials for development. Further she must intervene to correct certain errors and to smooth away insurmountable difficulties.

The child spontaneously chooses from different activities and materials. But at the same time, the Directress or the teacher must step in when the child is wrong. Montessori pointed out that the Directress should never be afraid of destroying what is evil.

Teachers or Directress

The teacher to Montessori was an observer and facilitator. She believed that the teachers should try to understand the children, and their needs, through observation. The teacher must first organize and prepare an environment of learning. The emphasis must be on the child. In the calm atmosphere the teacher must motivate, and encourage the child into a variety of activities. They should help the child to develop self-confidence and self-discipline.

Montessori shared her own experiences with the teachers. She trained the teachers on how to handle and help the children. Montessori believed that the children themselves were the "real teachers of the Montessori method" (Kramer 1988). This new role of teachers was a challenge for the teachers. Montessori worked out a way of teaching which her assistants followed. Teaching gradually progressed from simple to complicated perceptions and manifestations.

Positive Schooling Features as Reflected in the Schools Set by Rabindranath Tagore and Maria Montessori

Positive schooling is an approach in which children are provided with learning experiences that inculcate mutual trust and respect among the members of the school. In Positive schooling each member of the school contributes and work together to develop a healthy school environment.

The general factors that contribute to creating a positive school climate are

- Curriculum
- Methodology of teaching
- School Environment
- Student Teacher Interaction

Now let us explore the factors in Rabindranath Tagore's school at Santiniketan and Maria Montessori's 'Children's House'.

First, the curriculum and activities provided in the school should be of wide range. Both Tagore and Montessori stressed on activity-based curriculum.

Tagore's curricular goals emphasized personality development, fellow feeling, and intellectual spontaneity. The first criterion in Tagore's vision for relevant education was that it is locally relevant, but it must also be in touch with the wider world. He viewed curriculum not as subjects but as activities. He tried to provide a wide range of activities, like nature walks, excursions, craft, astronomy, sports, and many others. Tagore encouraged the students of Santiniketan to participate in festivals and plays which he created. At Santiniketan, the children were given a diverse atmosphere of learning different types of activities. The freedom and beauty of the natural setting at Santiniketan transformed the method of learning different subjects. Santiniketan to the students was like their own world; they reacted completely and freely to create. Festivals like *Basantotsab* and *Paushotsab* were also celebrated in different seasons to inculcate creativity, invention, and constructive efforts among students. Each student at Santiniketan created his or her own world and contributed to the creation of Santiniketan as a whole. Tagore opposed autocratic authority, as, according to him, children had their own place in school administration. Students were also free to participate at whatever level they liked and free to create their own learning agenda.

The curriculum, as proposed by Maria Montessori in 'The Montessori Method' was based on a true science of education, which involved information from the medical sciences, anthropology, and the clinical observation of children. The activities included in the Montessori Method focused on practical life skills, sensory ability, language skills, reading, writing, arithmetic, physical, social, cultural and moral skills, value and character formation. The practical life skills included a range of activities designed to develop the child's independence and self-reliance.

So we can see that both the educators tried to provide a wide range of activities for the students, to cater to the individual needs as well as the social needs which are important features of positive schooling. The first level of the Montessori curriculum was called "preparatory experiences" meant for children aged from 2½ to 4 years. The prepared environment at this inaugural level, scales the learning materials, furniture, and equipment in the classroom with the child's physical and mental ability. Sensory education materials train the senses of smell, hearing, touch, and so forth. Increasingly fine sensory discriminations are taught using materials that the children manipulate to learn textures and temperatures; language education focuses upon naming qualities of objects, recognizing the objects, and pronouncing their names. Academic learning begins at the age of 4 years and emphasizes writing, reading, and arithmetic. To round up the curriculum science, history, geography, geometry, and arithmetic are explored. Montessori did not include those aspects of the curriculum that she felt were obvious or already available in the classroom setting. Montessori saw the second plane of development (ages 6–12) as a time to gain knowledge about the universe. The child should be introduced to knowledge about the universe in the form of an epic story or the great lessons of Cosmic Education. So she stressed on integrated holistic lessons of various subjects instead of lessons in separate parts.

Second, developing appropriate teaching method is another important feature of positive schooling. Learning should be perceived as interesting, relevant, and important. All students are expected to learn and grow based on the individual abilities and skills.

The methodology adopted by Rabindranath Tagore was based on direct experience through nature. He believed in the practical training of the faculties of observation. Role-playing was another important method which he used to encourage independence and critical thought. Heuristic Method was also followed by Tagore. The Peripatetic Method, which believes in the integration of body and mind in order to establish a total rhythm and harmony in life was followed by Tagore. The children were given the freedom to explore and gain knowledge. He stressed on developing curiosity among the students. Maria Montessori believed in auto education. Both the educators talked about kinaesthetic education that is the education of the senses. Tagore believed more in '*Bodher Shikha*', that is education for feeling, while Maria Montessori stressed on the education of the senses. The methodology must be creatively implemented in a carefully selected environment by catering to the special needs of each particular child. The main element of Montessori's vision was that the mainspring of all children's efforts is their spontaneous interest in their surroundings and so there is no need for adults to use force or persuasion. Montessori asserted that her pedagogy was based on a system of logical, rational, and scientific inquiry. In the Montessori Method, the educational process is based on self-direction. In a prepared environment, the directress guides the child in a careful and respectful manner. The child responds to different learning situations at different phases. The most important aspect of Montessori pedagogy is independent work. The child chooses what he likes to do and for as long as he wants to work on it. In being able to freely decide, a child develops the discipline that exists within. Her pedagogy also encourages creative problem solving skills. The Montessori Method emphasizes problem solving, encourages creativity, independence, and develops self-control among children. The teacher is a facilitator. Both the educators tried to cater to the needs of the children and tried to make the learning experience an enjoyable and useful one. Positive schooling through favourable learning experiences was encouraged by both the educators.

Third, the school environment forms an important aspect of positive schooling. The school is perceived to be a place where children want to come. The physical environment of the school must be an ideal one.

At Santiniketan, the children were given diverse atmospheres of learning different types of activities. The freedom and beauty of the natural setting at Santiniketan transformed the method of learning different subjects. Subjects were learned in the open air, under the shade of trees; besides this, there were activities that served as expressions of life. These joyous exercises of inventive and constructive energies helped to build character. The pupils learnt to manage themselves and learnt to take responsibilities. The first important lesson to learn was improvisation, for learning was spontaneous and not imposed on them by external authorities. Students were also free to participate at whatever level they liked and were free to create their own learning agenda. Maria Montessori, on the other hand, tried to implement teaching reform with a disadvantaged population. *Casa dei Bambini* was a slum school, catering to Rome's disadvantaged children. Her educational methods were a form of social activism. Her school structure created a place where children could learn how to be self-directed, self-disciplined, and empowered them to be active members of society. She developed the didactic apparatus and believed in a prepared environment that would help children reach their full potential and help them to create a better world. Both Tagore and Montessori ensured an open, free, and spontaneous environment in their institutions so that the children could grow, experience, express their creativity, and realize their full potential. Freedom in the school environment was the key word for both these educators and they tried to realize them in their institutions. They tried to provide a non-threatening atmosphere for the children in their institutions which is one of the major feature of positive schooling.

Fourth, the student teacher interaction is an important aspect of positive schooling. Patterns of teacher-student interaction affect the child's development. Instruction that encourages high-level thinking promotes learning in children. At Santiniketan, Tagore considered Nature to be the first teacher of the students. To Tagore, the *Guru* or teacher is the one who dedicates his life for the students. The teacher's ability to recognize the potential of the students and guide them according to their capabilities was more important than following any particular method. He said that the teachers should follow their instincts while guiding the students. He was himself a teacher, and presented himself as role model to other teachers. Maria Montessori brought into being a new concept of teacher. She gave a new name to the teacher that is 'Directress'. She believed that a teacher in the Montessori Method needs to have a deep sense of respect for the child. She is the link between the environment and the child. She needs to create a positive situation for the child, so that it creates curiosity within the child. The Directress needs to possess the qualities of patience, sympathy, tact, and observation. Montessori believed in the principle of non-intervention but, at the same time, the teacher should interfere if the child is on the wrong path. Both Tagore and Montessori stressed on positive interactions between the students and teachers in their institutions.

Conclusion

The main features of the institutions established by Tagore and Montessori have been discussed. Both these educators established their institutions for different purposes, but they were similarly inspired by the deadness of the traditional education systems in their respective countries. Through their institutions, they tried to set examples for the world how to enliven the education system. In today's world, people have become immune to violence, and cruelty, and the total lack of gentleness to others. In this troubled world, it is necessary to look back at the values of 'universalism' and 'respect for diversity'. Rabindranath Tagore not only stressed on these values in his thoughts, but also practically implemented it in his life of action. Maria Montessori most passionately argued that education was the only means of eliminating war once and for all. She also stressed on the values of global citizenship and respect for diversity. She argued that all these values must form an important part of every child's education. She believed that through education, we can help more and more children grow up in a world and help them to live together in peace. Both Rabindranath Tagore and Maria Montessori were pioneers in peace education. They focused on the development of the whole child, the creative and critical thinking skills, along with inter-personal skills. These skills are so crucial that men and women would be both inspired and equipped to build a lasting peace, which is likely to have a special relevance in the present day education. Positive schooling plays an important role in developing these skills among children.

It is important to know what a school with positive school climate looks like and it is equally important to examine the process that can make it happen. Rabindranath Tagore and Maria Montessori have set examples of positive schooling. The main features of Tagore and Montessori's schools reflect an education system that cultivates the critical capacities of students, and fosters a complex understanding of the world and its people.

Advancement in technology and equipment, help in better monitoring of the school and develop a positive school climate. But, in order to create a positive climate in school in its true sense we need to look back at the ideals and practices of great educators. Rabindranath Tagore's poetic vision enabled him to devise a unique learning environment at Santiniketan. To him, his institution was a work of art and not a pedagogical laboratory. On the other hand, Maria Montessori's educational theory was based on science. Her institution was a pedagogical laboratory for her. Utilizing the scientific observation and experience of her medical career, and her work with differently abled children, she designed, in the Children's House, learning materials and a classroom environment that fostered children's natural desire to learn. As the world becomes more integrated and interdependent, the educational visions of Tagore and Montessori seem to emerge as more significant today.

References

Gardner, R. W. (1966). A psychologist looks at Montessori. In: J. L. Frost (Ed.), *Early childhood education rediscovered readings*. New York: Holt, Rinehart and Winston, Inc.

Hardy, M. C. (1917). The derivation of Montessori didactic apparatus. *The Elementary School Journal, 18*(4), 299.

Kramer, R. (1988). *Maria Montessori: A biography* (pp. 118–119). Reading Massachusetts: Perseus Books.

Montessori, M. (1964). *The Montessori method* (p. 28) (A. E. George, Trans.). New York: Schocken Books.

Tagore, R. (1961). The problem of education. In *Towards universal man* (p. 79). London: Asia Publishing House.

Tagore, R. (1962). *Reminiscences* (p. 141). Madras: Macmillan and Co.

Tagore, R. (2002). As cited in Chakraborti Mohit, *Pioneers in philosophy of education* (p. 45). New Delhi: Concept Publishing Company.

Tagore, R. (2012). As cited in Connell, K. M. (2012), *Rabindranath Tagore: The poet as educator* (p. 206) (2nd ed.). Kolkata: Visva-Bharati.

Standing, E. M. (1998). *Maria Montesssori, her life and work*. New York: Plume.

Spock, B., & Hathaway, M. L. (1967). Montessori and Traditional American Nursery Schools—How they are different, how they are alike. In J. L. Frost (Ed.), *Early childhood education rediscovered: Readings* (p. 75). New York: Holt, Rinehart and Winston, Inc.

The manufacturer's authorised representative in the EU is Springer Nature Customer Service Centre GmbH, Europaplatz 3, 69115 Heidelberg, Germany. If you have any concerns regarding our products, please contact ProductSafety@springernature.com

Printed and bound by CPI Group (UK) Ltd, Croydon, CR0 4YY

25/09/2026

02222884-0012